Respiratory Medicine

Series Editor:
Sharon I.S. Rounds

For further volumes:
http://www.springer.com/series/7665

Marc A. Judson

Editor

Pulmonary Sarcoidosis

A Guide for the Practicing Clinician

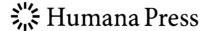 Humana Press

Editor
Marc A. Judson, M.D.
Division of Pulmonary
    and Critical Care Medicine
Department of Medicine
Albany Medical College
Albany, NY, USA

ISBN 978-1-4614-8926-9   ISBN 978-1-4614-8927-6 (eBook)
DOI 10.1007/978-1-4614-8927-6
Springer New York Heidelberg Dordrecht London

Library of Congress Control Number: 2013949139

Printed on acid-free paper

Humana Press is a brand of Springer
Springer is part of Springer Science+Business Media (www.springer.com)

*This book is dedicated to Sooyeon Kwon,
my beautiful, loving, and intelligent wife.
Her caring and support has made many
things possible in my life, including this work.*

Preface

Sarcoidosis is a disease with world-wide prevalence that affects all races, ethnic groups, individuals of all ages, and both sexes. The disease may affect any organ. Its severity may range from a radiographic or laboratory abnormality detected in a patient with no symptoms to a relentlessly progressive disease that is potentially life threatening. Despite the awareness of sarcoidosis as a specific disease entity for nearly one and one-half centuries, there is still no standard method of diagnosis, treatment approach, method of follow-up evaluation, or method to reliably predict prognosis.

Because sarcoidosis is a relatively rare disease, few clinicians have extensive clinical experience in its management. Furthermore, medical evidence concerning the clinical approach to sarcoidosis is scarce. Therefore, clinicians typically lack the necessary tools to make reliable treatment decisions concerning sarcoidosis patients.

The lung is the most common organ involved with sarcoidosis. Pulmonary manifestations of sarcoidosis include asymptomatic radiographic abnormalities, granulomatous inflammation of airways, and/or the lung interstitium causing pulmonary symptoms and fibrocystic disease that may result in severe pulmonary dysfunction and pulmonary hypertension.

This book will serve as a valuable resource for clinicians concerning the care of the pulmonary sarcoidosis patient. The focus of this book concerns issues of diagnosis, management, and prognosis of the disease. The authors are all clinicians with extensive experience in caring for these patients. Although they drew on their own expertise, the authors were encouraged to focus on the clinical data that are available. I hope that this book will serve as a practical guide for clinicians and thus improve the care of sarcoidosis patients.

Albany, NY, USA   Marc A. Judson, M.D.

Acknowledgments

I would like to acknowledge several individuals who were essential in the production of this book. I would like to thank the major effort of all the authors in writing these scholarly and clinically relevant chapters. I thank Springer, and in particular, Ms. Amanda Quinn and Mr. Michael Wilt, whose efforts were essential in the publication of this work. I thank all of my mentors, colleagues, and mentees who constantly educated me and questioned me over the years and helped me develop my passion for learning. In particular, I would like to thank Dr. Steven A. Sahn for his guidance concerning my academic career and writing skills. I would like to acknowledge all the sarcoidosis patients who I have treated over the years for their courage and their kindness. Finally, I thank my parents, my wife, and my children for their support and love.

Contents

Contributors

Robert P. Baughman, M.D. Department of Internal Medicine, University of Cincinnati Medical Center, Cincinnati, OH, USA

Marie Budev, D.O. Respiratory Institute, Cleveland Clinic, Cleveland, OH, USA

Daniel A. Culver, D.O. Respiratory Institute, Cleveland Clinic, Cleveland, OH, USA

Marjolein Drent, M.D., Ph.D. Department of Interstitial Lung Disease, Hospital Gelderse Vallei, Ede, The Netherlands

Faculty of Health, Medicine, and Life Sciences, (FHML), Maastricht University, Maastricht, The Netherlands

Andrew J. Goodwin, M.D., M.S.C.R. Division of Pulmonary, Critical Care, Allergy, and Sleep Medicine, Medical University of South Carolina, Charleston, SC, USA

Jan C. Grutters, M.D., Ph.D. Department of Pulmonology, St. Antonius Hospital, Nieuwegein, The Netherlands

Center of Interstitial Lung Diseases, St. Antonius Hospital, Nieuwegein, The Netherlands

Division Heart & Lungs, University Medical Center, Utrecht, The Netherlands

Marc A. Judson, M.D. Division of Pulmonary and Critical Care Medicine, Department of Medicine, Albany Medical College, Albany, NY, USA

Carlos E. Kummerfeldt, M.D. Division of Pulmonary, Critical Care, Allergy, and Sleep Medicine, Medical University of South Carolina, Charleston, SC, USA

Steven D. Nathan, M.D. Advanced Lung Disease and Transplant Program, Department of Medicine, Inova Fairfax Hospital, Falls Church, VA, USA

Efstratios Panselinas, M.D. Department of Pulmonary Medicine, General Army Hospital, Tripoli, Greece

Divya C. Patel, D.O. Respiratory Institute, Cleveland Clinic, Cleveland, OH, USA

Hiren V. Patel, M.D. Division of Pulmonary and Critical Care Medicine, University of Nevada School of Medicine, Las Vegas, NV, USA

Matthew P. Schreiber, M.D. Division of Pulmonary and Critical Care Medicine, University of Nevada School of Medicine, Las Vegas, NV, USA

Hidenobu Shigemitsu, M.D. Division of Pulmonary and Critical Care Medicine, University of Southern California Keck School of Medicine, Los Angeles, CA, USA

Division of Pulmonary and Critical Care Medicine, University of Nevada School of Medicine, Las Vegas, NV, USA

Oksana A. Shlobin, M.D. Advanced Lung Disease and Transplant Program, Department of Medicine, Inova Fairfax Hospital, Falls Church, VA, USA

Marcel Veltkamp, M.D., Ph.D. Department of Pulmonology, St. Antonius Hospital, Nieuwegein, The Netherlands

Center of Interstitial Lung Diseases, St. Antonius Hospital, Nieuwegein, The Netherlands

Athol U. Wells, M.D. Interstitial Lung Disease Unit, Royal Brompton Hospital, London, UK

Chapter 1
The Diagnosis of Sarcoidosis

Marc A. Judson

Abstract The diagnosis of sarcoidosis is never completely secure. The diagnosis can, rarely, be made on clinical grounds without biopsy confirmation if the clinical presentation is very specific for the disease. Otherwise, histological confirmation of granulomatous inflammation is required. However, identification of granulomatous inflammation is inadequate to make the diagnosis of sarcoidosis as this histological pattern is associated with many alternative diseases. Therefore, a diligent effort must be undertaken to exclude such diseases. This effort includes obtaining a detailed medical history as well as careful examination of the biopsied material. Because sarcoidosis is a multisystem granulomatous disease of unknown cause, additional efforts must be made to identify involvement in at least two organs to confirm the diagnosis. This chapter outlines the approach and potential pitfalls in establishing a diagnosis of sarcoidosis.

Keywords Sarcoidosis • Diagnosis • Etiology • Biopsy • Pathology

Introduction

Despite the claim that the method of diagnosis of sarcoidosis has been established [1], the reality is that the diagnosis is never completely secure. Certain clinical features are typical of sarcoidosis, but none of them are specific for the diagnosis. Sarcoidosis remains a diagnosis of exclusion, and it is impossible to exclude alternative diagnoses with complete confidence. This chapter reviews the diagnostic approach and potential pitfalls in establishing a diagnosis of sarcoidosis.

M.A. Judson, M.D. (✉)
Division of Pulmonary and Critical Care Medicine, Department of Medicine, Albany Medical College, Albany, NY, USA
e-mail: judsonm@mail.amc.edu

M.A. Judson (ed.), *Pulmonary Sarcoidosis: A Guide for the Practicing Clinician*,
Respiratory Medicine 17, DOI 10.1007/978-1-4614-8927-6_1,
© Springer Science+Business Media New York 2014

Definition

Sarcoidosis has been defined as multisystem granulomatous disorder of unknown cause [1]. With rare exceptions (vide infra), clinicoradiologic findings without histologic evidence of granulomatous inflammation are inadequate to render a diagnosis of sarcoidosis. Histologic evidence of granulomatous inflammation is also inadequate for the diagnosis of sarcoidosis because alternative causes of granulomatous inflammation need to be excluded. It is prudent to maintain a healthy degree of skepticism that an alternative diagnosis has been overlooked [2]. The fact that the disease is "multisystem" implies that there must be evidence of granulomatous inflammation in at least two organs for the diagnosis of sarcoidosis to be secure.

Diagnostic Approach

Figure 1.1 outlines the approach to the diagnosis to sarcoidosis. This is a multistep process that usually involves the collection of clinical information, histological examination of tissue for the presence of granulomatous inflammation, exclusion of

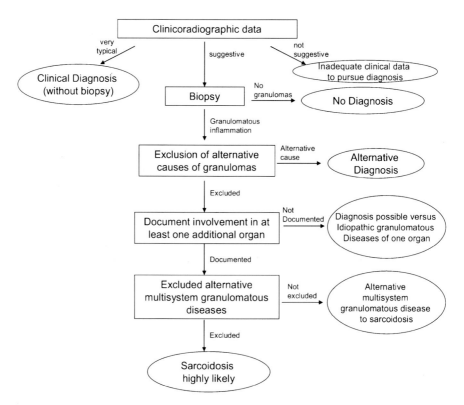

Fig. 1.1 The figure outlines the diagnostic algorithm for sarcoidosis. See text for details. Adapted from [2], with permission

Table 1.1 Clinicoradiographic data supporting or weakening the likelihood of sarcoidosis

	Supports	Weakens
Demographics	• US African American • Northern European	• Age < 18 years • Age > 50 years in male
Medical history	• Nonsmoking • No symptoms (in patients with CXR findings) • Positive family history of sarcoidosis • Symptoms involving ≥2 organs commonly involved with sarcoidosis (e.g., lung and eyes)	• Exposure to tuberculosis • Exposure to organic bioaerosol • Exposure to beryllium • Intravenous drug abuse
Laboratory data	• Elevated SACE, especially if >2× ULN	
Radiographic findings	• CXR: bilateral hilar adenopathy (especially if without symptoms) • HRCT: disease along the bronchovascular bundle	

CXR chest radiograph, *SACE* serum angiotensin-converting enzyme, *2× ULN* two times the upper limit of normal, *HRCT* high resolution computer tomography
Adapted from [2], with permission

known causes of this granulomatous inflammation, and documentation that the granulomatous inflammation is present in at least two organs [2]. This diagnostic approach will be discussed in detail in the sections that immediately follow.

Clinical Data Collection

As with most diseases, sarcoidosis can only be considered a potential diagnosis if clinical data have been collected that exceed a certain "threshold" such that the diagnosis is plausible. Certain clinical findings suggest the diagnosis of sarcoidosis, although none of them is pathognomonic [2]. This process involves weighing the clinical findings that support the diagnosis of sarcoidosis against the clinical findings that tend to refute it. If sufficient clinical evidence has accumulated suggesting that sarcoidosis is a reasonable consideration, a tissue biopsy is usually indicated. Table 1.1 outlines clinical findings that are often used to gauge the likelihood of the diagnosis of sarcoidosis.

Demographics

Sarcoidosis is rare before adulthood [3]. The disease usually presents before age 40, peaking in those aged 20–29 years old. There is a second smaller peak of increased incidence after age 50, especially in women [3]. The disease is slightly more frequent in women than men at a ratio of less than 2–1 [3, 4]. The disease is more prevalent in certain ethnicities such as African Americans and Northern Europeans [2–4].

Medical History

Patients with sarcoidosis often present with no symptoms [5]. This is especially common in white patients [6]. Therefore, sarcoidosis should be considered in asymptomatic patients with hilar adenopathy, mediastinal adenopathy, and/or diffuse parenchymal infiltrates on lung imaging [6, 7]. A family history should be elicited because the prevalence rate of sarcoidosis is much higher in first-degree relatives of sarcoidosis patients than in the general population [8]. A smoking history should be obtained as sarcoidosis is much more common in nonsmokers [9]. Potential sarcoidosis patients should be questioned about their occupational history, as the disease is common in certain occupations including firefighters [10].

In addition, patients should be questioned concerning potential exposures that may cause diseases that may mimic sarcoidosis. Specifically, a history of active tuberculosis, latent tuberculosis infection, and tuberculosis exposure should be obtained. Patients should be questioned concerning time spent in areas where certain fungi are endemic such as the Ohio River valley where histoplasmosis is common [11]. The possibility of beryllium exposure should be explored because chronic beryllium disease (CBD) can mimic sarcoidosis radiographically [12] and histologically [13, 14]. CBD has been misdiagnosed as sarcoidosis in up to 40 % of cases [2, 15]. As most patients are unaware of potential exposures to beryllium, it is important to ask about work industries where exposure to beryllium is plausible including aerospace, nuclear weapons, electronics, jewelry, sporting goods, ceramics, and dental [16]. Furthermore, minimal beryllium exposure may lead to significant disease [17, 18]. Hypersensitivity pneumonitis (HP) is a granulomatous pulmonary disease resulting from exposure to bioaerosols that may mimic sarcoidosis. A history of exposure to birds and hot tubs should be obtained as these are the most two common exposures causing HP in the USA [19, 20].

Evidence of Extrapulmonary Involvement

Because sarcoidosis is a systemic disease, evidence that a disorder is present in two or more organs supports a diagnosis of sarcoidosis [2]. At presentation, 95 % of sarcoidosis patients have clinical evidence of pulmonary involvement, and more than 40 % have evidence of involvement in the skin, liver, peripheral lymph node, or eye [21]. Therefore, sarcoidosis should be considered in patients with pulmonary disease and a concomitant disorder in one of these organs.

Radiographic Findings

Bilateral hilar adenopathy on chest radiograph suggests the diagnosis of sarcoidosis, especially if the patient has no fever, night sweats, or weight loss [2, 7, 22].

The chest radiograph often demonstrates bilateral enlargement the hilar lymph nodes as well as concomitant enlargement of the right paratracheal lymph nodes, which is described as the "1, 2, 3 sign" [23]. Findings on high resolution chest-computed tomography (HRCT) may be more specific for the diagnosis of sarcoidosis than those found on chest radiography, although they are inadequate for a diagnosis to be secured without biopsy confirmation. Typical HRCT findings that suggest sarcoidosis include parenchymal nodules and opacities that represent conglomerations of these nodules that have a perilymphatic distribution along the bronchovascular bundles as well as in subpleural locations [24–30].

Serum Angiotensin-Converting Enzyme

Angiotensin-converting enzyme (ACE) is produced in the epithelioid cell of the sarcoid granuloma [31], and serum ACE (SACE) levels reflect the total sarcoidosis granuloma burden [31]. Although SACE has been suggested as a diagnostic test for sarcoidosis, elevated SACE levels in isolation are inadequately sensitive or specific to reliably diagnose of exclude the disease [32]. In a review of 14 studies encompassing 4,195 patients concerning the diagnostic accuracy of SACE for sarcoidosis, the sensitivity was 77 % (range: 41–100 %) and the specificity was 93 % (range: 83–99 %) [33]. The likelihood of sarcoidosis increases in patients with higher SACE levels [33, 34], and SACE levels greater than 2 times the upper limits of normal are rarely seen in other diseases and not seen in cancer or lymphoma [32].

Making the Diagnosis of Sarcoidosis on Clinical Grounds Without a Tissue Biopsy

On rare occasions, the clinical presentation is so specific for sarcoidosis that the diagnosis can be made without a confirmatory tissue biopsy. These presentations are listed in Table 1.2. Even in these situations, the clinician should be diligent in terms of excluding possible, albeit unlikely, alternative diagnoses.

Selection of a Biopsy Site

With the exception of the rare instances where the clinical findings are highly specific for sarcoidosis (Table 1.2), the diagnosis requires a tissue biopsy (Fig. 1.1). It is in the patient's best interest for the biopsy to be minimally invasive and associated with the least morbidity. For these reasons, superficial biopsy sites are preferred compared to visceral organs [35]. Even in patients suspected to have sarcoidosis on the basis of obvious thoracic or abdominal disease, a thorough skin, conjunctival,

Table 1.2 Clinical presentations that may be assumed to be sarcoidosis without tissue confirmation provided additional data do not suggest an alternative diagnosis

- Lofgren's syndrome
  - Bilateral hilar adenopathy on chest radiograph
  - Erythema nodosum skin lesions
  - Fever (often)
  - (Ankle) arthralgias/arthritis (often)
- Herfort's syndrome
  - Uveitis
  - Parotitis
  - Fever (often)
- Bilateral hilar adenopathy on chest radiograph without symptoms
- Positive panda sign (parotid and lacrimal gland uptake) and lambda sign (bilateral hilar and right paratracheal lymph node uptake) on gallium-67 scan

Adapted from [2] with permission

lacrimal gland, and peripheral lymph node examination should be performed. The patient should be questioned about the presence of scars or tattoos, because sarcoidosis skin nodules have a predilection to form in these areas. The detection of a conjunctival nodule, palpable lacrimal gland, or palpable peripheral lymph node should prompt consideration of a biopsy for diagnosis.

When there is no clinical evidence that a superficial site is involved with sarcoidosis, a biopsy is usually attempted in an organ where sarcoidosis involvement is suspected. This is very often the lung, as pulmonary involvement occurs in more than 90 % of sarcoidosis patients early in the course of the disease [21]. The approach to lung biopsy for the diagnosis of pulmonary sarcoidosis continues to change with the advent of newer technologies. Although the diagnosis can almost always be made by mediastinoscopy when significant mediastinal adenopathy is present and by video-assisted thoracoscopic surgery when there is parenchymal lung disease, less invasive bronchoscopic procedures are usually preferred. The yield of transbronchial lung biopsy (TLB) for the diagnosis of pulmonary sarcoidosis ranges from 60 to 97 % depending on the number of biopsies taken and the presence of parenchymal disease on chest radiograph [36–42].

Endobronchial biopsy may be positive in more than 60 % of patients with pulmonary sarcoidosis [43]. Biopsies are more frequently positive in individuals with abnormal-appearing airways [43]. Furthermore, endobronchial biopsy can be performed with TLB and increases the yield for sarcoidosis above that using TLB alone [43].

Transbronchial needle aspiration under endobronchial ultrasound guidance (TBNA-EBUS) has been extensively evaluated as a diagnostic approach for pulmonary sarcoidosis over the last decade. The diagnostic yield is in the range of 80 % [44], and a positive result avoids the need for TLB and endobronchial biopsies if on-site cytopathology is performed. TBNA-EBUS has been shown to be superior to "blind" TBNA without ultrasound guidance for the diagnosis of sarcoidosis [45].

Examination of inflammatory cells from bronchoalveolar lavage fluid (BALF) is sometimes used as a complementary test for the diagnosis of pulmonary sarcoidosis.

Table 1.3 Causes of a lymphocytosis (≥15 % lymphocytes) in bronchoalveolar lavage fluid

Sarcoidosis
Granulomatous infectious diseases (mycobacteria, fungi)
Hypersensitivity pneumonitis
Viral pneumonitis
Drug-induced alveolitis
Lymphocytic interstitial pneumonitis (LIP)/lymphoma
Nonspecific interstitial pneumonitis (NSIP)
Cryptogenic organizing pneumonia (COP)
Chronic beryllium disease
Radiation pneumonitis

The diagnostic accuracy of the percentage of lymphocytes and the CD4/CD8 lymphocyte subpopulation ratio in BALF have been assessed. The sensitivity, specificity, positive and negative predictive values of these BALF analyses for the diagnosis of sarcoidosis have been variable, probably because of differences in the prevalence of sarcoidosis, the prevalence of other diseases associated with BALF lymphocytosis, and the cut-off values used. In general, BALF lymphocytosis (greater than 15 % lymphocytes) has a 90 % sensitivity for the diagnosis of sarcoidosis [46, 47], although the specificity is low [46]. Table 1.3 shows the differential diagnosis of BALF lymphocytosis, and this needs to be kept in mind in order to exclude alternative causes for this finding other than sarcoidosis. The BALF CD4/CD8 ratio is increased >3.5 in 50–60 % of pulmonary sarcoidosis patients. However, the specificity of the BALF CD4/CD8 ratio criterion has approached 95 % in some [48, 49] but not all [46] studies. Some have advocated that the BALF CD4/CD8 criterion is diagnostic of sarcoidosis when there are concomitant chest imaging findings compatible with sarcoidosis [47]; however, these criteria not been formally tested. At present, the role of BALF for the diagnosis of sarcoidosis is controversial and unsettled.

Granulomas can be detected histologically in any organ that is involved with sarcoidosis [35]. The biopsy of neural tissue and the heart are particularly problematic because of the potential morbidity associated with these procedures. Because patients with neurosarcoidosis will have extraneural sarcoidosis nearly 90 % of the time [50], most patients have extraneural disease from which a biopsy specimen can be obtained. Although endomyocardial biopsy is a fairly specific test for cardiac sarcoidosis in the proper clinical setting, its sensitivity is very low [51]. For this reason, endomyocardial biopsy is rarely performed for the diagnosis of sarcoidosis. Often, imaging studies are used surrogate tests for the diagnosis of neurosarcoidosis and cardiac sarcoidosis. Such studies should be interpreted cautiously as their specificity depends upon associated clinical evidence for sarcoidosis, which should almost always include previous biopsy confirmation of granulomatous inflammation of unknown cause in another organ (vide infra).

On some occasions, the diagnosis of sarcoidosis is suspected on clinical grounds, although no specific organ is identified to biopsy. There is no established approach for this situation. Total body imaging such as positron emission tomography (PET) [52] or gallium-67 scanning [53] has been proposed in such cases to identify an organ for biopsy, although no rigorous analysis of this approach has been undertaken. Another suggested approach in this situation is to biopsy organs that are commonly affected, even in the absence of symptoms or other clinical findings suggestive or sarcoidosis involvement of that organ. Conjunctival biopsies have performed in this situation, and the yield has ranged from 27 to 55 % in patient without ocular symptoms [54–60]. In vivo confocal microscopy of the conjunctiva can detect multinucleated giant cells without the need for a biopsy, and this has also been advocated to noninvasively confirm granulomatous inflammation in sarcoidosis patients [61]. Liver biopsy demonstrates granulomas in 24–78 % of sarcoidosis patients, even when they have no symptoms attributable to the liver and normal serum liver function tests [62–64]. However, hepatic granulomas are not specific for sarcoidosis so that clinical evidence of extrahepatic sarcoidosis must be present for the diagnosis to be secure [35]. Andonopoulos and colleagues found that gastrocnemius muscle biopsy revealed granulomas in 22 consecutive patients without muscle symptoms who had bilateral hilar adenopathy on chest radiograph [65]. However, most of these patients had strong clinical evidence of sarcoidosis; furthermore, this procedure is fairly invasive. Another invasive biopsy procedure for sarcoidosis is scalene lymph node biopsy [66], which has essentially been supplanted by diagnostic biopsy of more easily accessible sites.

Another test to consider when sarcoidosis is suspected on clinical grounds, although no specific organ is identified to biopsy is the Kveim test. This test involves the intradermal inoculation of a suspension of splenic tissue from spleen that was involved with sarcoidosis [67]. If a skin nodule develops at the inoculation site in 4–6 weeks, is biopsied, and reveals noncaseating granulomatous inflammation, this is highly specific for the diagnosis of sarcoidosis. Unfortunately, the Kveim test in not highly sensitive for the diagnosis of sarcoidosis; both the sensitivity and specificity of the test vary depending on the spleen that is used, and the suspension is not approved by the Food and Drug Administration. Therefore, the Kveim test is not approved as a standard diagnostic test for sarcoidosis.

Figure 1.2 shows our approach to the selection of a biopsy site for the diagnosis of sarcoidosis.

Pathology

Although granulomatous inflammation is necessary to establish a diagnosis of sarcoidosis in most cases, granulomas are nonspecific inflammatory reactions, and they are not diagnostic of sarcoidosis or any other granulomatous disease [2, 68]. Meticulous histological examination with appropriate staining of all biopsies should be performed to search for known causes of granulomatous inflammation, such as mycobacteria, fungi, parasites, and foreign material (e.g., talc).

Although there are no specific histological features that are diagnostic of sarcoid granulomas, there are certain features that suggest this diagnosis. The sarcoid granuloma usually consists of a compact (organized) collection of mononuclear phagocytes (macrophages and epithelioid cells) [69]. Typically, there is no necrosis within

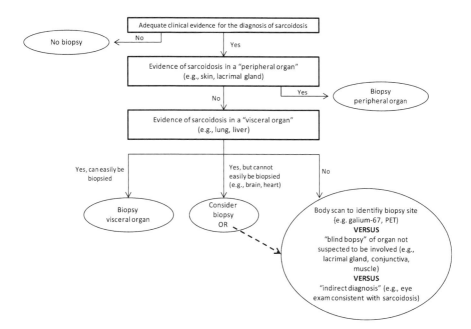

Fig. 1.2 The figure outlines the diagnostic approach to selecting a biopsy site for pathologic confirmation of granulomatous inflammation consistent with sarcoidosis. This approach emphasizes (a) selection of a relatively noninvasive biopsy site when possible; (b) biopsy of a site suspected to be clinically involved unless the biopsy would be highly invasive; (c) various approaches when no obvious organ involvement is demonstrated or only organs requiring very invasive biopsies demonstrate potential involvement

the sarcoid granuloma; however, on occasion, there is a small to moderate amount of necrosis. Usually, giant cells fuse within the sarcoid granuloma to form multinucleated giant cells. These granulomas are typically surrounded by lymphocytes in the periphery. A variety of inclusions may be present within the sarcoid granuloma including asteroid bodies, Schaumann's bodies, birefringent crystals, and Hamazaki–Wesenberg bodies; however these inclusions are not specific or diagnostic of sarcoidosis [68]. In particular, birefringent crystals within the sarcoid granuloma may lead to a misdiagnosis of talc granulomatosis [14]. Care must be taken to ensure that the crystal morphology and size are compatible with intravenously injected talc to ensure the diagnosis of talc granulomatosis [14].

Exclusion of Alternative Causes of Granulomatous Inflammation

Table 1.4 lists potential causes other than sarcoidosis for granulomatous inflammation based on the organ involved. The diagnosis of sarcoidosis requires that all these diagnoses have been excluded to a reasonable degree. As it is impossible to be

Table 1.4 Major pathologic differential diagnosis of sarcoidosis at biopsy

Lung	Lymph node	Skin	Liver	Bone marrow	Other biopsy sites
• Tuberculosis	• Tuberculosis	• Tuberculosis	• Tuberculosis	• Tuberculosis	• Tuberculosis
• Atypical mycobacteriosis	• Atypical mycobacteriosis	• Atypical mycobacteriosis	• Brucellosis	• Histoplasmosis	• Brucellosis
• Fungi	• Brucellosis	• Fungi	• Schistosomiasis	• Infectious mononucleosis	• Other infections
• Pneumocystis carinii	• Toxoplasmosis	• Reaction to foreign bodies: beryllium, zirconium, tattooing, paraffin, etc.	• Primary biliary cirrhosis	• Cytomegalovirus	• Crohn's disease
• Mycoplasma	• Granulomatous histiocytic necrotizing lymphadenitis (Kikuchi's disease)	• Rheumatoid nodules	• Crohn's disease	• Hodgkin's disease	• Giant cell myocarditis
• Hypersensitivity pneumonitis	• Cat-scratch disease		• Hodgkin's disease	• Non-Hodgkin's lymphomas	• GLUS syndrome
• Pneumoconiosis: beryllium (chronic beryllium disease), titanium, aluminum	• Sarcoid reaction in regional lymph nodes to carcinoma		• Non-Hodgkin's lymphomas	• Drugs	
• Drug reactions	• Hodgkin's disease		• GLUS syndrome	• GLUS syndrome	
• Aspiration of foreign materials	• Non-Hodgkin's lymphomas				
• Wegener's granulomatosis (sarcoid-type granulomas are rare)	• Granulomatous lesions of unknown significance (the GLUS syndrome)				
• Necrotizing sarcoid granulomatosis (NSG)					

Adapted from [2], with permission

completely assured that all these causes have been excluded, the diagnosis of sarcoidosis is never completely secure.

The exclusion of alternative causes of granulomatous inflammation requires a multifaceted approach [2]. A detailed medical history is essential to exclude potential exposure to infectious agents (e.g., tuberculosis and fungi), environmental exposures (e.g., organic bioaerosols generated from birds or hot tubs that may cause hypersensitivity pneumonitis), and occupational exposures (e.g., beryllium) (vide supra).

In addition to the medical history, the biopsy specimen must be meticulously examined for alternative causes of granulomatous inflammation [14]. This includes a search for infectious agents and foreign materials that could induce a granulomatous reaction. At a minimum, this should include appropriate stains of histologic material for mycobacteria and fungi, and usually, cultures for these organisms as well.

Verification of Sarcoidosis Involvement of a Second Organ

The presence of granulomatous inflammation of unknown cause in a single organ is inadequate for the diagnosis of sarcoidosis, as, by definition, multiple organs should be involved. Examples of such single organ granulomatous diseases that are distinguished from sarcoidosis include idiopathic granulomatous hepatitis [70], that is rarely found to be sarcoidosis (extrahepatic granulomas rarely develop over time) and idiopathic panuveitis, a granulomatous uveitis confined to the eye that is common in the southeastern USA [71].

Although granulomatous inflammation in an isolated organ is not diagnostic of sarcoidosis, treatment is usually identical to the treatment of sarcoidosis provided that alternative causes have been reasonably excluded. Therefore, it is usually not of clinical importance to search for additional organ involvement beyond a "general organ screen" as outlined in Table 1.5.

Although the diagnosis of sarcoidosis requires strong evidence that a second organ be involved, histological confirmation of involvement in a second organ is not always required. A consensus panel of sarcoidosis experts has established clinical criteria for "definite," "probable," and "possible" organ involvement with sarcoidosis for some organs without the need for a biopsy, provided alternative causes for this clinical finding has been reasonably excluded (Table 1.6) [72].

Table 1.5 Extent of workup for second organ involvement if a biopsy has revealed granulomatous inflammation consistent with sarcoidosis

Chest radiograph
Liver function tests
Complete blood count
Ophthalmologic examination
Electrocardiogram
Serum calcium
Urinalysis

Adapted from [2] with permission

Table 1.6 Clinical criteria for extrapulmonary sarcoidosis organ involvement in patients with biopsy-confirmed sarcoidosis in another organ[a]

Organ	Definite	Probable	Possible
Lungs	1. Chest roentgenogram with one or more of the following • Bilateral hilar adenopathy • Diffuse infiltrates • Upper lobe fibrosis 2. Restriction on pulmonary function tests	1. Lymphocytic alveolitis by bronchoalveolar lavage (BAL) 2. Any pulmonary infiltrates 3. Isolated reduced diffusing capacity for carbon monoxide	1. Any other adenopathy 2. Obstructive pulmonary function tests
Skin	1. Lupus pernio 2. Annular lesion 3. Erythema nodosum	1. Macular/papular 2. New nodules	1. Keloids 2. Hypopigmentation
Eyes	1. Lacrimal gland swelling 2. Uveitis 3. Optic neuritis	1. Blindness 2. Positive in vivo confocal microscopy	1. Glaucoma 2. Cataract
Liver	1. Liver function tests > three times the upper limit of normal	1. Compatible computed tomography (CT) scan 2. Elevated alkaline phosphate	
Hypercalcemia/ hypercalciuria/ nephrolithiasis	1. Increased serum calcium with no other cause	1. Increased urine calcium 2. Nephrolithiasis analysis showing calcium	1. Nephrolithiasis—no stone analysis 2. Nephrolithiasis with negative family history for stones
Neurologic	1. Positive magnetic resonance imaging (MRI) with uptake in meninges or brainstem 2. Cerebrospinal fluid with increased lymphocytes and/or protein 3. Diabetes insipidus 4. Bell's palsy 5. Cranial nerve dysfunction 6. Peripheral nerve biopsy 7. Positive positron emission tomography (PET) scan of CNS or spinal cord	1. Other abnormalities on magnetic resonance imaging (MRI) 2. Unexpected neuropathy 3. Positive electromyogram	1. Unexplained headaches 2. Peripheral nerve radiculopathy
Renal	1. Treatment responsive renal failure	1. Steroid responsive renal failure in patient with diabetes and/or hypertension	1. Renal failure in absence of other disease

Cardiac	1. Treatment responsive cardiomyopathy 2. Electrocardiogram showing intraventricular conduction defect or nodal block 3. Positive gallium scan of heart 4. Positive positron emission tomography (PET) scan of the heart	1. No other cardiac problem and either: • Ventricular arrhythmias • Cardiomyopathy 2. Positive thallium scan	1. In patient with diabetes and/or hypertension: • Cardiomyopathy • Ventricular arrhythmias
Non-thoracic lymph node		1. New palpable node above waist 2. Lymph node >2 cm by computed tomography (CT) scan	1. New palpable femoral lymph node
Bone marrow	1. Unexplained anemia 2. Leukopenia 3. Thrombocytopenia		1. Anemia with low mean corpuscular volume (MCV)
Spleen		1. Enlargement by: • Exam • Computed tomography (CT) scan • Radioisotope scan	
Bone/joints	1. Cystic changes on hand or feet radiographs	1. Asymmetric, painful clubbing	1. Arthritis with no other cause
Ear/nose/throat		1. Unexplained hoarseness with exam consistent with granulomatous involvement	1. New onset sinusitis 2. New onset dizziness
Parotid/salivary glands	1. Symmetrical parotitis with syndrome of mumps 2. Positive gallium scan (Panda sign)		1. Dry month
Muscles	1. Increased creatine phosphokinase (CK)/aldolase which decreases with treatment	1. Increased creatine phosphokinase (CK)/aldolase	1. Myalgias responding to treatment
Other organs			

aThere can be no other explanation for the clinical findings in this table for these criteria to be valid. In addition, biopsy of each of these organs would constitute "definite" involvement. Adapted from [72] with permission

Other Idiopathic Multiorgan Granulomatous Syndromes

There are other multiorgan granulomatous syndromes that are thought not to be sarcoidosis, but rather, separate clinical entities. This is a controversial issue because some consider these disorders under the penumbra of "sarcoidoses syndromes." Blau's syndrome consists of granulomatous iritis, arthritis, and skin rash [73]. The disease is a genetic disorder [74] and has an autosomal dominant pattern of inheritance with variable penetrance [73]. In contrast to sarcoidosis, most cases occur before 12 years of age. Blau's syndrome is considered a separate entity from childhood sarcoidosis on the basis of a lack of visceral (e.g., pulmonary) involvement and mode of inheritance [73].

In 1989, Brinker described a syndrome with: prolonged fever, granulomatous inflammation in the liver, spleen, bone marrow, and lymph nodes, a benign course and a tendency for recurrence. This entity has been described as the GLUS syndrome: granulomatous lesions of unknown significance. The GLUS syndrome is thought to be distinct from multisystem sarcoidosis because (1) elevated SACE levels are not found with the GLUS syndrome; (2) hypercalcemia is not found with the GLUS syndrome; (3) the Kveim test is negative in the GLUS syndrome; and (4) immunotyping of the T-lymphocytes in GLUS syndrome granulomas are different compared to those from sarcoidosis granulomas [75].

Necrotizing sarcoid granulomatosis (NSG) is a systemic granulomatous vasculitis [76]. Because of vascular involvement, necrosis is a prominent feature, unlike most cases of sarcoidosis. Although the lung is commonly involved, extrapulmonary involvement is also common [77]. It is debated whether NSG is a distinct clinical entity or a form of systemic sarcoidosis [77, 78].

The Future

Obviously, sarcoidosis has a cause. It may have one primary cause or there may be many causes of what we presently call, "sarcoidosis." Chronic beryllium disease was once thought to be sarcoidosis until its specific etiology was determined. It may be that, in the future, we will "pare off" additional specific causes of granulomatous inflammation that are now thought to be sarcoidosis. We may take a "splitter approach" and reclassify these diseases, attributing them to their specific cause rather than classifying them as sarcoidosis. Conversely, we may take a "lumper approach" and classify all these diseases as "the sarcoidoses." We may even prefer to lump chronic beryllium disease and even infectious granulomatous diseases under the sarcoidoses umbrella.

The development of sarcoidosis may depend not only on a specific cause but also on the host's immune system. It may be that specific causes of sarcoidosis depend on an interaction between an exposure and a genetically driven inflammatory response to that exposure [79]. There is mounting evidence that sarcoidosis, like many other granulomatous diseases, results from an antigen recognized and processed by an antigen-presenting cell that presents this antigen to a T-cell receptor via an HLA class II molecule [80]. It may be that specific antigenic causes of sarcoidosis depend on HLA class II polymorphisms that bind the antigen properly so that it can be presented to the T lymphocyte. In support of this contention, many HLA polymorphisms are associated with sarcoidosis [81], whereas others are protective [81]. In the future, causes of sarcoidosis may be determined by an analysis of the patient's immune response including analysis of their HLA genotype. It may even be possible to prevent the development of sarcoidosis by such an analysis so that specific antigenic exposures can be avoided.

Summary

The diagnosis of sarcoidosis is never secure. On the rare occasions, when certain clinical findings are present that are very specific for sarcoidosis, the diagnosis can be made on clinical grounds without performing a biopsy. In most cases, a biopsy revealing granulomatous inflammation is a necessary but insufficient criterion for the diagnosis of sarcoidosis. It is prudent to select the least invasive biopsy location based on the specific clinical presentation (e.g., skin). Because there are numerous infectious and noninfectious causes of granulomatous inflammation besides sarcoidosis, a diligent effort must be undertaken to exclude these possibilities. This effort includes taking a detailed history to inquire about potential infectious, environmental, and occupational exposures that could cause granulomatous inflammation (e.g., tuberculosis, beryllium exposure). This effort should also include a thorough examination of the pathological material to search for infectious agents and other material that could cause granulomatous inflammation. Although the pathologic characteristics of the biopsy are not definitive for the diagnosis nor can they exclude it, the presence of compact, non-necrotic granulomas would make the diagnosis much more likely. Because one can never been completely certain that all alternative causes of granulomatous inflammation have been excluded, the diagnosis of sarcoidosis is never completely secure. If sarcoidosis remains a reasonable possibility after a detailed medical history and pathological examination has been performed, a search should be undertaken for a second organ involved with sarcoidosis. The net result of this algorithm is not a definitive diagnosis of sarcoidosis but a statistical likelihood of the diagnosis [2].

References

1. Hunninghake GW, Costabel U, Ando M, et al. ATS/ERS/WASOG statement on sarcoidosis. American Thoracic Society/European Respiratory Society/World Association of Sarcoidosis and other Granulomatous Disorders. Sarcoidosis Vasc Diffuse Lung Dis. 1999;16:149–73.
2. Judson MA. The diagnosis of sarcoidosis. Clin Chest Med. 2008;29:415–27, viii.
3. Hosoda Y, Yamaguchi M, Hiraga Y. Global epidemiology of sarcoidosis. What story do prevalence and incidence tell us? Clin Chest Med. 1997;18:681–94.

4. Rybicki BA, Major M, Popovich Jr J, et al. Racial differences in sarcoidosis incidence: a 5-year study in a health maintenance organization. Am J Epidemiol. 1997;145:234–41.
5. Siltzbach LE, Fishman AP, editors. Sarcoidosis. New York: McGraw-Hill; 1980.
6. Sartwell PE, Edwards LB. Epidemiology of sarcoidosis in the U.S. Navy. Am J Epidemiol. 1974;99:250–7.
7. Reich JM, Brouns MC, O'Connor EA, et al. Mediastinoscopy in patients with presumptive stage I sarcoidosis: a risk/benefit, cost/benefit analysis. Chest. 1998;113:147–53.
8. Rybicki BA, Iannuzzi MC, Frederick MM, et al. Familial aggregation of sarcoidosis. A case-control etiologic study of sarcoidosis (ACCESS). Am J Respir Crit Care Med. 2001;164:2085–91.
9. Newman LS, Rose CS, Bresnitz EA, et al. A case control etiologic study of sarcoidosis: environmental and occupational risk factors. Am J Respir Crit Care Med. 2004;170:1324–30.
10. Prezant DJ, Dhala A, Goldstein A, et al. The incidence, prevalence, and severity of sarcoidosis in New York City firefighters. Chest. 1999;116:1183–93.
11. Edwards LB, Acquaviva FA, Livesay VT, et al. An atlas of sensitivity to tuberculin, PPD-B, and histoplasmin in the United States. Am Rev Respir Dis. 1969;99(Suppl):1–132.
12. Harris KM, McConnochie K, Adams H. The computed tomographic appearances in chronic berylliosis. Clin Radiol. 1993;47:26–31.
13. Newman LS, Kreiss K, King Jr TE, et al. Pathologic and immunologic alterations in early stages of beryllium disease. Re-examination of disease definition and natural history. Am Rev Respir Dis. 1989;139:1479–86.
14. Mukhopadhyay S, Gal AA. Granulomatous lung disease: an approach to the differential diagnosis. Arch Pathol Lab Med. 2010;134:667–90.
15. Muller-Quernheim J, Gaede KI, Fireman E, et al. Diagnoses of chronic beryllium disease within cohorts of sarcoidosis patients. Eur Respir J. 2006;27:1190–5.
16. Kreiss K, Day GA, Schuler CR. Beryllium: a modern industrial hazard. Annu Rev Public Health. 2007;28:259–77.
17. Taylor TP, Ding M, Ehler DS, et al. Beryllium in the environment: a review. J Environ Sci Health A Tox Hazard Subst Environ Eng. 2003;38:439–69.
18. Newman LS, Kreiss K. Nonoccupational beryllium disease masquerading as sarcoidosis: identification by blood lymphocyte proliferative response to beryllium. Am Rev Respir Dis. 1992;145:1212–4.
19. Yi ES. Hypersensitivity pneumonitis. Crit Rev Clin Lab Sci. 2002;39:581–629.
20. Glazer CS, Martyny JW, Lee B, et al. Nontuberculous mycobacteria in aerosol droplets and bulk water samples from therapy pools and hot tubs. J Occup Environ Hyg. 2007;4:831–40.
21. Baughman RP, Teirstein AS, Judson MA, et al. Clinical characteristics of patients in a case control study of sarcoidosis. Am J Respir Crit Care Med. 2001;164:1885–9.
22. Winterbauer RH, Belic N, Moores KD. Clinical interpretation of bilateral hilar adenopathy. Ann Intern Med. 1973;78:65–71.
23. Freiman DB, Miller WT. Sarcoidosis: a multisystem disease. Am Fam Physician. 1977;15:78–82.
24. Nishino M, Lee KS, Itoh H, et al. The spectrum of pulmonary sarcoidosis: variations of high-resolution CT findings and clues for specific diagnosis. Eur J Radiol. 2010;73:66–73.
25. Oberstein A, von Zitzewitz H, Schweden F, et al. Non invasive evaluation of the inflammatory activity in sarcoidosis with high-resolution computed tomography. Sarcoidosis Vasc Diffuse Lung Dis. 1997;14:65–72.
26. Leung AN, Brauner MW, Caillat-Vigneron N, et al. Sarcoidosis activity: correlation of HRCT findings with those of 67Ga scanning, bronchoalveolar lavage, and serum angiotensin-converting enzyme assay. J Comput Assist Tomogr. 1998;22:229–34.
27. Criado E, Sanchez M, Ramirez J, et al. Pulmonary sarcoidosis: typical and atypical manifestations at high-resolution CT with pathologic correlation. Radiographics. 2010;30:1567–86.
28. Hamper UM, Fishman EK, Khouri NF, et al. Typical and atypical CT manifestations of pulmonary sarcoidosis. J Comput Assist Tomogr. 1986;10:928–36.
29. Muller NL, Kullnig P, Miller RR. The CT findings of pulmonary sarcoidosis: analysis of 25 patients. AJR Am J Roentgenol. 1989;152:1179–82.

30. Dawson WB, Muller NL. High-resolution computed tomography in pulmonary sarcoidosis. Semin Ultrasound CT MR. 1990;11:423–9.
31. Sheffield EA. Pathology of sarcoidosis. Clin Chest Med. 1997;18:741–54.
32. O'Regan A, Berman JS. Sarcoidosis. Ann Intern Med. 2012;156:ITC5-1, ITC5-2, ITC5-3, ITC5-4, ITC5-5, ITC5-6, ITC5-7, ITC5-8, ITC5-9, ITC5-10, ITC15-11, ITC15-12, ITC15-13, ITC15-14, ITC15-15; quiz ITC15-16.
33. Bunting PS, Szalai JP, Katic M. Diagnostic aspects of angiotensin converting enzyme in pulmonary sarcoidosis. Clin Biochem. 1987;20:213–9.
34. De Smet D, Martens GA, Berghe BV, et al. Use of likelihood ratios improves interpretation of laboratory testing for pulmonary sarcoidosis. Am J Clin Pathol. 2010;134:939–47.
35. Teirstein AS, Judson MA, Baughman RP, et al. The spectrum of biopsy sites for the diagnosis of sarcoidosis. Sarcoidosis Vasc Diffuse Lung Dis. 2005;22:139–46.
36. Lynch 3rd JP, Kazerooni EA, Gay SE. Pulmonary sarcoidosis. Clin Chest Med. 1997;18:755–85.
37. Gilman MJ, Wang KP. Transbronchial lung biopsy in sarcoidosis. An approach to determine the optimal number of biopsies. Am Rev Respir Dis. 1980;122:721–4.
38. Koonitz CH, Joyner LR, Nelson RA. Transbronchial lung biopsy via the fiberoptic bronchoscope in sarcoidosis. Ann Intern Med. 1976;85:64–6.
39. Koerner SK, Sakowitz AJ, Appelman RI, et al. Transbronchinal lung biopsy for the diagnosis of sarcoidosis. N Engl J Med. 1975;293:268–70.
40. Mitchell DM, Mitchell DN, Collins JV, et al. Transbronchial lung biopsy through fibreoptic bronchoscope in diagnosis of sarcoidosis. Br Med J. 1980;280:679–81.
41. Poe RH, Israel RH, Utell MJ, et al. Probability of a positive transbronchial lung biopsy result in sarcoidosis. Arch Intern Med. 1979;139:761–3.
42. Roethe RA, Fuller PB, Byrd RB, et al. Transbronchoscopic lung biopsy in sarcoidosis. Optimal number and sites for diagnosis. Chest. 1980;77:400–2.
43. Shorr AF, Torrington KG, Hnatiuk OW. Endobronchial biopsy for sarcoidosis: a prospective study. Chest. 2001;120:109–14.
44. Agarwal R, Srinivasan A, Aggarwal AN, et al. Efficacy and safety of convex probe EBUS-TBNA in sarcoidosis: a systematic review and meta-analysis. Respir Med. 2012;106:883–92.
45. Tremblay A, Stather DR, Maceachern P, et al. A randomized controlled trial of standard vs endobronchial ultrasonography-guided transbronchial needle aspiration in patients with suspected sarcoidosis. Chest. 2009;136:340–6.
46. Nagai S, Izumi T. Bronchoalveolar lavage. Still useful in diagnosing sarcoidosis? Clin Chest Med. 1997;18:787–97.
47. Costabel U, Guzman J, Albera C, et al. Bronchoalveolar lavage in sarcoidosis. In: Baughman RP, editor. Lung biology in health and disease; sarcoidosis. New York: Informa; 2006. p. 399–414.
48. Winterbauer RH, Lammert J, Selland M, et al. Bronchoalveolar lavage cell populations in the diagnosis of sarcoidosis. Chest. 1993;104:352–61.
49. Costabel U, Zeiss AW, Guzman J. Sensitivity and specificity of BAL findings in sarcoidosis. Sarcoidosis. 1992;9:211–4.
50. Stern BJ, Krumholz A, Johns C, et al. Sarcoidosis and its neurological manifestations. Arch Neurol. 1985;42:909–17.
51. Uemura A, Morimoto S, Hiramitsu S, et al. Histologic diagnostic rate of cardiac sarcoidosis: evaluation of endomyocardial biopsies. Am Heart J. 1999;138:299–302.
52. Teirstein AS, Machac J, Almeida O, et al. Results of 188 whole-body fluorodeoxyglucose positron emission tomography scans in 137 patients with sarcoidosis. Chest. 2007;132:1949–53.
53. Sulavik SB, Palestro CJ, Spencer RP, et al. Extrapulmonary sites of radiogallium accumulation in sarcoidosis. Clin Nucl Med. 1990;15:876–8.
54. Chung YM, Lin YC, Huang DF, et al. Conjunctival biopsy in sarcoidosis. J Chin Med Assoc. 2006;69:472–7.
55. Khan F, Wessely Z, Chazin SR, et al. Conjunctival biopsy in sarcoidosis: a simple, safe, and specific diagnostic procedure. Ann Ophthalmol. 1977;9:671–6.

56. Nichols CW, Eagle Jr RC, Yanoff M, et al. Conjunctival biopsy as an aid in the evaluation of the patient with suspected sarcoidosis. Ophthalmology. 1980;87:287–91.
57. Leavitt JA, Campbell RJ. Cost-effectiveness in the diagnosis of sarcoidosis: the conjunctival biopsy. Eye (Lond). 1998;12(Pt 6):959–62.
58. Spaide RF, Ward DL. Conjunctival biopsy in the diagnosis of sarcoidosis. Br J Ophthalmol. 1990;74:469–71.
59. Bornstein JS, Frank MI, Radner DB. Conjunctival biopsy in the diagnosis of sarcoidosis. N Engl J Med. 1962;267:60–4.
60. Crick R, Hoyle C, Mather G. Conjunctival biopsy in sarcoidosis. Br Med J. 1955;2:1180–1.
61. Wertheim MS, Mathers WD, Suhler EB, et al. Histopathological features of conjunctival sarcoid nodules using noninvasive in vivo confocal microscopy. Arch Ophthalmol. 2005;123: 274–6.
62. Lehmuskallio E, Hannuksela M, Halme H. The liver in sarcoidosis. Acta Med Scand. 1977;202:289–93.
63. Hercules HD, Bethlem NM. Value of liver biopsy in sarcoidosis. Arch Pathol Lab Med. 1984;108:831–4.
64. Bilir M, Mert A, Ozaras R, et al. Hepatic sarcoidosis: clinicopathologic features in thirty-seven patients. J Clin Gastroenterol. 2000;31:337–8.
65. Andonopoulos AP, Papadimitriou C, Melachrinou M, et al. Asymptomatic gastrocnemius muscle biopsy: an extremely sensitive and specific test in the pathologic confirmation of sarcoidosis presenting with hilar adenopathy. Clin Exp Rheumatol. 2001;19:569–72.
66. Truedson H, Stjernberg N, Thunell M. Scalene lymph node biopsy. A diagnostic method in sarcoidosis. Acta Chir Scand. 1985;151:121–3.
67. Siltzbach LE. The Kveim test in sarcoidosis. A study of 750 patients. JAMA. 1961;178:476–82.
68. Rosen Y. Pathology of sarcoidosis. Semin Respir Crit Care Med. 2007;28:36–52.
69. Adams DO. The biology of the granuloma. In: Ioachim HL, editor. Pathology of granulomas. New York: Raven; 1983. p. 1–20.
70. Israel HL, Goldstein RA. Hepatic granulomatosis and sarcoidosis. Ann Intern Med. 1973;79:669–78.
71. Merrill PT, Kim J, Cox TA, et al. Uveitis in the southeastern United States. Curr Eye Res. 1997;16:865–74.
72. Judson MA, Baughman RP, Teirstein AS, et al. Defining organ involvement in sarcoidosis: the ACCESS proposed instrument. ACCESS Research Group. A case control etiologic study of sarcoidosis. Sarcoidosis Vasc Diffuse Lung Dis. 1999;16:75–86.
73. Manouvrier-Hanu S, Puech B, Piette F, et al. Blau syndrome of granulomatous arthritis, iritis, and skin rash: a new family and review of the literature. Am J Med Genet. 1998;76:217–21.
74. Kurokawa T, Kikuchi T, Ohta K, et al. Ocular manifestations in Blau syndrome associated with a CARD15/Nod2 mutation. Ophthalmology. 2003;110:2040–4.
75. Brinker H. Granulomatous lesions of unknown significance: the GLUS syndrome. In: James DG, editor. Sarcoidosis and other granulomatous disorders. Philadelphia: W.B. Saunders; 1994. p. 69–86.
76. Churg A, Carrington CB, Gupta R. Necrotizing sarcoid granulomatosis. Chest. 1979;76:406–13.
77. Quaden C, Tillie-Leblond I, Delobbe A, et al. Necrotising sarcoid granulomatosis: clinical, functional, endoscopical and radiographical evaluations. Eur Respir J. 2005;26:778–85.
78. Lazzarini LC, de Fatima do Amparo Teixeira M, Souza Rodrigues R, et al. Necrotizing sarcoid granulomatosis in a family of patients with sarcoidosis reinforces the association between both entities. Respiration. 2008;76:356–60.
79. Rossman MD, Thompson B, Frederick M, et al. HLA and environmental interactions in sarcoidosis. Sarcoidosis Vasc Diffuse Lung Dis. 2008;25:125–32.
80. Baughman RP, Culver DA, Judson MA. A concise review of pulmonary sarcoidosis. Am J Respir Crit Care Med. 2011;183:573–81.
81. Martinetti M, Luisetti M, Cuccia M. HLA and sarcoidosis: new pathogenetic insights. Sarcoidosis Vasc Diffuse Lung Dis. 2002;19:83–95.

Chapter 2
The Pulmonary Manifestations of Sarcoidosis

Marcel Veltkamp and Jan C. Grutters

Abstract The pulmonary manifestation of sarcoidosis has a great variability and is notorious for mimicking many other interstitial lung diseases. Knowledge of pulmonary manifestations is important in diagnosing saroidosis because thoracic involvement is present in over 90 % of patients. In this chapter, classical findings on chest X-ray and HRCT are described as well as multiple uncommon findings in radiology. The most common findings are bilateral hilar lymphadenopathy, reticulonodular pattern, perilymphatic distribution of nodules, and predominant upper- and middle lobe parenchymal abnormalities. Uncommon findings are unilateral lymphadenopathy, reticular pattern, excessive ground glass opacities, pleural disease, solitary mass, and predominant lower lobe parenchymal abnormalities. Furthermore, the appearance of pulmonary hypertension and necrotizing sarcoid granulomatosis will be described. Finally, imaging of pulmonary sarcoidosis with positron emission tomography with ^{18}F-Fluordeoxyglucose (^{18}F-FDG PET) will be discussed.

Keywords Sarcoidosis • Intrathoracic manifestations • Lymphadenopathy • Parenchymal involvement • Pulmonary fibrosis • Chest X-ray • HRCT • PET

M. Veltkamp, M.D., Ph.D. (✉)
Department of Pulmonology, St. Antonius Hospital, Koekoekslaan 1, 3435 CM Nieuwegein, The Netherlands

Center of Interstitial Lung Diseases, St. Antonius Hospital, Koekoekslaan 1, 3435 CM Nieuwegein, The Netherlands
e-mail: m.veltkamp@antoniusziekenhuis.nl

J.C. Grutters, M.D., Ph.D.
Department of Pulmonology, St. Antonius Hospital, Koekoekslaan 1, 3435 CM Nieuwegein, The Netherlands

Center of Interstitial Lung Diseases, St. Antonius Hospital, Koekoekslaan 1, 3435 CM Nieuwegein, The Netherlands

Division Heart & Lungs, University Medical Center, Utrecht, The Netherlands
e-mail: j.grutters@antoniusziekenhuis.nl

M.A. Judson (ed.), *Pulmonary Sarcoidosis: A Guide for the Practicing Clinician*,
Respiratory Medicine 17, DOI 10.1007/978-1-4614-8927-6_2,
© Springer Science+Business Media New York 2014

Abbreviations

BHL   Bilateral hilar lymphadenopathy
COP   Cryptogenic organizing pneumonia
HRCT   High resolution computed tomography
LIP   Lymphocytic interstitial pneumonia
NSG   Necrotizing sarcoid angiitis and granulomatosis
PET   Positron emission tomography
SPL   Secondary pulmonary lobule
SURT   Sarcoidosis of the upper respiratory tract

Introduction

Clinical Manifestations

The clinical manifestations of sarcoidosis are highly variable and often nonspecific. Every organ can be affected, but thoracic involvement occurs in more than 90 % of patients. It is important to state that an estimated 40 % of sarcoidosis patients are asymptomatic, with incidental findings on chest radiographs [1–3]. Dyspnea, dry cough, or chest pain occurs in approximately 50 % of all patients. Massive hilar and/ or mediastinal lymphadenopathy is often asymptomatic, but may cause fatigue, retrosternal pain, or dysphagia in some patients [4, 5]. In pulmonary sarcoidosis, chest physical findings are usually minimal. Even in patients where radiographic abnormalities are extensive, crackles are present in less than 20 % of sarcoidosis patients. Finger clubbing is also uncommon in sarcoidosis [2].

Radiographic Scoring Systems: Scadding Staging

Sarcoidosis is commonly staged according to its appearance on the chest radiograph following the Scadding criteria (Table 2.1) [6]. Stage 0 indicates no visible intrathoracic findings. Stage I represents bilateral hilar lymphadenopathy, which may be accompanied by paratracheal lymphadenopathy. Stage II represents bilateral hilar lymphadenopathy accompanied by parenchymal infiltration. Stage III represents parenchymal infiltration without hilar lymphadenopathy. Stage IV consists of advanced fibrosis with evidence of honeycombing, hilar retraction, bullae, cysts, and emphysema. Despite the nomenclature, patients do not all progress through stages I–IV and these stages have no sequential order. For example, a patient may present with stage III which normalizes during follow-up. Also, it can be seen that a patient who initially presents with stage I disease that normalizes can present later on with parenchymal disease only (stage III) [7]. Hillerdal and colleagues found

Table 2.1 Radiographic staging of sarcoidosis patients at presentation according to the Scadding criteria. The estimated frequency at presentation is given as well as the probability of spontaneous resolution during disease course [8–10]

Radiographic stage	Chest X-ray	Frequency (%)	Resolution (%)
0	Normal	5–15	
I	BHL	25–65	60–90
II	BHL and pulmonary infiltrates	20–40	40–70
III	Pulmonary infiltrates without BHL	10–15	10–20
IV	Advanced pulmonary fibrosis	5	0

BHL bilateral hilar lymphadenopathy

that in a cohort of patients presenting with stage I disease 9 % progressed to stage II compared to 1.6 % who progressed to stage III or IV. Of patients presenting with stage II disease only 5.5 % progressed to stage III or IV disease [1].

An interesting feature of the above mentioned Scadding criteria is the fact that is gives prognostic information [8–10]. In stage I disease, spontaneous resolution occurs in 60–90 % of patients. Spontaneous resolution occurs in 40–70 % of patients with stage II disease and in 10–20 % of patients with stage III disease. The majority of spontaneous remissions occur within the first 2 years of disease presentation. There is no spontaneous resolution in patients with stage IV pulmonary sarcoidosis. An important limitation of the Scadding criteria is the great interobserver variability, especially between stages II and III, and III and IV [7].

Pulmonary Function Test

All varieties of abnormalities in pulmonary function tests can be seen in sarcoidosis: obstructive, restrictive, diffusion impairment, or combinations of these. However, in sarcoidosis patients with abnormal lung function testing, a decreased diffusion capacity and a restrictive ventilatory defect are most often seen. Almost 50 % of patients also have obstructive airway disease [9]. Furthermore, bronchial hyper responsiveness is seen in up to 20 % of patients and is associated with the presence of microscopic non-necrotizing granulomas in the endobronchial mucosa [11–13].

Large Airway Involvement

Sarcoidosis of the upper respiratory tract (SURT) may involve the nose, sinuses, larynx, oral cavity, ear, trachea, and bronchi [14, 15]. The incidence of SURT is approximately 5 % [16]. During bronchoscopy common lesions in the trachea as well as in the bronchi are erythema, thickening of the mucosa, and a "cobblestone appearance" (Fig. 2.1), which yields a high number of granulomas on biopsy. In a small study by Shorr and colleagues it was shown that 71 % of sarcoidosis patients

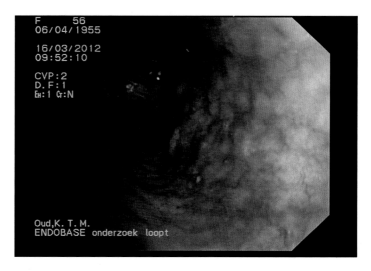

F   56
06/04/1955

16/03/2012
09:52:10

CVP:2
D. F:1
Eн:1 Gr:N

Oud,K. T. M.
ENDOBASE onderzoek loopt

Fig. 2.1 Endobronchial "cobblestone" appearance in a 57-year-old sarcoidosis patient. Biopsy proved multiple non-necrotizing granulomas. Courtesy of Dr. A.C. Verschoof, Hospital Gelderse Vallei, Ede, The Netherlands

undergoing bronchoscopy had bronchial abnormalities [17]. Severe endoluminal stenosis of the trachea or main bronchi is rare in sarcoidosis, estimated to be less than 1 % [18]. It is important to state when diagnosing sarcoidosis that even in patients with a normal appearing airway, granulomas can be identified in almost 30 % of patients [17].

Mediastinal and Hilar Lymphadenopathy

Lymphadenopathy is the most common intrathoracic manifestation of sarcoidosis occurring in approximately 80 % of patients during their illness, irrespectively of radiographic staging [19–25]. An overview of common and uncommon sites of thoracic lymphadenopathy in sarcoidosis is given in Table 2.2. In most cases bilateral hilar lymphadenopathy is present (Fig. 2.2), with unilateral hilar adenopathy occurring in only 3–5 % of patients [19, 26, 27]. When present, unilateral hilar lymphadenopathy is more common on the right side as on the left side. Furthermore, besides the hilar region, lymphadenopathy in sarcoidosis is also seen in the right paratracheal, aortopulmonary window, and tracheobronchial regions [22–25, 28]. A typical example of bilateral lymphadenopathy and right paratracheal lymphnode enlargement in sarcoidosis is known as Garland's triad or 1-2-3 sign.

The groups of Niimi and Patil demonstrated that the most commonly involved nodal stations are Naruke 4R (right lower paratracheal), Naruke 10R (right hilar), Naruke 7 (sub-carinal), Naruke 5 (aortopulmonary window), Naruke 11R (right interlobular), and Naruke 11L (left interlobular) [23, 24] (Table 2.2).

Table 2.2 Classical versus more uncommon features of pulmonary sarcoidosis at HRCT. The features are also divided in potentially reversible versus irreversible

Classical findings, potentially reversible
Lymphadenopathy: bilateral hilar, mediastinal, right paratracheal, subcarinal, aortopulmonary
Reticulonodular pattern: micronodules (2–4 mm, well defined, bilateral distribution)
Perilymphatic distribution of nodules (peribronchovascular, subpleural, interlobular septal)
Predominant upper- and middle zones parenchymal abnormalities
Uncommon findings, potentially reversible
Lymphadenopathy: unilateral, isolated, anterior and posterior mediastinal, paracardiac
Reticular pattern
Isolated cavitations
Isolated ground glass opacities without micronodules
Mosaic attenuation pattern
Pleural disease (effusion, pleural thickening, chylothorax, pneumothorax)
Mycetoma
Macronodules (>5 mm, coalescing). Galaxy sign and cluster sign
Classical findings reflecting irreversible fibrosis or chronic disease
Reticular opacities, predominantly middle and upper zones
Architectural distortion
Traction bronchiectasis
Volume loss, predominantly upper lobes
Calcified lymphnodes
Fibrocystic changes
Uncommon findings reflecting irreversible fibrosis or chronic disease
Honeycomb-like changes
Reticular opacities in predominantly lower lobes

The differential diagnosis of hilar and mediastinal lymphadenopathy is broad, with the major diagnostic alternatives being lymphoma, metastatic disease, and infections (especially tuberculosis). An important feature of lymphadenopathy in sarcoidosis is the symmetrical distribution, being rather unusual in the abovementioned diagnostic alternatives. Lymphadenopathy can also be seen in other interstitial lung diseases such as (idiopathic) interstitial pneumonitis and hypersensitivity pneumonitis. However, in diseases other than sarcoidosis, usually only one or two nodes are enlarged and their maximal short axis diameter is mostly <15 mm [24]. Mediastinal lymphadenopathy without hilar involvement is uncommon and a biopsy-proven diagnosis is warranted.

Lymph node calcification is visible at presentation in approximately 20 % of patients, increasing to 44 % during disease course [29]. The morphology of calcified lymph nodes is variable and nonspecific. Sometimes, the calcification can have an

Fig. 2.2 Characteristic
distribution of bilateral hilar
lymphadenopathy in stage I
sarcoidosis on a chest X-ray

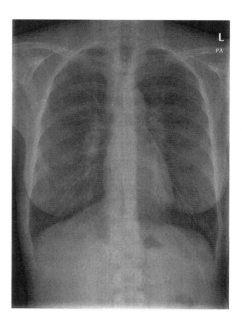

Fig. 2.2 Characteristic distribution of bilateral hilar lymphadenopathy in stage I sarcoidosis on a chest X-ray

eggshell appearance [30]. Calcification of lymph nodes is linked to the duration of disease and can be seen in other granulomatous disorders like tuberculosis or histoplasmosis as well. When comparing calcified lymph nodes in sarcoidosis and tuberculosis it was found that in sarcoidosis their diameter was significantly larger, calcium deposition more focal, and hilar distribution more bilaterally (65 % vs. 8 %) [25].

Parenchymal Involvement

Basic Anatomic Patterns in Interstitial Lung Disease

When interpreting a chest X-ray or HRCT in interstitial lung disease, knowledge of microscopic lung anatomy is essential. In microscopic lung anatomy there are primary as well as secondary pulmonary lobules. A primary pulmonary lobule is defined as the area of the lung distal to the respiratory bronchioles. It is smaller than an acinus and is composed of alveolar ducts, alveolar sacs, and alveoli. The primary pulmonary lobule is rarely used in HRCT imaging, but is the reason the secondary pulmonary lobule (SPL) has its name. The SPL is the smallest part of the lung that is surrounded by connective tissue septa. (Fig. 2.3a). It measures 1–2.5 cm in diameter and is made up of approximately 12 pulmonary acini [31]. Interpretation of HRCT in interstitial lung diseases depends, among other things, on the type of involvement of the SPL. The center of each SPL is named the centrilobular area and contains a small terminal bronchiole, a pulmonary artery branch, and pulmonary

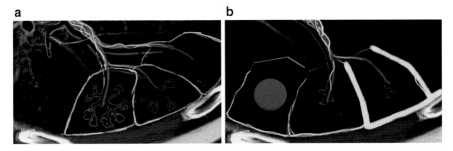

Fig. 2.3 Overview of the pulmonary secondary lobule. (**a**) The terminal bronchiole in the center divides into respiratory bronchioles with acini that contain alveoli. Branches of the pulmonary artery are in *blue*, branches of pulmonary veins are colored *red*. Lymphatic vessels are depicted in *yellow*. (**b**) The *blue circle* indicates the centrilobular area (*left*). The perilymphatic area is shown in *yellow* (*right*). Publication with permission from http://www.radiologyassistant.nl

lymphatics. The margins of the SPL are made up of the interlobular septa containing connective tissue, a pulmonary vein, and pulmonary lymphatics (Fig. 2.3b). The term perilymphatic defines the distribution of lymphatics along the peribronchovascular bundles, the centrilobular area, the interlobular septa, and the subpleural interstitium including the fissures. Within the SPL there are also intralobular septa, which are delicate strands of connective tissue separating adjacent pulmonary acini and primary pulmonary lobules. They are continuous with the interlobular septa.

Radiological Patterns in Parenchymal Sarcoidosis

The HRCT appearance of pulmonary sarcoidosis has a great variability and is notorious for mimicking many other interstitial lung diseases. The most important two radiological patterns in sarcoidosis with involvement of the lung parenchyma are the nodular pattern and the reticulonodular pattern. The distribution of nodules on HRCT can follow three different patterns; random distribution, centrilobular distribution, and perilymphatic distribution (Fig. 2.4).

Nodular and Reticulonodular Pattern

The nodular pattern is seen in almost 90 % of sarcoidosis patients with parenchymal involvement [32, 33]. Sarcoid granulomas are microscopic in size but can aggregate to form small nodules which can be seen on HRCT. These small nodules are 1–10 mm in diameter, usually have irregular margins, and are predominantly present in the mid and upper zones of the lungs. The nodules are frequently found along the bronchovascular bundles and in the subpleural region (Fig. 2.5) following a perilymphatic distribution. Aggregated subpleural nodules account for the fissural

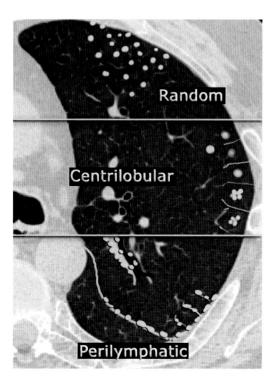

Fig. 2.4 Different nodal distribution patterns in interstitial lung diseases. In most cases, small nodules can be placed into one of three categories: random, centrilobular, or perilymphatic distribution. In sarcoidosis, small nodules typically follow a perilymphatic distribution. *Random distribution*: Randomly distributed nodules do not follow a particular pattern of involvement with respect to the pulmonary architecture and the secondary pulmonary lobule. These nodules affect the fissures, peribronchovascular structures, and the center of the secondary pulmonary nodules. However they lack a predominance in any of these areas since they are randomly distributed. *Centrilobular*: Centrilobular nodules exist predominantly in the center of the secondary lobule around the small airways. Centrilobular nodules spare the subpleural surface. They are typically at least 5–10 mm away from the pleural surfaces. *Perilymphatic*: Nodules that are distributed with a perilymphatic predominance are seen near the fissures, subpleural location, and the peribronchovascular structures. Publication with permission from http://www.radiologyassistant.nl

thickening that can be seen on HRCT. The nodules adjacent to interfaces of vessels, airways, and septa give these structures an irregular or beaded appearance, implicating to be pathognomonic for sarcoidosis. This pattern is also seen in histological specimens, where granulomas are found in association with lymphatics along vessels, airways, and in the subpleural area [34]. This distribution of granulomas can also explain the high rate of success in diagnosing sarcoidosis by bronchial and transbronchial biopsy. Frequently, sarcoidosis causes nodular septal thickening defining the reticulonodular pattern. A reticular pattern is a descriptive term (reticulum meaning network) with several morphological variations ranging from generalized thickening of interlobular septa to honeycomb lung destruction. A pure reticular pattern is rarely seen in sarcoidosis [35].

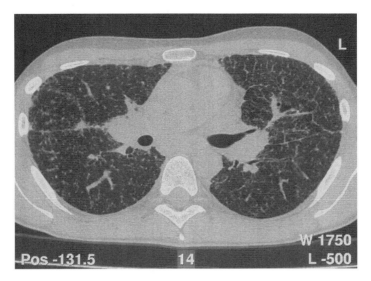

Fig. 2.5 HRCT with the classical perilymphatic distribution of nodules in a patient with sarcoidosis. Note the occurrence of small nodules along subpleural surface and fissures, along interlobular septa and the peribronchovascular bundles giving these structures a "beaded" appearance. This is thought to be pathognomonic for sarcoidosis

Large Nodules and Alveolar Sarcoidosis

Sarcoid nodules can aggregate into pulmonary nodules (no greater than 3 cm in diameter) or large masses (Fig. 2.6). Such a presentation is uncommon in sarcoidosis and estimated to be 2.4–4 % [19, 27, 36–38]. In a retrospective analysis in African-American patients, it was found that 82 % had multiple masses/nodules and only 18 % had a solitary lesion [39]. An air bronchogram was seen in 58 % of the cases and the nodules tend to be more peripheral. The margins of the nodules are often irregular and hazy [37]. The nodules can remain stable for years; however, partial or complete regression has been described [36]. Cavitation is rarely seen in large pulmonary masses and is usually benign, however, hemoptysis can occur [40, 41]. In approximately 10–20 % of patients, massive consolidation with air bronchograms develops [42–45] (Fig. 2.7). The pathologic mechanism is loss of alveolar air due to compression of the alveoli by coalescent granulomas in the interstitium [26]. The alveolar opacities are usually present in the peripheral middle zones of the lung [26, 37].

Galaxy Sign, Cluster Sign, and (Reversed) Halo Sign

Recently, three CT signs have been reviewed in sarcoidosis involving a more atypical distribution of large and small nodules [46]. The "sarcoid galaxy sign" represents a large pulmonary nodule or mass surrounded by many small satellite nodules

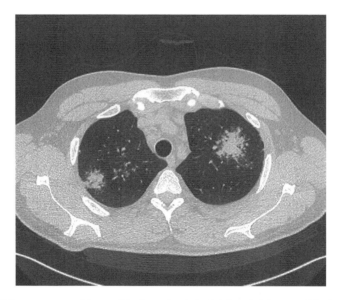

Fig. 2.6 Pulmonary mass with sarcoid galaxy sign in both left and right upper lobe in a 28-year-old sarcoidosis patient. In both upper lobes the mass is surrounded by multiple small satellite nodules. Courtesy of Dr. K. Cuppens, University Hospital Leuven, Belgium

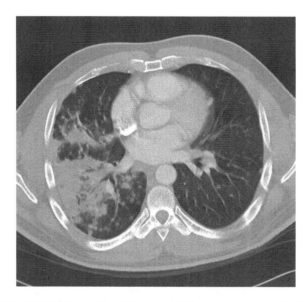

Fig. 2.7 Alveolar consolidation in the middle and right lower lobe of a sarcoidosis patient. Note the presence of air bronchograms in the major consolidation in the right lower lobe. Furthermore, multiple nodules with a mildly irregular outline are seen bilaterally

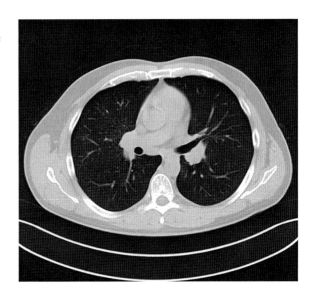

Fig. 2.8 Sarcoid cluster sign in sarcoidosis. Note the subtle clustering of micronodules without confluence in the right parahilar region. Courtesy of Prof. dr. J. Verschakelen and Prof. dr. W. Wuyts, University Hospital Leuven, Belgium

(Fig. 2.6). It is named after a galaxy, where the stars are known to be more concentrated to the galactic center than in the periphery. The "sarcoid cluster sign" is also characterized by clusters of multiple small nodules forming a pulmonary mass but, in contrast to the galaxy sign, the nodules do not tend to coalesce in the center (Fig. 2.8). The most important differential diagnosis for "sarcoid galaxy sign" or "sarcoid cluster sign" is tuberculosis. However, clusters of small nodules can also be seen in cryptococcus infection and silicosis [46]. The "reversed halo sign" is a far more nonspecific sign and describes a focal area of ground glass opacity surrounded by an almost complete ring of consolidation (Fig. 2.9). It was first described as a specific finding in patients with cryptogenic organizing pneumonia (COP) [47]. Later on, multiple authors described the "reversed halo sign" in various diseases such as tuberculosis, aspergillosis, Wegener's granulomatosis, and adenocarcinoma in situ (formerly known as bronchoalveolar carcinoma) [48]. The "reversed halo sign" is also known as the "atoll sign" due to its resemblance of a ring shaped coral reef that encloses a lagoon with shallow water [49]. A true "halo sign," describing a pulmonary mass with a surrounding area of ground glass has been rarely described in sarcoidosis [50].

Ground Glass Opacities

Ground glass attenuation in HRCT is defined as areas of hazy increased attenuation with preservation of bronchial and vascular margins. In sarcoidosis patients, the prevalence of ground glass opacities is estimated to be 40 % ranging from 16 to 83 % [29, 42, 45, 51, 52]. Historically, it was believed to represent active alveolitis, but now it is thought to be caused by small interstitial granulomas or fibrotic lesions

Fig. 2.9 Reversed halo sign in both lower lobes in a 32-year-old patient clinically and radiologically suspected of sarcoidosis. There is a focal area of ground glass opacity surrounded by an almost complete ring of consolidation. Lung biopsy of the mass in the right lower lobe revealed a histopathological diagnosis of lymphocytic interstitial pneumonia (LIP)

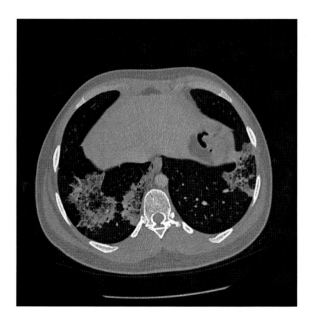

beyond the resolution of CT [34]. Ground glass is multifocal and often accompanied by subtle micronodularity [53]. Furthermore, it is most frequently seen at disease presentation [43]. The response to steroids depends on the presence of underlying fibrosis, with clearance being more likely if it is of short duration [45].

Fibrotic Sarcoidosis

At presentation, approximately 5 % of sarcoidosis patients have fibrotic changes on their chest X-ray [9, 10]. However, in an estimated 10–20 % of patients fibrosis develops or becomes more prominent during disease course [54]. On the chest X-ray, linear opacities radiating laterally from the hilum into the middle and upper zones is a characteristic finding [26]. The hila are shifted upward and vessels and fissures are distorted (Fig. 2.10) [19]. Due to compensatory hyperinflation, the lower lobes are sometimes transradiant. On HRCT, fibrotic changes are represented by fibrous bands, hilar retraction, displacement of fissures, traction bronchiectasis, honeycomb cysts, bullae, and irregular reticular opacities including intralobular lines and irregular septal thickening. Fibrosis is seen predominantly in the upper and middle lobes in a patchy distribution. A common feature of fibrotic sarcoidosis is the presence of conglomerated masses surrounding and encompassing vessels and bronchi. It occurs in 60 % of fibrotic sarcoidosis and is associated with bronchial distortion [44].

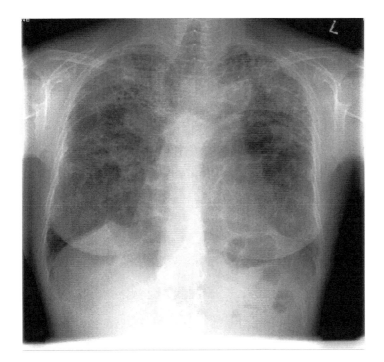

Fig. 2.10 Pulmonary fibrosis on a chest X-ray in a 46-year-old sarcoidosis patient. Note that the hila are shifted upward

Fibrotic cysts, bullae, traction bronchiectasis, and paracicatricial emphysema (air space enlargement and lung destruction developing adjacent to areas of pulmonary scarring) represent advanced fibrotic sarcoidosis (Fig. 2.11). Cystic abnormalities are particularly common in the upper lobes in advanced fibrotic sarcoidosis [55]. Honeycombing (subpleural clustering of cystic airspaces) is thought to be less common in sarcoidosis compared to other end-stage lung diseases [56]. If present, honeycomb-like cysts are most commonly found in the upper lobes but can also be seen in the lower lobes mimicking idiopathic pulmonary fibrosis [35].

Mosaic Attenuation Pattern and Airtrapping

Mosaic attenuation is defined as a patchwork of regions with varied attenuation on HRCT. This pattern can represent patchy interstitial disease, vascular disease, or small airway disease. In patients with sarcoidosis, the presence of mosaic attenuation frequently results from small airway involvement by granulomas or fibrosis [57, 58]. To verify that mosaic attenuation is caused by small airway disease,

Fig. 2.11 Fibrotic pulmonary sarcoidosis on HRCT. The CT demonstrates parenchymal distortion and destruction. Multiple honeycomb cysts are noted throughout the upper lobes bilaterally

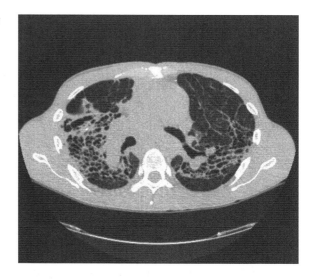

inspiratory images on CT must be compared with the parenchymal appearance on expiratory images in order to identify airtrapping. Airtrapping is a common but nonspecific feature of pulmonary sarcoidosis occurring in 95 % of patients [57, 59].

Mycetomas

The formation of mycetomas occurs in approximately 2 % of sarcoidosis patients, especially in stage IV cystic disease [60]. Fungal balls can develop in pre-existing bullae or cysts which are colonized by fungi, usually *Aspergillus* species. The characteristic appearance of a pulmonary aspergilloma consists of a mobile opacity occupying part or most of the cavity. It is surrounded by a peripheral rim of air known as the air crescent sign or Monod sign (Fig. 2.12) [61]. A common symptom in patients with aspergillomas is hemoptysis and, when massive, can be life threatening.

Pleural Involvement

Pleural Effusion

In sarcoidosis, granulomas can be found on both visceral and parietal pleura. This pleural localization as well as blockage of lymphatic channels by granulomas can result in pleural effusion. However, pleural effusion is an uncommon manifestation of sarcoidosis with an estimated incidence of 0.7–10 % on chest X-ray [62–67]. In a more recent study, the occurrence of pleural effusion was studied with ultrasonography in 181 patients with sarcoidosis presenting at the outpatient clinic of a

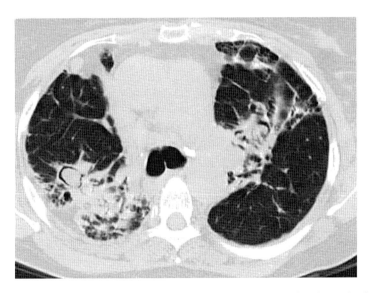

Fig. 2.12 Aspergilloma in the right upper lobe of a 57-year-old patient with advanced pulmonary sarcoidosis. The aspergilloma is surrounded by a peripheral rim of air known as the air crescent sign or Monod sign

University Hospital [68]. In 2.8 % of patients pleural fluid was detected, with some patients having a parapneumonic effusion and congestive heart failure. Therefore, in this study only 1.1 % of patients had sarcoidosis-related pleural effusion demonstrated by biopsy-proven sarcoid pleural involvement. Sarcoidosis-related pleural effusion occurs more often in the right side of the lung compared to the left (45 % vs. 33 %, respectively) [67]. It mostly resolves spontaneously within 6 months [69], sometimes leaving residual pleural thickening [26, 65].

Chylothorax

The development of chylothorax is an exceptionally rare complication of sarcoidosis, with only a few case reports in the literature [70–73]. In one case report, chylothorax was the presenting feature of sarcoidosis [71].

Pneumothorax

It has been estimated that pneumothorax has a 2–3 % prevalence in sarcoidosis patients [74, 75]. Cases of spontaneous pneumothorax may develop due to rupture of a subpleural bleb, particularly in patients with advanced fibrocystic disease [67]. Bilateral pneumothorax in sarcoidosis has also been reported [76].

Necrotizing Sarcoid Granulomatosis

Necrotizing sarcoid angiitis and granulomatosis (NSG) is a rare entity and seen as a variant of sarcoidosis [77], however, with some uncertainty. It is debated whether NSG is a manifestation of systemic sarcoidosis with necrotizing granulomata or a form of necrotizing angiitis with a sarcoid-like reaction [78]. NSG is defined by a granulomatous vasculitis, confluent non-necrotizing granulomas, and foci of infarct-like necrosis with variable degrees of fibrosis [77, 79]. Since the first paper in 1973 [80], approximately 135 cases have been described [81]. The clinical features of NSG are nonspecific. The lungs are primarily affected; however, other organs can also be affected. Radiographic features are similar to the nodular presentation with large pulmonary nodules or masses as described in section "Parenchymal Involvement."

Pulmonary Hypertension

It is estimated that 1–6 % of patients with sarcoidosis have pulmonary hypertension, most patients having advanced stages on chest radiography (Scadding stages III and IV) [82, 83]. However, fibrosis or extensive parenchymal abnormalities are not always present and the absence should not exclude further evaluation for pulmonary hypertension [84]. Clinical characteristics are often atypical but some symptoms can suggest underlying pulmonary hypertension; dyspnea more severe compared to functional impairment, chest pain, and near syncope on exertion. Also, almost 25 % of sarcoidosis patients with pulmonary hypertension present with signs of right-sided heart failure [83, 84]. Diagnosing pulmonary hypertension in sarcoidosis solely with the use of CT is difficult and merely impossible. However, severe pulmonary hypertension is likely to be present when the diameter of the main pulmonary artery at the level of its bifurcation is clearly greater than that of the adjacent ascending aorta or more than 29 mm [85]. In a study by Nunes and colleagues, a higher frequency of ground glass attenuation and septal lines was found in sarcoidosis patients with pulmonary hypertension compared to sarcoidosis patients without pulmonary hypertension [84].

Positron Emission Tomography

In the last 10–15 years, positron emission tomography (PET) with ^{18}F-Fluordeoxyglucose (^{18}F-FDG PET) has emerged as a powerful tool to visualize the intensity and extent of sarcoidosis activity throughout the body [86–88]. This seems important for clinicians dealing with sarcoidosis patients with unexplained,

Fig. 2.13 ^{18}F-FDG PET in a 50-year-old patient with active pulmonary and extrapulmonary sarcoidosis. Note the high uptake in the right upper lobe representing a massive consolidation. Due to a high uptake in both skeleton and bone marrow a biopsy of the right crista iliaca was performed revealing multiple non-necrotizing granulomas and fibrosis

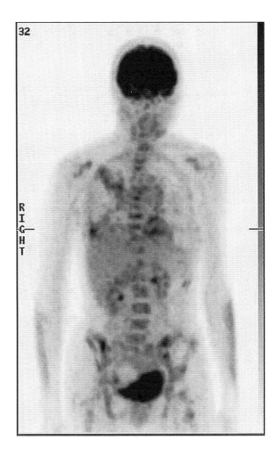

persistent, and disabling symptoms not coinciding with pulmonary function tests and radiographic features. It has been demonstrated that ^{18}F-FDG PET is a more sensitive technique in detecting disease activity in sarcoidosis compared to genotype-corrected ACE en sIL-2R [87, 89]. Pulmonary disease activity can be demonstrated with ^{18}F-FDG PET in patients with either a normal chest X-ray or signs of extensive fibrosis (Scadding stage IV). This observation has two important implications. First, when screening for pulmonary involvement in patients presenting with extrapulmonary sarcoidosis, a normal chest X-ray does not exclude pulmonary involvement. Second, in a majority of patients with Scadding stage IV persistent parenchymal disease activity can be detected using ^{18}F-FDG PET [89]. ^{18}F-FDG PET has been demonstrated to asses to possible functional improvement that can be achieved by immunosuppressive therapy [90] Therefore in some patients with stage IV disease anti-inflammatory therapy might be appropriate. An example of ^{18}F-FDG PET in active pulmonary sarcoidosis is given in Fig. 2.13.

References

1. Hillerdal G, Nou E, Osterman K, Schmekel B. Sarcoidosis: epidemiology and prognosis. A 15-year European study. Am Rev Respir Dis. 1984;130(1):29–32.
2. Lynch 3rd JP, Kazerooni EA, Gay SE. Pulmonary sarcoidosis. Clin Chest Med. 1997;18(4): 755–8.
3. Reich JM. Mortality of intrathoracic sarcoidosis in referral vs population-based settings: influence of stage, ethnicity, and corticosteroid therapy. Chest. 2002;121(1):32–9.
4. Hendrick DJ, Blackwood RA, Black JM. Chest pain in the presentation of sarcoidosis. Br J Dis Chest. 1976;70(3):206–10.
5. Cappell MS. Endoscopic, radiographic, and manometric findings in dysphagia associated with sarcoid due to extrinsic esophageal compression from subcarinal lymphadenopathy. Am J Gastroenterol. 1995;90(3):489–92.
6. Scadding JG. Prognosis of intrathoracic sarcoidosis in England. A review of 136 cases after five years' observation. Br Med J. 1961;2(5261):1165–72.
7. Grutters JC, Drent M, Van den Bosch JMM. European Respiratory Society Monograph 2009; 46(Interstitial Lung Diseases):126-54. doi:10.1183/1025448x.00046008.
8. Statement on sarcoidosis. Joint Statement of the American Thoracic Society (ATS), the European Respiratory Society (ERS) and the World Association of Sarcoidosis and Other Granulomatous Disorders (WASOG) adopted by the ATS Board of Directors and by the ERS Executive Committee, February 1999. Am J Respir Crit Care Med. 1999;160(2):736–55.
9. Baughman RP, Teirstein AS, Judson MA, Rossman MD, Yeager Jr H, Bresnitz EA, et al. Clinical characteristics of patients in a case control study of sarcoidosis. Am J Respir Crit Care Med. 2001;164(10 Pt 1):1885–9.
10. Nunes H, Brillet PY, Valeyre D, Brauner MW, Wells AU. Imaging in sarcoidosis. Semin Respir Crit Care Med. 2007;28(1):102–20.
11. Bechtel JJ, Starr 3rd T, Dantzker DR, Bower JS. Airway hyperreactivity in patients with sarcoidosis. Am Rev Respir Dis. 1981;124(6):759–61.
12. Marcias S, Ledda MA, Perra R, Severino C, Rosetti L. Aspecific bronchial hyperreactivity in pulmonary sarcoidosis. Sarcoidosis. 1994;11(2):118–22.
13. Shorr AF, Torrington KG, Hnatiuk OW. Endobronchial involvement and airway hyperreactivity in patients with sarcoidosis. Chest. 2001;120(3):881–6.
14. Baughman RP, Lower EE, Tami T. Upper airway. 4: Sarcoidosis of the upper respiratory tract (SURT). Thorax. 2010;65(2):181–6.
15. James DG, Barter S, Jash D, MacKinnon DM, Carstairs LS. Sarcoidosis of the upper respiratory tract (SURT). J Laryngol Otol. 1982;96(8):711–8.
16. Panselinas E, Halstead L, Schlosser RJ, Judson MA. Clinical manifestations, radiographic findings, treatment options, and outcome in sarcoidosis patients with upper respiratory tract involvement. South Med J. 2010;103(9):870–5.
17. Shorr AF, Torrington KG, Hnatiuk OW. Endobronchial biopsy for sarcoidosis: a prospective study. Chest. 2001;120(1):109–14.
18. Chambellan A, Turbie P, Nunes H, Brauner M, Battesti JP, Valeyre D. Endoluminal stenosis of proximal bronchi in sarcoidosis: bronchoscopy, function, and evolution. Chest. 2005;127(2): 472–81.
19. Kirks DR, McCormick VD, Greenspan RH. Pulmonary sarcoidosis. Roentgenologic analysis of 150 patients. Am J Roentgenol Radium Ther Nucl Med. 1973;117(4):777–86.
20. James DG, Neville E, Siltzbach LE. A worldwide review of sarcoidosis. Ann N Y Acad Sci. 1976;278:321–34.
21. Siltzbach LE, James DG, Neville E, Turiaf J, Battesti JP, Sharma OP, et al. Course and prognosis of sarcoidosis around the world. Am J Med. 1974;57(6):847–52.
22. Sider L, Horton Jr ES. Hilar and mediastinal adenopathy in sarcoidosis as detected by computed tomography. J Thorac Imaging. 1990;5(2):77–80.

23. Patil SN, Levin DL. Distribution of thoracic lymphadenopathy in sarcoidosis using computed tomography. J Thorac Imaging. 1999;14(2):114–7.
24. Niimi H, Kang EY, Kwong JS, Carignan S, Muller NL. CT of chronic infiltrative lung disease: prevalence of mediastinal lymphadenopathy. J Comput Assist Tomogr. 1996;20(2):305–8.
25. Gawne-Cain ML, Hansell DM. The pattern and distribution of calcified mediastinal lymph nodes in sarcoidosis and tuberculosis: a CT study. Clin Radiol. 1996;51(4):263–7.
26. Rabinowitz JG, Ulreich S, Soriano C. The usual unusual manifestations of sarcoidosis and the "hilar haze" – a new diagnostic aid. Am J Roentgenol Radium Ther Nucl Med. 1974;120(4):821–3.
27. Romer FK. Presentation of sarcoidosis and outcome of pulmonary changes. Dan Med Bull. 1982;29(1):27–32.
28. Spann RW, Rosenow 3rd EC, DeRemee RA, Miller WE. Unilateral hilar or paratracheal adenopathy in sarcoidosis: a study of 38 cases. Thorax. 1971;26(3):296–9.
29. Murdoch J, Muller NL. Pulmonary sarcoidosis: changes on follow-up CT examination. AJR Am J Roentgenol. 1992;159(3):473–7.
30. McLoud TC, Putman CE, Pascual R. Eggshell calcification with systemic sarcoidosis. Chest. 1974;66(5):515–7.
31. Webb WR. Thin-section CT, of the secondary pulmonary lobule: anatomy and the image – the 2004 Fleischner lecture. Radiology. 2006;239(2):322–38.
32. McLoud TC, Epler GR, Gaensler EA, Burke GW, Carrington CB. A radiographic classification for sarcoidosis: physiologic correlation. Invest Radiol. 1982;17(2):129–38.
33. Israel HL, Karlin P, Menduke H, DeLisser OG. Factors affecting outcome of sarcoidosis. Influence of race, extrathoracic involvement, and initial radiologic lung lesions. Ann N Y Acad Sci. 1986;465:609–18.
34. Nishimura K, Itoh H, Kitaichi M, Nagai S, Izumi T. Pulmonary sarcoidosis: correlation of CT and histopathologic findings. Radiology. 1993;189(1):105–9.
35. Padley SP, Padhani AR, Nicholson A, Hansell DM. Pulmonary sarcoidosis mimicking cryptogenic fibrosing alveolitis on CT. Clin Radiol. 1996;51(11):807–10.
36. Sharma OP, Hewlett R, Gordonson J. Nodular sarcoidosis: an unusual radiographic appearance. Chest. 1973;64(2):189–92.
37. Battesti JP, Saumon G, Valeyre D, Amouroux J, Pechnick B, Sandron D, et al. Pulmonary sarcoidosis with an alveolar radiographic pattern. Thorax. 1982;37(6):448–52.
38. McNicol MW, Luce PJ. Sarcoidosis in a racially mixed community. J R Coll Physicians Lond. 1985;19(3):179–83.
39. Malaisamy S, Dalal B, Bimenyuy C, Soubani AO. The clinical and radiologic features of nodular pulmonary sarcoidosis. Lung. 2009;187(1):9–15.
40. Edelman RR, Johnson TS, Jhaveri HS, Kim D, Kasdon E, Frank HA, et al. Fatal hemoptysis resulting from erosion of a pulmonary artery in cavitary sarcoidosis. AJR Am J Roentgenol. 1985;145(1):37–8.
41. Loh GA, Lettieri CJ, Shah AA. Bronchial arterial embolisation for massive haemoptysis in cavitary sarcoidosis. BMJ Case Rep. 2013. doi:10.1136/bcr-2012-008268.
42. Leung AN, Brauner MW, Caillat-Vigneron N, Valeyre D, Grenier P. Sarcoidosis activity: correlation of HRCT findings with those of 67Ga scanning, bronchoalveolar lavage, and serum angiotensin-converting enzyme assay. J Comput Assist Tomogr. 1998;22(2):229–34.
43. Brauner MW, Grenier P, Mompoint D, Lenoir S, de Cremoux H. Pulmonary sarcoidosis: evaluation with high-resolution CT. Radiology. 1989;172(2):467–71.
44. Abehsera M, Valeyre D, Grenier P, Jaillet H, Battesti JP, Brauner MW. Sarcoidosis with pulmonary fibrosis: CT patterns and correlation with pulmonary function. AJR Am J Roentgenol. 2000;174(6):1751–7.
45. Remy-Jardin M, Giraud F, Remy J, Wattinne L, Wallaert B, Duhamel A. Pulmonary sarcoidosis: role of CT in the evaluation of disease activity and functional impairment and in prognosis assessment. Radiology. 1994;191(3):675–80.
46. Marchiori E, Zanetti G, Barreto MM, de Andrade FT, Rodrigues RS. Atypical distribution of small nodules on high resolution CT studies: patterns and differentials. Respir Med. 2011;105(9):1263–7.

47. Voloudaki AE, Bouros DE, Froudarakis ME, Datseris GE, Apostolaki EG, Gourtsoyiannis NC. Crescentic and ring-shaped opacities. CT features in two cases of bronchiolitis obliterans organizing pneumonia (BOOP). Acta Radiol. 1996;37(6):889–92.
48. Marchiori E, Zanetti G, Mano CM, Hochhegger B, Irion KL. The reversed halo sign: another atypical manifestation of sarcoidosis. Korean J Radiol. 2010;11(2):251–2.
49. Zompatori M, Poletti V, Battista G, Diegoli M. Bronchiolitis obliterans with organizing pneumonia (BOOP), presenting as a ring-shaped opacity at HRCT (the atoll sign). A case report. Radiol Med. 1999;97(4):308–10.
50. Marten K, Rummeny EJ, Engelke C. The CT halo: a new sign in active pulmonary sarcoidosis. Br J Radiol. 2004;77(924):1042–5.
51. Grenier P, Chevret S, Beigelman C, Brauner MW, Chastang C, Valeyre D. Chronic diffuse infiltrative lung disease: determination of the diagnostic value of clinical data, chest radiography, and CT and Bayesian analysis. Radiology. 1994;191(2):383–90.
52. Grenier P, Valeyre D, Cluzel P, Brauner MW, Lenoir S, Chastang C. Chronic diffuse interstitial lung disease: diagnostic value of chest radiography and high-resolution CT. Radiology. 1991;179(1):123–32.
53. Martin SG, Kronek LP, Valeyre D, Brauner N, Brillet PY, Nunes H, et al. High-resolution computed tomography to differentiate chronic diffuse interstitial lung diseases with predominant ground-glass pattern using logical analysis of data. Eur Radiol. 2010;20(6):1297–310.
54. Moller DR. Pulmonary fibrosis of sarcoidosis. New approaches, old ideas. Am J Respir Cell Mol Biol. 2003;29(3 Suppl):S37–41.
55. Freundlich IM, Libshitz HI, Glassman LM, Israel HL. Sarcoidosis. Typical and atypical thoracic manifestations and complications. Clin Radiol. 1970;21(4):376–83.
56. Primack SL, Hartman TE, Hansell DM, Muller NL. End-stage lung disease: CT findings in 61 patients. Radiology. 1993;189(3):681–6.
57. Davies CW, Tasker AD, Padley SP, Davies RJ, Gleeson FV. Air trapping in sarcoidosis on computed tomography: correlation with lung function. Clin Radiol. 2000;55(3):217–21.
58. Hansell DM, Milne DG, Wilsher ML, Wells AU. Pulmonary sarcoidosis: morphologic associations of airflow obstruction at thin-section CT. Radiology. 1998;209(3):697–704.
59. Bartz RR, Stern EJ. Airways obstruction in patients with sarcoidosis: expiratory CT scan findings. J Thorac Imaging. 2000;15(4):285–9.
60. Pena TA, Soubani AO, Samavati L. Aspergillus lung disease in patients with sarcoidosis: a case series and review of the literature. Lung. 2011;189(2):167–72.
61. Pesle GD, Monod O. Bronchiectasis due to asperigilloma. Dis Chest. 1954;25(2):172–83.
62. Chusid EL, Siltzbach LE. Sarcoidosis of the pleura. Ann Intern Med. 1974;81(2):190–4.
63. Sharma OP, Gordonson J. Pleural effusion in sarcoidosis: a report of six cases. Thorax. 1975;30(1):95–101.
64. Beekman JF, Zimmet SM, Chun BK, Miranda AA, Katz S. Spectrum of pleural involvement in sarcoidosis. Arch Intern Med. 1976;136(3):323–30.
65. Wilen SB, Rabinowitz JG, Ulreich S, Lyons HA. Pleural involvement in sarcoidosis. Am J Med. 1974;57(2):200–9.
66. Tommasini A, Di Vittorio G, Facchinetti F, Festi G, Schito V, Cipriani A. Pleural effusion in sarcoidosis: a case report. Sarcoidosis. 1994;11(2):138–40.
67. Soskel NT, Sharma OP. Pleural involvement in sarcoidosis. Curr Opin Pulm Med. 2000;6(5):455–68.
68. Huggins JT, Doelken P, Sahn SA, King L, Judson MA. Pleural effusions in a series of 181 outpatients with sarcoidosis. Chest. 2006;129(6):1599–604.
69. Littner MR, Schachter EN, Putman CE, Odero DO, Gee JB. The clinical assessment of roentgenographically atypical pulmonary sarcoidosis. Am J Med. 1977;62(3):361–8.
70. Aberg H, Bah M, Waters AW. Sarcoidosis: complicated by chylothorax. Minn Med. 1966;49(7):1065–70.
71. Jarman PR, Whyte MK, Sabroe I, Hughes JM. Sarcoidosis presenting with chylothorax. Thorax. 1995;50(12):1324–5.

72. Lengyel RJ, Shanley DJ. Recurrent chylothorax associated with sarcoidosis. Hawaii Med J. 1995;54(12):817–8.
73. Parker JM, Torrington KG, Phillips YY. Sarcoidosis complicated by chylothorax. South Med J. 1994;87(8):860–2.
74. Hours S, Nunes H, Kambouchner M, Uzunhan Y, Brauner MW, Valeyre D, et al. Pulmonary cavitary sarcoidosis: clinico-radiologic characteristics and natural history of a rare form of sarcoidosis. Medicine (Baltimore). 2008;87(3):142–51.
75. Froudarakis ME, Bouros D, Voloudaki A, Papiris S, Kottakis Y, Constantopoulos SH, et al. Pneumothorax as a first manifestation of sarcoidosis. Chest. 1997;112(1):278–80.
76. Akelsson IG, Eklund A, Skold CM, Tornling G. Bilateral spontaneous pneumothorax and sarcoidosis. Sarcoidosis. 1990;7(2):136–8.
77. Popper HH, Klemen H, Colby TV, Churg A. Necrotizing sarcoid granulomatosis – is it different from nodular sarcoidosis? Pneumologie. 2003;57(5):268–71.
78. Koss MN, Hochholzer L, Feigin DS, Garancis JC, Ward PA. Necrotizing sarcoid-like granulomatosis: clinical, pathologic, and immunopathologic findings. Hum Pathol. 1980;11(5 Suppl):510–9.
79. Rosen Y. Pathology of sarcoidosis. Semin Respir Crit Care Med. 2007;28(1):36–52.
80. Liebow AA. The J. Burns Amberson lecture – pulmonary angiitis and granulomatosis. Am Rev Respir Dis. 1973;108(1):1–18.
81. Yeboah J, Afkhami M, Lee C, Sharma OP. Necrotizing sarcoid granulomatosis. Curr Opin Pulm Med. 2012;18(5):493–8.
82. Handa T, Nagai S, Miki S, Fushimi Y, Ohta K, Mishima M, et al. Incidence of pulmonary hypertension and its clinical relevance in patients with sarcoidosis. Chest. 2006;129(5):1246–52.
83. Sulica R, Teirstein AS, Kakarla S, Nemani N, Behnegar A, Padilla ML. Distinctive clinical, radiographic, and functional characteristics of patients with sarcoidosis-related pulmonary hypertension. Chest. 2005;128(3):1483–9.
84. Nunes H, Humbert M, Capron F, Brauner M, Sitbon O, Battesti JP, et al. Pulmonary hypertension associated with sarcoidosis: mechanisms, haemodynamics and prognosis. Thorax. 2006;61(1):68–74.
85. Nunes H, Uzunhan Y, Freynet O, Humbert M, Brillet PY, Kambouchner M, et al. Pulmonary hypertension complicating sarcoidosis. Presse Med. 2012;41(6 Pt 2):e303–16.
86. Braun JJ, Kessler R, Constantinesco A, Imperiale A. 18F-FDG PET/CT in sarcoidosis management: review and report of 20 cases. Eur J Nucl Med Mol Imaging. 2008;35(8):1537–43.
87. Keijsers RG, Verzijlbergen FJ, Oyen WJ, van den Bosch JM, Ruven HJ, van Velzen-Blad H, et al. 18F-FDG PET, genotype-corrected ACE and sIL-2R in newly diagnosed sarcoidosis. Eur J Nucl Med Mol Imaging. 2009;36(7):1131–7.
88. Teirstein AS, Machac J, Almeida O, Lu P, Padilla ML, Iannuzzi MC. Results of 188 whole-body fluorodeoxyglucose positron emission tomography scans in 137 patients with sarcoidosis. Chest. 2007;132(6):1949–53.
89. Mostard RL, Voo S, van Kroonenburgh MJ, Verschakelen JA, Wijnen PA, Nelemans PJ, et al. Inflammatory activity assessment by F18 FDG-PET/CT in persistent symptomatic sarcoidosis. Respir Med. 2011;105(12):1917–24.
90. Keijsers RG, Verzijlbergen EJ, van den Bosch JM, Zanen P, van de Garde EM, Oyen WJ, et al. 18F-FDG PET as a predictor of pulmonary function in sarcoidosis. Sarcoidosis Vasc Diffuse Lung Dis. 2011;28(2):123–9.

Chapter 3
The Treatment of Pulmonary Sarcoidosis

Robert P. Baughman and Marjolein Drent

Abstract Decisions regarding treatment of sarcoidosis rely on several factors. These include symptoms, organ involvement, signs of functional impairment, and current and prior therapy. Over the years, the treatment options for sarcoidosis have increased. While this has allowed the clinician to tailor therapy for the individual patient, it also has led to the need to consider risk and benefit each individual patient. Not all therapy is equally effective in sarcoidosis. The benefits from an individual therapy may be more apparent within a few weeks, such as with glucocorticoids and anti-TNF biologic agents, whereas cytotoxic drugs such as methotrexate (MTX) may take up to 6 months or longer to demonstrate their effectiveness. Some drugs such as pentoxifylline seem only to be useful as steroid-sparing agents for pulmonary disease. In addition drugs such as chloroquine and thalidomide may be effective for cutaneous disease but not pulmonary disease.

Keywords Sarcoidosis • Prednisone • Methotrexate • Azathioprine • Leflunomide • Hydroxychloroquine • Infliximab • Adalimumab

R.P. Baughman, M.D. (✉)
Department of Internal Medicine, University of Cincinnati Medical Center, Cincinnati, OH, USA
e-mail: baughmrp@ucmail.uc.edu

M. Drent, M.D., Ph.D.
Department of Interstitial Lung Disease, Hospital Gelderse Vallei, Ede, The Netherlands

Faculty of Health, Medicine and Life Sciences (FHML), Maastricht University, Maastricht, The Netherlands

M.A. Judson (ed.), *Pulmonary Sarcoidosis: A Guide for the Practicing Clinician*, Respiratory Medicine 17, DOI 10.1007/978-1-4614-8927-6_3, © Springer Science+Business Media New York 2014

Introduction

Decisions regarding treatment of sarcoidosis rely on several factors. These include symptoms, organ involvement, signs of functional impairment, and current and prior therapy. Over the years, the treatment options for sarcoidosis have increased. While this has allowed the clinician to tailor therapy for the individual patient, it also has led to the need to consider risk and benefit each individual patient.

Not all therapy is equally effective in sarcoidosis. The benefits from an individual therapy may be more apparent within a few weeks, such as with glucocorticoids and anti-TNF biologic agents [1, 2], whereas cytotoxic drugs such as methotrexate (MTX) may take up to 6 months or longer to demonstrate their effectiveness [3]. Some drugs such as pentoxifylline seem only to be useful as steroid-sparing agents for pulmonary disease [4, 5]. In addition, drugs such as chloroquine and thalidomide may be effective for cutaneous disease but not pulmonary disease [6, 7].

Despite our increasing number of agents for treating sarcoidosis, there is evidence to suggest that the rate of hospitalization and death from sarcoidosis is rising [8, 9]. There are several possible reasons for this, including increased recognition of the disease as a cause of mortality, complications of the disease such as pulmonary hypertension [10, 11], and complications of treatment such as infection [12]. As we add more potent treatments, we may be increasing the overall risk for the patient. Another limitation to treatment decisions is the relatively few well controlled double blind placebo-controlled trials [13, 14]. This is in part because of the diverse presentation of sarcoidosis. Nevertheless, evidence recommendations can often be given for individual patient situations [15]. In this chapter, we will review the indications for therapy, current treatment options, and propose guidelines for treatment and monitoring with various agents.

Indication for Therapy

Table 3.1 lists those indications proposed as relative and absolute indications for therapy [16]. For many patients, the decision to treat will be based upon the level of symptoms and presence of functional impairment [17]. This is especially true for pulmonary and cutaneous disease. For example, a small skin lesion on the arm or back may not warrant any treatment. However, lupus pernio and hypercalcemia will often be treated with systemic therapy [18].

Pulmonary disease is the most common manifestation of sarcoidosis. However, not all patients with pulmonary disease require systemic therapy. Dyspnea and cough are the major indications for therapy. In the USA, about half of patients with pulmonary disease require systemic therapy [19, 20]. A smaller percentage of patients seem to require systemic therapy for pulmonary disease in Europe and Asia [21, 22]. However, advanced pulmonary disease is encountered throughout the

Table 3.1 Indications for treatment in sarcoidosis

Absolute	Relative[a]
Neurologic	Pulmonary
Cardiac	Cutaneous
Ocular	Hepatosplenomegaly
Hypercalcemia	Nephrolithiasis
Organ failure[b]	Systemic inflammatory response
	Fatigue
	Small fiber neuropathy and autonomic dysfunction

[a]Treatment indicated if patient symptomatic
[b]Such as renal or liver failure

Table 3.2 Parameters to monitor in pulmonary sarcoidosis

	Validated	Reproducible	Sarcoidosis specific	Low cost
Forced vital capacity (FVC)	3+[a, b]	3+	No	Yes
Forced expiratory volume in 1 s (FEV-1)	3+[b]	3+	No	Yes
FEV-1/FVC	3+[b]	3+	No	Yes
Diffusion lung carbon monoxide (DLCO)	3+[b]	2+	No	Yes
6-min walk distance (6MWD) [29]	2+[b]	1+	No	Yes
Chest X-ray: Scadding [33]	No	1+	Yes	Yes
Chest X-ray: Muers [35]	No	2+	Yes	Yes
HRCT Score [38]	Yes	1+	Yes	No
Positron emission tomography (PET) [40, 130]	No	Not tested	No	No
Saint George Respiratory Questionnaire (SGRQ)	3+[b]	2+	No	Yes
Short form-36 (SF-36)	3+[b]	2+	No	Yes
Sarcoidosis Health Questionnaire [131]	3+	2+	Yes	Yes
King's Sarcoidosis Questionnaire [132]	3+	2+	Yes	Yes
Fatigue Assessment Score [43]	3+	2+	Yes	Yes

Adapted from Baughman et al. [25]
[a]Scale: No, 1–3+, unknown
[b]Not validated for sarcoidosis

world. This includes pulmonary fibrosis, which can lead to significant morbidity and some mortality [23, 24].

For pulmonary disease, several parameters have been proposed to initially assess and monitor disease [25] and are summarized in Table 3.2. These include those obtained with pulmonary function testing, especially the forced vital capacity (FVC). Changes in FVC are the most widely used measure of response to therapy [26]. However, other static pulmonary function tests, including the DLCO may change with therapy [27]. Exercise capacity can be assessed by the 6-min walk test, which allows one to determine the 6-min walk distance (6MWD). While changes in 6MWD may be a reflection of changes in lung function, there are several other factors which can affect 6MWD [28]. These include other conditions such as pulmonary hypertension as well as other factors, such as fatigue [29] and impaired muscle strength [30]. Full cardiopulmonary exercise testing does provide information not obtained from routine spirometry [31, 32]. However, the variability of performing the test across centers has led to limited use in clinical trials of treatments.

Chest imaging has also been used to assess response to therapy. The Scadding staging system has proved a useful way of characterizing the majority of patients with pulmonary disease [33]. There are problems with reproducibility of the staging system [34]. In addition, most studies fail to show significant changes in stage with therapy. Muers et al. devised a detailed radiographic score similar to what has been used in pneumoconiosis [35]. Significant improvement in the Muers' score were seen with prednisone therapy [27] and infliximab [34] compared to placebo. The Muers' score is time consuming and others have reported that a simple comparison of chest X-ray before and after therapy has been useful [36, 37]. However, this method was not able to differentiate patients treated with infliximab versus those treated with placebo [34].

CT scanning, including high resolution CT (HRCT) imaging, has proved useful in identifying manifestations of sarcoidosis as well as complications of the disease such as bronchiectasis, fibrosis, and aspergillomas. Scoring systems for HRCT have been proposed [38, 39]. To date, no study assessing response to treatment in a systematic way of the utility of HRCT is published.

Positron emission tomography using fluor-18 fluorodeoxyglucose (PET) scanning of sarcoidosis has demonstrated that increased activity may be seen in the lungs with parenchymal lung disease. A negative correlation between $^{18F\text{-}FDG}$ PET activity and FVC has been found [40]. Mostard et al. demonstrated that the severity of the pulmonary involvement, assessed by HRCT features and lung function parameters, appeared to be associated with PET activity in sarcoidosis [40]. The majority of patients with fibrotic changes demonstrated inflammatory activity at pulmonary and extra-thoracic sites. In addition, improvement in lung function and PET activity in the lung has been shown after several treatments [41, 42].

Finally several measures of quality of life (QOL) have been reported in the treatment of sarcoidosis. For the most part, the studies have failed to show convincing evidence of change, but this may be due to study design. Also, many of the questionnaires are not sarcoidosis specific. The fatigue assessment scale (FAS) was developed for sarcoidosis patients [43]. Minimal clinically important differences have been determined for this scale [44]. The FAS scale has been shown to significantly improve with neurostimulants [45] and neurostimulant-like [46] drugs.

Figures 3.1 and 3.2 summarize an approach to treating sarcoidosis. In Fig. 3.1, the level of disease is determined based on pulmonary function studies and level of symptoms. In some cases, patients with normal pulmonary function may still have an advanced level of disease because of extra pulmonary disease, such as ocular or neurologic disease. Also, patients with symptoms and normal lung function should lead to investigation of alternative causes of dyspnea. These would include cardiac or muscle disease or complications such as pulmonary hypertension. Figure 3.2 is a guide to the usual therapy for each of these levels of disease.

	FVC>80%	FVC 60-79%	FVC<60%
No symptoms	A	A	Look for other causes of restriction
Mild/moderate symptoms And/or Significant extra-pulmonary disease	B	B	C
Oxygen supplementation 6 minute walk <150 m	Look for alternative causes*	C	D
Significant neurologic or cardiac disease	D	D	D

Fig. 3.1 The level of disease is determined based on pulmonary function studies and level of symptoms. In some cases, patients with normal pulmonary function may still have an advanced level of disease because of extra pulmonary disease, such as ocular or neurologic disease. Also, patients with symptoms and normal lung function should lead to investigation of alternative causes of dyspnea. *Alternative causes would include cardiac or muscle disease or complications such as pulmonary hypertension

Level of Disease	Standard Therapy	May Consider
A	No treatment	Inhaled corticosteroids or NSAIDs
B	Oral corticosteroids	Anti-malarial drugs Cytotoxic agents for patients with persistent disease or steroid associated toxicity
C	Low dose oral corticosteroids and/or cytotoxic therapy	Combination cytotoxic therapy Use of biologic agents for patients with chronic symptoms and/or treatment associated toxicity
D	Anti-TNF-alpha therapy plus cytotoxic therapy and/or low dose corticosteroids*	Other biologic agents Referral for lung transplant if no response to therapy

Fig. 3.2 A guide to the usual therapy for each of these levels of disease determined in Fig. 3.1. *Anti-TNF agents should be used in caution in patients with moderate to severe cardiomyopathy

Individual Treatments

Glucocorticoids: The most widely used treatment for sarcoidosis remains glucocorticoids [47]. This is based on the observation that these drugs can be quite effective for the disease. In addition, several trials have demonstrated a significant improvement in FVC, DLCO, or chest roentgenogram [27, 48]. The drug has also been used effectively in all other manifestations of sarcoidosis, including neurologic [49], cutaneous [18], cardiac [50], and ocular disease [51].

Several case series have demonstrated that corticosteroids are the preferred first drug for sarcoidosis patients. The overall frequency of initial corticosteroid therapy use is about 50 %, but varies from 30 to 80 % (Fig. 3.3) [20, 52–54]. In addition, some underlying conditions may be more likely to treat with corticosteroids. For example, neurological and cardiac involvement is almost always treated initially with corticosteroids. In one report of a large sarcoidosis population in the USA, the most common reason to use corticosteroid therapy was cardiac disease, while lung disease was the third most common, even though the overall prevalence of pulmonary disease was 18 times higher than cardiac disease [19]. For patients with cardiac or neurologic disease, a combination of corticosteroids and cytotoxic agents (such as MTX or azathioprine) are often used for initial therapy, although there is no specific trial demonstrating superiority of this approach over corticosteroids alone.

A bigger question is what dose to begin therapy. The usual dose is 20–40 mg a day. Tapering of corticosteroids is often over a prolonged period. One group did demonstrate a more rapid response to lower doses of prednisone and usually tapered over 2–6 weeks. However, this was more for an acute decompensation of the disease,

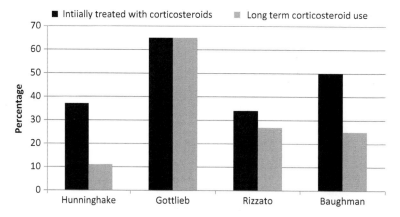

Fig. 3.3 Percentage of patients treated with corticosteroids within the first 6 months of diagnosis and percentage of overall patients who were on corticosteroids long term (at least 2 years from initial evaluation) [20, 52–54]

Fig. 3.4 Average prednisone dose at various time intervals for patients with acute pulmonary sarcoidosis receiving either placebo or methotrexate. There was a significant difference in the average prednisone dose after 6 months of therapy [59]

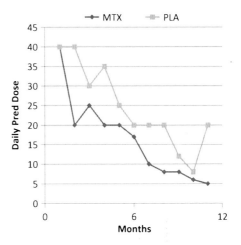

not for standard management of the underlying condition. Figure 3.4 demonstrates the average daily prednisone dosage from one study comparing MTX to placebo for acute pulmonary sarcoidosis. The dose of prednisone was reviewed every 1–2 months, but significant reduction was not seen until 6 months of therapy. After that point, half of the placebo patients required an increase in their prednisone dosage.

The approach to reduction of prednisone is almost as variable as the initial dose. In one multicenter trial, a steroid-tapering regimen was proposed and was able to be applied to over 80 % of visits. A modified version of this schedule evaluates the patient after the first 6–8 weeks of therapy. If the patient has improved, the dose of prednisone is halved. If the patient is stable, the dose is not changed for another 6–8 weeks. At the next and all subsequent visits, the dose is halved if the patient is stable or improved. If the patient relapses, the dose is doubled. For patients in whom the dose cannot be kept below 10 mg within 4–6 months, a steroid sparing alternative is added.

Unfortunately, once a patient begins corticosteroids, they may require long-term treatment. Figure 3.3 also demonstrates the percentage of patients who require long-term therapy in four large studies [20, 52–54]. These studies highlight that there is a subset of patients with chronic disease who are often considered for steroid sparing agent. These would be for patients with level B, C, or D symptoms. At most sarcoidosis centers, these patients represent the majority of patients who are still being followed 2–5 years after their initial diagnosis [55].

The toxicity of prednisone includes weight gain, mood swings, diabetes, cataracts, glaucoma, acne, and increased bruising. Osteopenia and osteoporosis are particular problems with long-term glucocorticosteroid use. Guidelines for preventing osteoporosis have been proposed by the American College of Rheumatology. These include supplemental calcium and vitamin D for sarcoidosis patients; there is an increased rate of hypercalcemia and hypercalcuria based on autonomous 1-alpha hydroxylase activity in the granulomas and increased levels of 1,25-diOH-vitamin D3, especially in patients with chronic sarcoidosis [56]. Therefore, modifications of the ACR recommendations have been made and are summarized in Table 3.3 [57].

Table 3.3 Recommendations regarding osteoporosis prevention for sarcoidosis patients on chronic corticosteroid therapy

- Obtain baseline bone density
- Check serum calcium and 25-OH and 1,25-di[OH]-vitamin D3 levels
- If bone density normal
  - Serum calcium and 1,25-di[OH] low
    (a) Calcium and vitamin D supplement
  - Serum calcium normal and 1,25-di[OH] normal or elevated
    (b) Calcium supplement alone
  - Serum calcium elevated or history of hypercalcemia or hypercalcuria[a]
    (c) No calcium or vitamin D supplement
- If bone density low treat with bisphosphonate and
  - Serum calcium and 1,25-di[OH] low
    (a) Calcium and vitamin D supplement
  - Serum calcium normal and 1,25-di[OH] normal or elevated
    (b) Calcium supplement alone
  - Serum calcium elevated or history of hypercalcemia or hypercalcuria[a]
    (c) No calcium or vitamin D supplement

Adapted from Sweiss et al. [57]
[a]Patients with history of nephrocalcinosis should have 24-h urine to look for hypercalcuria

Methotrexate: This drug is the most commonly prescribed steroid-sparing cytotoxic agent for chronic sarcoidosis [47]. Initial reports suggested approximately two-thirds of patients will respond to the drug after 6 months of therapy [58]. It has been shown to be steroid sparing as compared to placebo in a double blind placebo-controlled trial [59]. The drug has been reported as effective in pulmonary [58], cutaneous [60], ocular [51], and neurologic disease [49]. Guidelines for MTX dosage and monitoring have mostly derived from those developed for rheumatoid arthritis and psoriasis. However, since bone marrow involvement is common in sarcoidosis [61], the dose used in sarcoidosis is often only 10–15 mg a week. In some cases, we have used as little as 2.5 mg a week in patients with significant leukopenia due to their sarcoidosis. In addition, liver involvement is common in sarcoidosis. Surveillance liver biopsies have been performed in sarcoidosis patients on prolonged courses of MTX [62]. However, it appears that routine liver function testing can be useful to detect potential MTX hepatotoxicity. This is especially true with changes in the transaminase levels over time. Folic and folinic acid supplementation may be useful to reduce MTX toxicity [63, 64]. Dosage and evidence-based recommendations for monitoring while prescribing MTX is provided in Table 3.4. These recommendations have been adapted from those made by an expert panel [65].

Table 3.4 Evidence-based recommendations for use of pharmacologic therapy for sarcoidosis

Cytotoxic agents		
Azathioprine	50–200 mg oral daily	*Monitoring blood work*: Complete blood count and hepatic function should be monitored every 1–3 months as long as patients are on therapy *Monitoring of drug clearance*: Measurement of TPMT is useful to detect patients at risk for leucopenia from azathioprine, especially those who will receive higher doses or have a history suggestive of TPMT deficiency [133]. The dose may need adjustment according to creatinine clearance *Monitoring for drug/drug interaction*: Allopurinol inhibits the xanthine oxidase pathway. Patients should not receive azathioprine if they are on allopurinol	For patients who will undergo concurrent therapy with azathioprine and allopurinol, a reduction in dose of azathioprine is recommended. (Grade 1A) For patients who will undergo azathioprine therapy, obtaining complete blood counts and renal/hepatic profiles every 1–3 months is recommended. (Grade 1B)
Cyclophosphamide	50–200 mg oral daily OR 500–1,500 mg intravenously every 2–4 weeks	*Monitoring blood work*: A complete blood count and creatinine should be obtained when commencing cyclophosphamide therapy and repeated at least every 4–6 weeks. Patients treated with intermittent intravenous dosing should have a complete blood count prior to the next intravenous dosing. Urine analysis should be performed every 4–8 weeks to look for evidence of hemorrhagic cystitis. In patients with persistent, unexplained hematuria, cystoscopy should be strongly considered to evaluate for possible bladder cancer. Since CYC can induce sterility in men and women, counseling regarding ovarian and/or sperm harvesting prior to initiation of therapy should be considered. In women, gonadotropin releasing hormone given prior to initiation of CYC may prevent premature menopause *Monitoring of drug clearance*: Cyclophosphamide is cleared by the kidneys and direct toxicity to the bladder is the proposed mechanism for hemorrhagic cystitis and bladder cancer. Patients should be well hydrated on the day of dosing, with the recommendation of eight glasses of water as a rule of thumb. For patients at risk for bladder toxicity, co-administration of MESNA may reduce toxicity *Monitoring for drug/drug interaction*: Cyclophosphamide will cause increased rate of bone marrow suppression when used with other cytotoxic drugs. An increased rate of neutropenia may also be seen when used with rituximab	For patients who will undergo cyclophosphamide therapy, monitoring of complete blood count, renal profile, and urinalysis, at least monthly for dose adjustment is recommended (Grade 1B) For patients who will undergo cyclophosphamide therapy, increased fluid intake (e.g., 2 l in addition to normal intake in adults; additional volume given to children needs to be calculated on the basis of body weight) on the days of therapy is recommended (Grade 1C) For patients who undergo or have undergone cyclophosphamide therapy and develop hematuria, further evaluation is recommended (Grade 1B)

(continued)

Table 3.4 (continued)

| Leflunomide | 10–20 mg daily | *Monitoring blood work:* A complete blood count, liver function panel, phosphate, and creatinine should be obtained when commencing leflunomide therapy and repeated every 4–6 weeks for the first 6 months of treatment. After 6 months, if stable, these parameters can be checked every 6–12 weeks. Clinical monitoring for infections and signs of hepatotoxicity is also recommended. If leflunomide is co-administered with MTX, laboratory should be obtained every 1–3 months on an indefinite basis *Monitoring of drug clearance:* Leflunomide is renally cleared and dose modification should be considered for moderate to severe renal disease. The half-life of the drug is quite prolonged and for patients with toxicity, cholestyramine should be used for rapid elimination *Monitoring for drug/drug interaction:* Leflunomide will interact with MTX and trimethoprim/sulfamethoxazole. However the drugs can be given concurrently, but may require more frequent monitoring of the complete blood count. There is insufficient data for leflunomide, but based on published information regarding methotrexate, screening for the excessive use of alcohol or prior history of hepatitis C is recommended | For patients who will undergo leflunomide therapy, screening for the use of alcohol and chronic viral hepatitis prior to treatment are recommended (Grade 2C) For patients who undergo leflunomide therapy, performance of liver function tests and complete blood counts are recommended (Grade 1C) For patients who undergo leflunomide therapy and develop new or worsening signs or symptoms of lung disease, further evaluation is recommended (Grade 1C) For patients who undergo leflunomide therapy and develop neuropathic symptoms, prompt consideration of discontinuing therapy and washing out with cholestyramine are recommended (Grade 1C) |
| Methotrexate (MTX) | 2.5–15 mg once a week | *Monitoring blood work:* Patients should be monitored with a complete blood count, liver function panel, phosphate, and creatinine when commencing MTX therapy and the tests repeated every 4–12 weeks. Clinical monitoring for infections and signs of hepatotoxicity is also recommended. Patients with baseline transaminases or bilirubin of greater than three times upper limit of normal should be more carefully monitored and initial dose should perhaps be lower, such as 2.5–5 mg once a week *Monitoring of drug clearance:* MTX is cleared by the kidney and the dose may require modification even with mild renal impairment. Patients with moderate to severe renal impairment (GFR <30 ml/min) normally should not be treated with MTX. Folic acid supplementation of 1 mg a day has been used *Monitoring for drug/drug interaction:* MTX will interact with leflunomide and trimethoprim/sulfamethoxazole; however the drugs can be given concurrently, but may require more frequent monitoring of the complete blood count. There is a mild interaction with penicillin-based antibiotics and non steroidals such as naprosyn which can lead to mild elevation (<10 %) of the MTX level. Screening for the excessive use of alcohol or prior history of hepatitis C is recommended | For patients who will undergo MTX therapy, screening for the use of alcohol and chronic viral hepatitis prior to treatment are recommended (Grade 2C) For patients who undergo MTX therapy, performance of liver function tests and complete blood counts are recommended (Grade 1C) For patients who undergo MTX therapy, folic acid supplementation is recommended (Grade 1A) For patients who undergo MTX therapy and develop new or worsening signs or symptoms of lung disease, further evaluation is recommended (Grade 1B) For patients who undergo MTX therapy and develop persistently elevated liver transaminases above their own baseline, cessation of treatment or evaluation by liver biopsy is recommended (Grade 1B) For patients with renal insufficiency, ascites, or pleural effusions who undergo methotrexate therapy, decreased MTX clearance may be present and dose reduction may be required (Grade 2C) |

Mycophenolate	500–2,000 mg twice a day	*Monitoring blood work*: Complete blood count should be monitored every 1–3 months as long as patients are on therapy *Monitoring of drug clearance*: Mycophenolate blood levels may be obtained if signs and symptoms of gastrointestinal intolerance develop (e.g., diarrhea). High blood levels suggest that mycophenolate may be a cause of diarrhea *Monitoring for drug/drug interaction*: Live vaccines should be avoided while patients are being treated with mycophenolate. Concomitant use of azathioprine should be avoided	For patients who undergo mycophenolic acid therapy and develop adverse GI affects, including diarrhea, interruption of therapy or reduction in dose is recommended (Grade 1B) For patients who undergo mycophenolic acid therapy and develop signs or symptoms of progressive multifocal leukoencephalopathy, cessation of treatment is suggested (Grade 2C)
Chloroquine/ hydroxychloroquine	Chloroquine 250 mg daily Hydroxychloroquine 200–400 mg daily	*Monitoring blood work*: Studies of chloroquine and hydroxychloroquine therapy have suggested a complete blood count and liver function study initially and every 6–12 months. Patients should undergo an ocular examination at least once a year. Since these drugs can cause heart block and cardiomyopathy, patients with unexplained cardiac symptoms should be considered for echocardiogram and electrocardiogram *Monitoring of drug clearance*: Chloroquine and hydroxychloroquine are both cleared by the kidneys. They have prolonged half-lives (more than 1 month) *Monitoring for drug/drug interaction*: Chloroquine and hydroxychloroquine have potentially significant interactions with D-penicillamine and cimetidine leading to higher levels of drug	For patients receiving hydroxychloroquine and chloroquine an eye examination at least once per year is suggested (Grade 2B)

Adapted from Baughman et al. [65]

Azathioprine: The cytotoxic agent azathioprine was most frequently used as a steroid-sparing agent for solid organ transplantation. It had been reported as effective for pulmonary sarcoidosis [66]. It has been used as an alternative to MTX in chronic sarcoidosis. Some groups use the agent because of familiarity with the drug [47]. Since azathioprine has less hepatotoxicity than MTX, it is often used in treating symptomatic hepatic disease [67, 68]. It also may be an alternative agent for patients who develop pulmonary toxicity from MTX. It is associated with a higher frequency of nausea and leukopenia than MTX [69] and therefore is not a likely candidate when those complications rise from MTX treatment. Azathioprine is associated with an increased rate of skin cancers and infections [70]. In a recent trial of idiopathic pulmonary fibrosis, azathioprine therapy was associated with an increased mortality compared to placebo treated patients [71]. Dosage and evidence-based recommendations for monitoring while prescribing azathioprine is provided in Table 3.4. These recommendations have been adapted from those made by an expert panel [65].

Leflunomide: Developed as an alternative to MTX for rheumatoid arthritis [72], leflunomide has been reported as effective in treating chronic sarcoidosis [73, 74]. In one series, treatment was associated with a significant improvement in forced vital capacity compared to pretreatment values [73]. While the drug has similar toxicity as MTX, the frequency of nausea is less. In addition, pulmonary toxicity is much less frequent with leflunomide, although it can still occur [75]. Leflunomide is associated with systemic hypertension and peripheral neuropathy [75, 76], toxicities not associated with MTX. Dosage and evidence-based recommendations for monitoring while prescribing leflunomide is provided in Table 3.4. These recommendations have been adapted from those made by an expert panel [65].

Mycophenolate: While not as commonly used as other cytotoxic agents, mycophenolate appears to be effective at least in some patients with chronic sarcoidosis. It has been reported in small case reports as effective in treating cutaneous [77], ocular [78], and neurologic disease [79]. While the drug has not been used that frequently in sarcoidosis, it appears to have some advantages over other cytotoxic agents. This includes a lower rate of leukopenia, an important issue in sarcoidosis patients who may have bone marrow involvement from the underlying disease [61, 80]. There is an increased rate of infection and cutaneous malignancies similar to that seen with azathioprine [81, 82]. Dosage and evidence-based recommendations for monitoring while prescribing mycophenolate is provided in Table 3.4. These recommendations have been adapted from those made by an expert panel [65].

Antimalarial agents: Chloroquine and hydroxychloroquine represent the two antimalarial drugs that have been used in treating sarcoidosis [6, 83]. These agents have been reported as effective in both cutaneous and pulmonary disease. These drugs appear to be more effective for cutaneous than pulmonary disease [6, 84]. However one study did find chloroquine was superior to placebo in treating patients with chronic pulmonary disease [85]. The major toxicity of these drugs is ocular and routine eye examinations are recommended for both agents [86]. Hydroxychloroquine is associated with low risk of ocular toxicity, especially when low doses that are adjusted for patient's weight are employed [87]. However, eye examinations on a regular basis should still be considered [88]. Dosage and evidence based recommendations for monitoring while prescribing the antimalarial agents is provided in Table 3.4. These recommendations have been adapted from those made by an expert panel [65].

Tumor Necrosis Factor Inhibitors

Tumor necrosis factor (TNF) was found to be secreted in high levels from alveolar macrophages of some patients with sarcoidosis [89]. Alveolar macrophages from patients with chronic sarcoidosis with worsening disease despite corticosteroid therapy still released high levels of TNF [90]. These observations suggested that inhibition of TNF may be a target of therapy in sarcoidosis patients [91]. When the chimeric monoclonal anti-TNF antibody infliximab became available for clinical use, there were a large number of case series demonstrating the effectiveness of some of these drugs in refractory sarcoidosis [92–94]. These drugs proved effective for cutaneous lesions, such as lupus pernio [95], neurologic [96], and other forms of refractory disease [97, 98]. Subsequently, two double-blind placebo were performed. Both of these found infliximab was superior to placebo in treating refractory pulmonary disease [2, 99]. In the larger of these studies, infliximab treatment was also superior to placebo in treating extra pulmonary disease [100]. Dosage and evidence-based recommendations for monitoring for infliximab and adalimumab are provided in Table 3.5. These recommendations have been adapted from those made by an expert panel [65].

Examining the various reports regarding the use of TNF-alpha inhibitors for sarcoidosis, guidelines have been proposed (Table 3.6) [101]. Analysis of the two randomized trials using infliximab for pulmonary sarcoidosis provides some insight regarding who is more likely to respond to treatment. However, these two studies have some major differences. The study led by Rossman included only 19 patients. Analysis was performed after only 6 weeks of therapy. The study led by Baughman consisted of 138 patients. Analysis was performed after 24 weeks of therapy. In the larger randomized trial comparing infliximab to placebo, the median FVC was 69 %. Subgroup analysis of response to infliximab found that those patients with a FVC > 69 % had no significant response to infliximab therapy compared to placebo, while there was significantly larger response for those whose FVC was less than 69 % [2]. In the other randomized trial, there was an even larger response to infliximab compared to placebo (Fig. 3.5). The median FVC for that study was 60 % [99]. These studies support the concept that more severe patients are more likely to respond to therapy.

Not all patients with chronic pulmonary sarcoidosis will respond to infliximab therapy [102]. There is little evidence to support that these drugs would be effective for patients with severe fibrosis [23]. There have been two markers which were

Table 3.5 Evidence-based recommendations for use of biologic agents for sarcoidosis

TNF-alpha inhibitors	Usual dosage	Clinical recommendations	Evidence-based recommendations
Adalimumab	40 mg subcutaneously every 1–2 weeks	*Assessing risk for tuberculosis:* Tuberculin skin testing and chest radiograph should be obtained and reviewed prior to therapy. In addition, one should consider the risk for histoplasmosis, blastomycosis, or coccidioidomycosis for patients living in or visiting endemic areas	A chest X-ray is recommended prior to treatment (Grade 1C)
			A tuberculin skin test is recommended to screen for latent tuberculosis prior to treatment (Grade 1C)
Infliximab	3–5 mg/kg intravenously initially, 2 weeks later than every 4–8 weeks	*Assessing risk for hepatitis:* Hepatitis serology should be obtained prior to onset of therapy. Use of drug should be avoided if active viral hepatitis is present	For patients with a chest X-ray consistent with prior tuberculosis or a positive tuberculin skin test, and/or are high risk individuals, active tuberculosis infection should be excluded prior to treatment with adalimumab (Grade 1C) or infliximab (Grade 1B)
		Monitoring blood work: Patients with a history of viral hepatitis or chronic carrier states should be monitored for viral hepatitis reactivation as long as patients are on therapy. Anti-dsDNA antibodies can be measured if lupus-like symptoms develop during therapy	For patients with latent *M. tuberculosis*, active prophylactic treatment following published guidelines before initiation of anti-TNF-alpha therapy is recommended (Grade 1B)
		Monitoring for drug/drug interaction: Live vaccines should be avoided while patients are being treated with adalimumab	For patients with latent *M. tuberculosis*, close monitoring for tuberculosis is recommended for up to 6 months after discontinuing therapy (Grade 1C)
			For patients who develop symptoms indicative of tuberculosis, prompt evaluation for active disease is recommended (Grade 1C)
			For patients with known grade III or IV New York Heart Association class heart failure, administration of adalimumab (Grade 1C) or infliximab (Grade 1B) is not recommended
			For patients with a history of congestive heart failure (CHF) who undergo anti-TNF alpha therapy, close observation for CHF exacerbation is recommended (Grade 1C)
			For patients with a history of demyelinating disease, administration is not suggested (Grade 2C)
			For patients with no history of demyelinating disease who experience symptoms or display signs of a demyelinating process, discontinuation of therapy is suggested (Grade 2C)
			For patients who develop symptoms of a lupus-like disorder, discontinuation of therapy is suggested (Grade 2C)
			For patients who are at risk for viral hepatitis, serologic screening for hepatitis B is recommended prior to treatment (Grade 1C)
			For patients who have hepatitis B virus infection, anti-TNF-alpha therapy should not be administered (Grade 1C)
			For patients who develop unresolved infections, discontinuation of treatment until the infection is resolved is recommended (Grade 1B)
			For patients who are pregnant, administration of anti-TNF alpha therapy is used only if alternatives are not able to be used (Grade 2C)
Rituximab	1 g intravenously every 2–4 weeks	*Monitoring blood work:* Complete blood count should be checked prior to each treatment. Patients should have serology checked for viral hepatitis prior to initiating therapy	For patients who undergo anti-lymphocyte antibody therapy, monitoring for infusion reactions is recommended (Grade 1B)
		Monitoring of drug clearance: No specific recommendations	
		Monitoring for drug/drug interaction: Rituximab can be used in combination with other immunosuppressive agents and as such additive or synergistic suppression of host immunity particularly lymphocyte-based defenses can occur during use of this agent. There is also the potential for more neutropenia when the drug is given with cytotoxic agents, including cyclophosphamide	

Adapted from Baughman et al. [65]

Table 3.6 Features predictive of response to anti-TNF therapy for chronic sarcoidosis

Feature	Response	Studies
FVC < 70 %	Increased response compared to placebo of 3.3[a] to 5.9 %	Baughman et al. [2] Rossman et al. [99]
Dyspnea > 1 on Medical Research Council scale	Increased response to compared to placebo 3.8 %[b]	Baughman et al. [2]
Disease duration > 2 years	Increased response to compared to placebo 3.2 %[a]	Baughman et al. [2]
Elevated C reactive protein	Increased response to compared to placebo 5.1 %[b]	Sweiss et al. [103]
Reticulonodular infiltrate on chest X-ray	Patients with >5 % improvement in FVC after treatment: Infliximab: 47 % Placebo: 11 %[a]	Baughman et al. [34]
Lupus pernio	Resolution or near resolution of skin lesions: Infliximab 77 % All other regimens: 29 %[c]	Stagaki et al. [18]
Neurologic disease	Patients failing other regimens all responded	Moravan [79] Sodhi [105]
Chronic ocular disease	Patients failing other regimens responded to either adalimumab or infliximab	Baughman [106] Baughman [51] Erckens [107]
Extra pulmonary sarcoidosis	Patients with chronic extra pulmonary disease more likely to improve with infliximab than placebo based on physician organ specific assessment[c]	Judson [100]

[a]Compared to placebo, $p < 0.05$
[b]Compared to placebo, $p < 0.02$
[c]Compared to placebo, $p < 0.002$

identified retrospectively from a randomized trial of patients with treated with infliximab. An elevated C reactive protein (CRP) was associated with a significantly higher rate of response to infliximab compared to control [103]. Patients with reticulonodular infiltrates on chest roentgenogram were also more likely to respond to therapy [34]. That study also identified a inflammatory profile which was associated with an enhanced response to therapy [104]. These markers need to be studied prospectively before they can be applied in standard practice.

Anti-TNF therapy has been employed in refractory extra pulmonary disease as well. In one study, the overall response of extra-pulmonary disease responded better to infliximab compared to placebo [100]. That study employed a physician assessment of each organ and comparisons were made before and after therapy. Specific organ involvement has also been reported. In a study of over a hundred treatment regimens for patients with *lupus pernio*, Stagaki et al. found that infliximab was associated with significantly higher rate of resolution or near completed rate of resolution compared to any other regimen employed [18]. In patients with

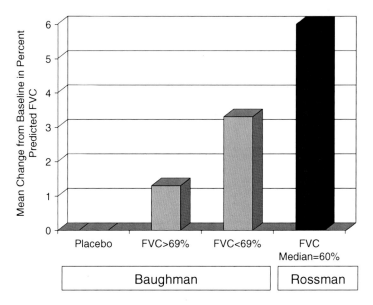

Fig. 3.5 The mean change in FVC compared to placebo after 6 weeks (Rossman) or 24 weeks (Baughman) of therapy [2, 99]. For Baughman study, the study median was 69 %. For those patients whose pretreatment FVC was less than 69 %, there was a significant change in FVC compared to placebo ($p < 0.05$)

refractory neurosarcoidosis failing other regimens, two case series reported responses in all patients treated with infliximab [79, 105]. For ocular sarcoidosis, both infliximab [51, 106] and adalimumab [51, 107] have been reported as successful in treating patients who have failed other regimens.

Other Agents

Rituximab has been reported as effective in treating refractory cases of sarcoidosis. These include joint and eye disease [108, 109]. It is a monoclonal antibody which leads to B cell depletion and has proved useful in treating refractory rheumatoid arthritis [110]. It has a significantly different toxicity profile than the TNF-alpha inhibitors. Dosage and evidence-based recommendations for monitoring while administering rituximab is provided in Table 3.5. These recommendations have been adapted from those made by an expert panel [65].

The phosphodiesterase 4 (PDE-4) inhibitors have been reported as effective in some cases of sarcoidosis. These drugs inhibit TNF release by alveolar macrophages [111, 112]. Pentoxifylline was the first drug in this class reported as effective in treating sarcoidosis [113]. In a randomized, placebo-controlled trial, pentoxifylline was steroid sparing compared to placebo, but was not associated with significant improvement in lung function [5]. Aprelimast is a more selective PDE-4 inhibitor.

In an open label trial of chronic cutaneous sarcoidosis, it was shown to be effective [114]. The major toxicity of this class of drugs has been nausea and tachycardia.

The antioxidants may have a role in treating some patients with sarcoidosis. Quercetin has been shown to reduce oxidant stress in sarcoidosis patients [115]. Its role in improving outcome in sarcoidosis is currently under study. Another antioxidant, N-acetyl cysteine (NAC), has been suggested as a potential treatment for pulmonary fibrosis. This was based on its effectiveness as a supplemental agent to azathioprine in patients with idiopathic pulmonary fibrosis [116]. The effectiveness of NAC in the treatment of sarcoidosis is also under study.

Special Considerations in Sarcoidosis

There are several clinical problems associated with sarcoidosis which do not always respond to just anti-inflammatory therapy. These conditions may respond to specific therapy for these complications. However, that specific therapy may not be effective for other aspects of the disease. Examples of this include sarcoidosis associated pulmonary hypertension, fatigue, and small fiber neuropathy. For all three of these conditions, alternative therapies have been reported as effective.

Sarcoidosis-associated pulmonary hypertension (SAPH) can occur in 5–15 % of unselected sarcoidosis patients an up to 50 % of persistently dyspneic sarcoidosis patients [10, 117, 118]. As noted in Fig. 3.1, SAPH can lead to hypoxia and/or significant dyspnea in patients with normal pulmonary function studies and no evidence of parenchymal lung disease. Diagnosis and treatment of this condition will be discussed elsewhere in this book.

Significant fatigue associated with sarcoidosis has been reported in over half of patients [119–121]. It may occur for years after all other evidence of disease activity has resolved [122]. In some cases, the fatigue may be due to sleep disturbances, which are common in sarcoidosis [123, 124]. In some cases, treatment of the underlying disease with TNF inhibitors has improved fatigue [125]. Neurostimulants have been reported as useful in treating sarcoidosis associated fatigue (SAF) [126]. Specific pharmacologic treatment for SAF has been studied using double blind, crossover design studies. The neurostimulant D-methylphenidate was found to be superior to placebo in treating SAF [45]. In that study, patients were receiving one or more systemic therapy for their sarcoidosis but still had clinically significant fatigue. In another report, r-modafinil was found to be superior to placebo in treating SAF [46]. That study found that there was no difference in improvement for fatigue in those patients with daytime hypersomnulence versus those without, as assessed by multiple sleep latency time. This would suggest these neurostimulants work for fatigue in patients with or without sleep disturbance.

Small fiber neuropathy is a clinical problem encountered in sarcoidosis [127]. Intravenous immunoglobulin therapy was reported as effective in a small case series [128]. A recent report suggests that ARA 290 may provide a novel solution to this problem [129].

Recently, Heij et al. demonstrated in a pilot study that ARA 290 reduced small fiber neuropathy-related symptoms including fatigue, autonomic dysfunction, and pain. ARA 290 (a peptide designed to activate the innate repair receptor that arrests injury and initiates cytoprotection, anti-inflammation, and healing) reduces allodynia in preclinical neuropathy models. Moreover, they found a significant improvement from baseline in the pain and physical functioning dimensions of the SF-36 QOL questionnaire [129].

Conclusion

While not all patients with sarcoidosis require treatment, a significant percent of patients do require systemic therapy. An approach to treatment based on lung function and other relevant clinical parameters including and the level of symptoms (see also Fig. 3.1) can lead to a step wise approach to therapy (Fig. 3.2). In patients placed on systemic therapy, the treating physician must monitor for toxicity.

References

1. McKinzie BP, Bullington WM, Mazur JE, Judson MA. Efficacy of short-course, low-dose corticosteroid therapy for acute pulmonary sarcoidosis exacerbations. Am J Med Sci. 2010;339(1):1–4.
2. Baughman RP, Drent M, Kavuru M, Judson MA, Costabel U, Du BR, et al. Infliximab therapy in patients with chronic sarcoidosis and pulmonary involvement. Am J Respir Crit Care Med. 2006;174(7):795–802.
3. Lower EE, Baughman RP. The use of low dose methotrexate in refractory sarcoidosis. Am J Med Sci. 1990;299:153–7.
4. Judson MA, Silvestri J, Hartung C, Byars T, Cox CE. The effect of thalidomide on corticosteroid-dependent pulmonary sarcoidosis. Sarcoidosis Vasc Diffuse Lung Dis. 2006;23(1):51–7.
5. Park MK, Fontana JR, Babaali H, Gilbert-McClain LI, Joo J, Moss J, et al. Steroid sparing effects of pentoxifylline in pulmonary sarcoidosis. Sarcoidosis Vasc Diffuse Lung Dis. 2009;26:121–31.
6. Siltzbach LE, Teirstein AS. Chloroquine therapy in 43 patients with intrathoracic and cutaneous sarcoidosis. Acta Med Scand. 1964;425:302S–8.
7. Baughman RP, Judson MA, Teirstein AS, Moller DR, Lower EE. Thalidomide for chronic sarcoidosis. Chest. 2002;122:227–32.
8. Gerke AK, Yang M, Tang F, Cavanaugh JE, Polgreen PM. Increased hospitalizations among sarcoidosis patients from 1998 to 2008: a population-based cohort study. BMC Pulm Med. 2012;12:19. doi:10.1186/1471-2466-12-19.:19-12.
9. Swigris JJ, Olson AL, Huie TJ, Fernandez-Perez ER, Solomon J, Sprunger D, et al. Sarcoidosis-related mortality in the United States from 1988 to 2007. Am J Respir Crit Care Med. 2011;183(11):1524–30.
10. Baughman RP, Engel PJ, Taylor L, Lower EE. Survival in sarcoidosis associated pulmonary hypertension: the importance of hemodynamic evaluation. Chest. 2010;138:1078–85.
11. Shorr AF, Davies DB, Nathan SD. Predicting mortality in patients with sarcoidosis awaiting lung transplantation. Chest. 2003;124(3):922–8.

12. Baughman RP, Lower EE. Fungal infections as a complication of therapy for sarcoidosis. QJM. 2005;98:451–6.
13. Paramothayan NS, Lasserson TJ, Jones PW. Corticosteroids for pulmonary sarcoidosis. Cochrane Database Syst Rev. 2005;(2):CD001114.
14. Paramothayan S, Lasserson T, Walters EH. Immunosuppressive and cytotoxic therapy for pulmonary sarcoidosis. Cochrane Database Syst Rev. 2003;(3):CD003536.
15. Baughman RP, Nunes H. Therapy for sarcoidosis: evidence-based recommendations. Expert Rev Clin Immunol. 2012;8(1):95–103.
16. Hunninghake GW, Costabel U, Ando M, Baughman R, Cordier JF, Du BR, et al. ATS/ERS/WASOG statement on sarcoidosis. American Thoracic Society/European Respiratory Society/World Association of Sarcoidosis and other Granulomatous Disorders. Sarcoidosis Vasc Diffuse Lung Dis. 1999;16(Sep):149–73.
17. Baughman RP, Costabel U, du Bois RM. Treatment of sarcoidosis. Clin Chest Med. 2008;29(3):533–48.
18. Stagaki E, Mountford WK, Lackland DT, Judson MA. The treatment of lupus pernio: results of 116 treatment courses in 54 patients. Chest. 2009;135(2):468–76.
19. Judson MA, Boan AD, Lackland DT. The clinical course of sarcoidosis: presentation, diagnosis, and treatment in a large white and black cohort in the United States. Sarcoidosis Vasc Diffuse Lung Dis. 2012;29:119–27.
20. Baughman RP, Judson MA, Teirstein A, Yeager H, Rossman M, Knatterud GL, et al. Presenting characteristics as predictors of duration of treatment in sarcoidosis. QJM. 2006; 99(5):307–15.
21. Pietinalho A, Ohmichi M, Hiraga Y, Lofroos AB, Selroos O. The mode of presentation of sarcoidosis in Finland and Hokkaido, Japan. A comparative analysis of 571 Finnish and 686 Japanese patients. Sarcoidosis. 1996;13:159–66.
22. Loddenkemper R, Kloppenborg A, Schoenfeld N, Grosser H, Costabel U. Clinical findings in 715 patients with newly detected pulmonary sarcoidosis – results of a cooperative study in former West Germany and Switzerland. WATL Study Group. Wissenschaftliche Arbeitsgemeinschaft fur die Therapie von Lungenkrankheitan. Sarcoidosis Vasc Diffuse Lung Dis. 1998;15(2):178–82.
23. Nardi A, Brillet PY, Letoumelin P, Girard F, Brauner M, Uzunhan Y, et al. Stage IV sarcoidosis: comparison of survival with the general population and causes of death. Eur Respir J. 2011;38(6):1368–73.
24. Baughman RP, Winget DB, Bowen EH, Lower EE. Predicting respiratory failure in sarcoidosis patients. Sarcoidosis. 1997;14:154–8.
25. Baughman RP, Drent M, Culver DA, Grutters JC, Handa T, Humbert M, et al. Endpoints for clinical trials of sarcoidosis. Sarcoidosis Vasc Diffuse Lung Dis. 2012;29:90–8.
26. Keir G, Wells AU. Assessing pulmonary disease and response to therapy: which test? Semin Respir Crit Care Med. 2010;31(4):409–18.
27. Gibson GJ, Prescott RJ, Muers MF, Middleton WG, Mitchell DN, Connolly CK, et al. British Thoracic Society Sarcoidosis study: effects of long term corticosteroid treatment. Thorax. 1996;51(3):238–47.
28. Baughman RP, Lower EE. Six-minute walk test in managing and monitoring sarcoidosis patients. Curr Opin Pulm Med. 2007;13(5):439–44.
29. Baughman RP, Sparkman BK, Lower EE. Six-minute walk test and health status assessment in sarcoidosis. Chest. 2007;132(1):207–13.
30. Marcellis RG, Lenssen AF, Elfferich MD, De VJ, Kassim S, Foerster K, et al. Exercise capacity, muscle strength and fatigue in sarcoidosis. Eur Respir J. 2011;38(3):628–34.
31. Marcellis RG, Lenssen AF, de Vries GJ, Baughman RP, van der Grinten CP, Verschakelen JA, et al. Is there an added value of cardiopulmonary exercise testing in sarcoidosis patients? Lung. 2013;191(1):43–52.
32. Wallaert B, Talleu C, Wemeau-Stervinou L, Duhamel A, Robin S, Aguilaniu B. Reduction of maximal oxygen uptake in sarcoidosis: relationship with disease severity. Respiration. 2011;82(6):501–8.

33. Scadding JG. Prognosis of intrathoracic sarcoidosis in England. Br Med J. 1961;4:1165–72.
34. Baughman RP, Shipley R, Desai S, Drent M, Judson MA, Costabel U, et al. Changes in chest roentgenogram of sarcoidosis patients during a clinical trial of infliximab therapy: comparison of different methods of evaluation. Chest. 2009;136:526–35.
35. Muers MF, Middleton WG, Gibson GJ, Prescott RJ, Mitchell DN, Connolly CK, et al. A simple radiographic scoring method for monitoring pulmonary sarcoidosis: relations between radiographic scores, dyspnoea grade and respiratory function in the British Thoracic Society Study of Long-Term Corticosteroid Treatment. Sarcoidosis Vasc Diffuse Lung Dis. 1997;14(1):46–56.
36. Zappala CJ, Desai SR, Copley SJ, Spagnolo R, Cramer D, Sen D, et al. Optimal scoring of serial change on chest radiography in sarcoidosis. Sarcoidosis Vasc Diffuse Lung Dis. 2011;28(2):130–8.
37. Judson MA, Gilbert GE, Rodgers JK, Greer CF, Schabel SI. The utility of the chest radiograph in diagnosing exacerbations of pulmonary sarcoidosis. Respirology. 2008;13(1):97–102.
38. Drent M, de Vries J, Lenters M, Lamers RJ, Rothkranz-Kos S, Wouters EF, et al. Sarcoidosis: assessment of disease severity using HRCT. Eur Radiol. 2003;13(11):2462–71.
39. Oberstein A, von Zitzewitz H, Schweden F, Muller-Quernheim J. Non invasive evaluation of the inflammatory activity in sarcoidosis with high-resolution computed tomography. Sarcoidosis Vasc Diffuse Lung Dis. 1997;14(1):65–72.
40. Mostard RL, Verschakelen JA, van Kroonenburgh MJ, Nelemans PJ, Wijnen PA, Voo S, et al. Severity of pulmonary involvement and (18)F-FDG PET activity in sarcoidosis. Respir Med. 2012;12:10.
41. Sobic-Saranovic D, Grozdic I, Videnovic-Ivanov J, Vucinic-Mihailovic V, Artiko V, Saranovic D, et al. The utility of 18F-FDG PET/CT for diagnosis and adjustment of therapy in patients with active chronic sarcoidosis. J Nucl Med. 2012;53(10):1543–9.
42. Keijsers RG, Verzijlbergen EJ, van den Bosch JM, Zanen P, van de Garde EM, Oyen WJ, et al. 18F-FDG PET as a predictor of pulmonary function in sarcoidosis. Sarcoidosis Vasc Diffuse Lung Dis. 2011;28(2):123–9.
43. de Vries J, Michielsen H, van Heck GL, Drent M. Measuring fatigue in sarcoidosis: the Fatigue Assessment Scale (FAS). Br J Health Psychol. 2004;9(Pt 3):279–91.
44. de Kleijn WP, De VJ, Wijnen PA, Drent M. Minimal (clinically) important differences for the Fatigue Assessment Scale in sarcoidosis. Respir Med. 2011;105(9):1388–95.
45. Lower EE, Harman S, Baughman RP. Double-blind, randomized trial of dexmethylphenidate hydrochloride for the treatment of sarcoidosis-associated fatigue. Chest. 2008;133(5):1189–95.
46. Lower EE, Malhotra A, Surdulescu V, Baughman RP. Armodafinil for sarcoidosis-associated fatigue: a double-blind, placebo-controlled, crossover trial. J Pain Symptom Manage. 2013;45(2):159–69.
47. Schutt AC, Bullington WM, Judson MA. Pharmacotherapy for pulmonary sarcoidosis: a Delphi consensus study. Respir Med. 2010;104(5):717–23.
48. Pietinalho A, Tukiainen P, Haahtela T, Persson T, Selroos O, the Finnish Pulmonary Sarcoidosis Study Group. Early treatment of stage II sarcoidosis improves 5-year pulmonary function. Chest. 2002;121:24–31.
49. Lower EE, Broderick JP, Brott TG, Baughman RP. Diagnosis and management of neurologic sarcoidosis. Arch Intern Med. 1997;157:1864–8.
50. Chapelon-Abric C, de Zuttere D, Duhaut P, Veyssier P, Wechsler B, Huong DL, et al. Cardiac sarcoidosis: a retrospective study of 41 cases. Medicine (Baltimore). 2004;83(6):315–34.
51. Baughman RP, Lower EE, Ingledue R, Kaufman AH. Management of ocular sarcoidosis. Sarcoidosis Vasc Diffuse Lung Dis. 2012;29:26–33.
52. Gottlieb JE, Israel HL, Steiner RM, Triolo J, Patrick H. Outcome in sarcoidosis. The relationship of relapse to corticosteroid therapy. Chest. 1997;111(3):623–31.
53. Hunninghake GW, Gilbert S, Pueringer R, Dayton C, Floerchinger C, Helmers R, et al. Outcome of the treatment for sarcoidosis. Am J Respir Crit Care Med. 1994;149(4 Pt 1):893–8.

54. Rizzato G, Montemurro L, Colombo P. The late follow-up of chronic sarcoid patients previously treated with corticosteroids. Sarcoidosis. 1998;15:52–8.
55. Baughman RP, Nagai S, Balter M, Costabel U, Drent M, Du BR, et al. Defining the clinical outcome status (COS) in sarcoidosis: results of WASOG Task Force. Sarcoidosis Vasc Diffuse Lung Dis. 2011;28(1):56–64.
56. Kavathia D, Buckley JD, Rao D, Rybicki B, Burke R. Elevated 1, 25-dihydroxyvitamin D levels are associated with protracted treatment in sarcoidosis. Respir Med. 2010;104(4): 564–70.
57. Sweiss NJ, Lower EE, Korsten P, Niewold TB, Favus MJ, Baughman RP. Bone health issues in sarcoidosis. Curr Rheumatol Rep. 2011;13(3):265–72.
58. Lower EE, Baughman RP. Prolonged use of methotrexate for sarcoidosis. Arch Intern Med. 1995;155:846–51.
59. Baughman RP, Winget DB, Lower EE. Methotrexate is steroid sparing in acute sarcoidosis: results of a double blind, randomized trial. Sarcoidosis Vasc Diffuse Lung Dis. 2000;17: 60–6.
60. Webster GF, Razsi LK, Sanchez M, Shupack JL. Weekly low-dose methotrexate therapy for cutaneous sarcoidosis. J Am Acad Dermatol. 1991;24:451–4.
61. Lower EE, Smith JT, Martelo OJ, Baughman RP. The anemia of sarcoidosis. Sarcoidosis. 1988;5:51–5.
62. Baughman RP, Koehler A, Bejarano PA, Lower EE, Weber Jr FL. Role of liver function tests in detecting methotrexate-induced liver damage in sarcoidosis. Arch Intern Med. 2003;163(5):615–20.
63. Morgan SL, Baggott JE, Vaughn WH, Austin JS, Veitch TA, Lee JY, et al. Supplementation with folic acid during methotrexate therapy for rheumatoid arthritis. Ann Intern Med. 1994;121:833–41.
64. van Ede AE, Laan RF, Rood MJ, Huizinga TW, van de Laar MA, van Denderen CJ, et al. Effect of folic or folinic acid supplementation on the toxicity and efficacy of methotrexate in rheumatoid arthritis: a forty-eight week, multicenter, randomized, double-blind, placebo-controlled study. Arthritis Rheum. 2001;44(7):1515–24.
65. Baughman RP, Meyer KC, Nathanson I, Angel L, Bhorade SM, Chan KM, et al. Monitoring of nonsteroidal immunosuppressive drugs in patients with lung disease and lung transplant recipients: American College of Chest Physicians evidence-based clinical practice guidelines. Chest. 2012;142(5):e1S–111.
66. Muller-Quernheim J, Kienast K, Held M, Pfeifer S, Costabel U. Treatment of chronic sarcoidosis with an azathioprine/prednisolone regimen. Eur Respir J. 1999;14:1117–22.
67. Kennedy PT, Zakaria N, Modawi SB, Papadopoulou AM, Murray-Lyon I, du Bois RM, et al. Natural history of hepatic sarcoidosis and its response to treatment. Eur J Gastroenterol Hepatol. 2006;18(7):721–6.
68. Cremers JP, Drent M, Baughman RP, Wijnen PA, Koek GH. Therapeutic approach of hepatic sarcoidosis. Curr Opin Pulm Med. 2012;18(5):472–82.
69. McKendry RJR, Cyr M. Toxicity of methotrexate compared with azathioprine in the treatment of rheumatoid arthritis: a case-control study of 131 patients. Arch Intern Med. 1989;149:685–9.
70. Wang K, Zhang H, Li Y, Wei Q, Li H, Yang Y, et al. Safety of mycophenolate mofetil versus azathioprine in renal transplantation: a systematic review. Transplant Proc. 2004;36(7): 2068–70.
71. Raghu G, Anstrom KJ, King Jr TE, Lasky JA, Martinez FJ. Prednisone, azathioprine, and N-acetylcysteine for pulmonary fibrosis. N Engl J Med. 2012;366(21):1968–77.
72. Emery P, Breedveld FC, Lemmel EM, Kaltwasser JP, Dawes PT, Gomor B, et al. A comparison of the efficacy and safety of leflunomide and methotrexate for the treatment of rheumatoid arthritis. Rheumatology (Oxford). 2000;39(6):655–65.
73. Sahoo DH, Bandyopadhyay D, Xu M, Pearson K, Parambil JG, Lazar CA, et al. Effectiveness and safety of leflunomide for pulmonary and extrapulmonary sarcoidosis. Eur Respir J. 2011;38:1145–50.

74. Baughman RP, Lower EE. Leflunomide for chronic sarcoidosis. Sarcoidosis Vasc Diffuse Lung Dis. 2004;21:43–8.

75. Alcorn N, Saunders S, Madhok R. Benefit-risk assessment of leflunomide: an appraisal of leflunomide in rheumatoid arthritis 10 years after licensing. Drug Saf. 2009;32(12): 1123–34.

76. Osiri M, Shea B, Robinson V, Suarez-Almazor M, Strand V, Tugwell P, et al. Leflunomide for the treatment of rheumatoid arthritis: a systematic review and metaanalysis. J Rheumatol. 2003;30(6):1182–90.

77. Kouba DJ, Mimouni D, Rencic A, Nousari HC. Mycophenolate mofetil may serve as a steroid-sparing agent for sarcoidosis. Br J Dermatol. 2003;148(1):147–8.

78. Bhat P, Cervantes-Castaneda RA, Doctor PP, Anzaar F, Foster CS. Mycophenolate mofetil therapy for sarcoidosis-associated uveitis. Ocul Immunol Inflamm. 2009;17(3):185–90.

79. Moravan M, Segal BM. Treatment of CNS sarcoidosis with infliximab and mycophenolate mofetil. Neurology. 2009;72(4):337–40.

80. Browne PM, Sharma OP, Salkin D. Bone marrow sarcoidosis. JAMA. 1978;240:43–50.

81. Bichari W, Bartiromo M, Mohey H, Afiani A, Burnot A, Maillard N, et al. Significant risk factors for occurrence of cancer after renal transplantation: a single center cohort study of 1265 cases. Transplant Proc. 2009;41(2):672–3.

82. Eisen HJ, Kobashigawa J, Keogh A, Bourge R, Renlund D, Mentzer R, et al. Three-year results of a randomized, double-blind, controlled trial of mycophenolate mofetil versus aza-thioprine in cardiac transplant recipients. J Heart Lung Transplant. 2005;24(5):517–25.

83. Chloroquine in the treatment of sarcoidosis. A report from the Research Committee of the British Tuberculosis Association. Tubercle. 1967;48(4):257–72.

84. Baughman RP, Lower EE. Evidence-based therapy for cutaneous sarcoidosis. Clin Dermatol. 2007;25(3):334–40.

85. Baltzan M, Mehta S, Kirkham TH, Cosio MG. Randomized trial of prolonged chloroquine therapy in advanced pulmonary sarcoidosis. Am J Respir Crit Care Med. 1999;160(1):192–7.

86. Leecharoen S, Wangkaew S, Louthrenoo W. Ocular side effects of chloroquine in patients with rheumatoid arthritis, systemic lupus erythematosus and scleroderma. J Med Assoc Thai. 2007;90(1):52–8.

87. Yam JC, Kwok AK. Ocular toxicity of hydroxychloroquine. Hong Kong Med J. 2006;12(4):294–304.

88. Elder M, Rahman AM, McLay J. Early paracentral visual field loss in patients taking hydroxychloroquine. Arch Ophthalmol. 2006;124(12):1729–33.

89. Baughman RP, Strohofer SA, Buchsbaum J, Lower EE. Release of tumor necrosis factor by alveolar macrophages of patients with sarcoidosis. J Lab Clin Med. 1990;115:36–42.

90. Ziegenhagen MW, Rothe E, Zissel G, Muller-Quernheim J. Exaggerated TNFalpha release of alveolar macrophages in corticosteroid resistant sarcoidosis. Sarcoidosis Vasc Diffuse Lung Dis. 2002;19:185–90.

91. Baughman RP, Iannuzzi M. Tumour necrosis factor in sarcoidosis and its potential for tar-geted therapy. BioDrugs. 2003;17(6):425–31.

92. Baughman RP, Lower EE. Infliximab for refractory sarcoidosis. Sarcoidosis Vasc Diffuse Lung Dis. 2001;18:70–4.

93. Pettersen JA, Zochodne DW, Bell RB, Martin L, Hill MD. Refractory neurosarcoidosis responding to infliximab. Neurology. 2002;59(10):1660–1.

94. Meyerle JH, Shorr A. The use of infliximab in cutaneous sarcoidosis. J Drugs Dermatol. 2003;2(4):413–4.

95. Doty JD, Mazur JE, Judson MA. Treatment of sarcoidosis with infliximab. Chest. 2005;127(3):1064–71.

96. Sollberger M, Fluri F, Baumann T, Sonnet S, Tamm M, Steck AJ, et al. Successful treatment of steroid-refractory neurosarcoidosis with infliximab. J Neurol. 2004;251(6):760–1.

97. Sweiss NJ, Welsch MJ, Curran JJ, Ellman MH. Tumor necrosis factor inhibition as a novel treatment for refractory sarcoidosis. Arthritis Rheum. 2005;53(5):788–91.

98. Saleh S, Ghodsian S, Yakimova V, Henderson J, Sharma OP. Effectiveness of infliximab in treating selected patients with sarcoidosis. Respir Med. 2006;100(11):2053–9.

99. Rossman MD, Newman LS, Baughman RP, Teirstein A, Weinberger SE, Miller WJ, et al. A double-blind, randomized, placebo-controlled trial of infliximab in patients with active pulmonary sarcoidosis. Sarcoidosis Vasc Diffuse Lung Dis. 2006;23:201–8.

100. Judson MA, Baughman RP, Costabel U, Flavin S, Lo KH, Kavuru MS, et al. Efficacy of infliximab in extrapulmonary sarcoidosis: results from a randomised trial. Eur Respir J. 2008;31(6):1189–96.

101. Baughman RP, Lower EE, Drent M. Inhibitors of tumor necrosis factor (TNF) in sarcoidosis: who, what, and how to use them. Sarcoidosis Vasc Diffuse Lung Dis. 2008;25: 76–89.

102. Maneiro JR, Salgado E, Gomez-Reino JJ, Carmona L. Efficacy and safety of TNF antagonists in sarcoidosis: data from the Spanish registry of biologics BIOBADASER and a systematic review. Semin Arthritis Rheum. 2012;42(1):89–103.

103. Sweiss NJ, Barnathan ES, Lo K, Judson MA, Baughman R. C-reactive protein predicts response to infliximab in patients with chronic sarcoidosis. Sarcoidosis Vasc Diffuse Lung Dis. 2010;27:49–56.

104. Loza MJ, Brodmerkel C, du Bois RM, Judson MA, Costabel U, Drent M, et al. Inflammatory profile and response to anti-TNF therapy in patients with chronic pulmonary sarcoidosis. Clin Vaccine Immunol. 2011;18:931–9.

105. Sodhi M, Pearson K, White ES, Culver DA. Infliximab therapy rescues cyclophosphamide failure in severe central nervous system sarcoidosis. Respir Med. 2009;103(2):268–73.

106. Baughman RP, Bradley DA, Lower EE. Infliximab for chronic ocular inflammation. Int J Clin Pharmacol Ther. 2005;43:7–11.

107. Erckens RJ, Mostard RL, Wijnen PA, Schouten JS, Drent M. Adalimumab successful in sarcoidosis patients with refractory chronic non-infectious uveitis. Graefes Arch Clin Exp Ophthalmol. 2012;250(5):713–20.

108. Belkhou A, Younsi R, El Bouchti I, El Hassani S. Rituximab as a treatment alternative in sarcoidosis. Joint Bone Spine. 2008;75(4):511–2.

109. Lower EE, Baughman RP, Kaufman AH. Rituximab for refractory granulomatous eye disease. Clin Ophthalmol. 2012;6:1613–8. doi:10.2147/OPTH.S35521.

110. Higashida J, Wun T, Schmidt S, Naguwa SM, Tuscano JM. Safety and efficacy of rituximab in patients with rheumatoid arthritis refractory to disease modifying antirheumatic drugs and anti-tumor necrosis factor-alpha treatment. J Rheumatol. 2005;32(11):2109–15.

111. Spatafora M, Chiappara G, Merendino AM, D'Amico D, Bellia V, Bonsignore G. Theophylline suppresses the release of tumour necrosis factor-alpha by blood monocytes and alveolar macrophages. Eur Respir J. 1994;7(2):223–8.

112. Tong Z, Dai H, Chen B, Abdoh Z, Guzman J, Costabel U. Inhibition of cytokine release from alveolar macrophages in pulmonary sarcoidosis by pentoxifylline: comparison with dexamethasone. Chest. 2003;124(4):1526–32.

113. Zabel P, Entzian P, Dalhoff K, Schlaak M. Pentoxifylline in treatment of sarcoidosis. Am J Respir Crit Care Med. 1997;155:1665–9.

114. Baughman RP, Judson MA, Ingledue R, Craft NL, Lower EE. The safety and efficacy of apremilast in chronic cutaneous sarcoidosis. Arch Dermatol. 2012;148(2):262–4.

115. Boots AW, Drent M, de Boer VC, Bast A, Haenen GR. Quercetin reduces markers of oxidative stress and inflammation in sarcoidosis. Clin Nutr. 2011;30(4):506–12.

116. Demedts M, Behr J, Buhl R, Costabel U, Dekhuijzen R, Jansen HM, et al. High-dose acetylcysteine in idiopathic pulmonary fibrosis. N Engl J Med. 2005;353(21):2229–42.

117. Bourbonnais JM, Samavati L. Clinical predictors of pulmonary hypertension in sarcoidosis. Eur Respir J. 2008;32(2):296–302.

118. Palmero V, Sulica R. Sarcoidosis-associated pulmonary hypertension: assessment and management. Semin Respir Crit Care Med. 2010;31(4):494–500.

119. de Kleijn WP, Elfferich MD, de Vries J, Jonker GJ, Lower EE, Baughman RP, et al. Fatigue in sarcoidosis: American versus Dutch patients. Sarcoidosis Vasc Diffuse Lung Dis. 2009;26(2):92–7.

120. de Kleijn WP, de Vries J, Lower EE, Elfferich MD, Baughman RP, Drent M. Fatigue in sarcoidosis: a systematic review. Curr Opin Pulm Med. 2009;15(5):499–506.

121. Gvozdenovic BS, Mihailovic-Vucinic V, Ilic-Dudvarski A, Zugic V, Judson MA. Differences in symptom severity and health status impairment between patients with pulmonary and pulmonary plus extrapulmonary sarcoidosis. Respir Med. 2008;102(11):1636–42.
122. Korenromp IH, Heijnen CJ, Vogels OJ, van den Bosch JM, Grutters JC. Characterization of chronic fatigue in sarcoidosis in clinical remission. Chest. 2011;140(2):441–7.
123. Verbraecken J, Hoitsma E, van der Grinten CP, Cobben NA, Wouters EF, Drent M. Sleep disturbances associated with periodic leg movements in chronic sarcoidosis. Sarcoidosis Vasc Diffuse Lung Dis. 2004;21(2):137–46.
124. Turner GA, Lower EE, Corser BC, Gunther KL, Baughman RP. Sleep apnea in sarcoidosis. Sarcoidosis. 1997;14:61–4.
125. Elfferich MD, Nelemans PJ, Ponds RW, de Vries J, Wijnen PA, Drent M. Everyday cognitive failure in sarcoidosis: the prevalence and the effect of anti-TNF-alpha treatment. Respiration. 2010;80:212–9.
126. Wagner MT, Marion SD, Judson MA. The effects of fatigue and treatment with methylphenidate on sustained attention in sarcoidosis. Sarcoidosis Vasc Diffuse Lung Dis. 2005;22(3):235.
127. Hoitsma E, Marziniak M, Faber CG, Reulen JP, Sommer C, De Baets M, et al. Small fibre neuropathy in sarcoidosis. Lancet. 2002;359(9323):2085–6.
128. Parambil JG, Tavee JO, Zhou L, Pearson KS, Culver DA. Efficacy of intravenous immunoglobulin for small fiber neuropathy associated with sarcoidosis. Respir Med. 2011;105(1):101–5.
129. Heij L, Niesters M, Swartjes M, Hoitsma E, Drent M, Dunne A, et al. Safety and efficacy of ARA290 in sarcoidosis patients with symptoms of small fiber neuropathy: a randomized, double blind, pilot study. Mol Med. 2013;18:1430–6.
130. Keijsers RG, Verzijlbergen JF, van Diepen DM, van den Bosch JM, Grutters JC. 18F-FDG PET in sarcoidosis: an observational study in 12 patients treated with infliximab. Sarcoidosis Vasc Diffuse Lung Dis. 2008;25(2):143–9.
131. Cox CE, Donohue JF, Brown CD, Kataria YP, Judson MA. The sarcoidosis health questionnaire. A new measure of health-related quality of life. Am J Respir Crit Care Med. 2003;168:323–9.
132. Patel AS, Siegert RJ, Creamer D, Larkin G, Maher TM, Renzoni EA, et al. The development and validation of the King's Sarcoidosis Questionnaire for the assessment of health status. Thorax. 2013;68(1):57–65.
133. Hagaman JT, Kinder BW, Eckman MH. Thiopurine S-methyltranferase testing in idiopathic pulmonary fibrosis: a pharmacogenetic cost-effectiveness analysis. Lung. 2010;188(2):125–32.

Chapter 4
Acute Pulmonary Exacerbation of Sarcoidosis

Efstratios Panselinas and Marc A. Judson

Abstract Sarcoidosis patients frequently experience an acute exacerbation of pulmonary sarcoidosis (APES). Despite the frequent occurrence of APES, there is a paucity of information regarding its definition, diagnostic criteria, diagnosis, and treatment. APES is a significant clinical problem that adversely affects the quality of life of sarcoidosis patients. We propose the following clinical criteria for the diagnosis of APES: the development or worsening of pulmonary symptoms over at least a 1-month period in patients with known sarcoidosis that cannot be not explained by an alternative cause, combined with a decline in spirometry ($\geq$10 % from previous baseline FVC and/or FEV1). Risk factors for APES include previous treatment with corticosteroids, Black race, and fibrocystic sarcoidosis. The pathogenesis of APES may involve direct or indirect effects of pulmonary granulomatous inflammation. Although relatively low-dose corticosteroid (20 mg of daily prednisone equivalent) for a relatively short time (3 weeks duration) is usually adequate to resolve APES, the corticosteroid tapering schedule and the prognosis of APES are unknown. We believe that further attention to APES will improve the quality of life of sarcoidosis patients.

Keywords Sarcoidosis • Pulmonary exacerbation • Definition • Risk factors • Diagnosis • Differential diagnosis • Treatment • Corticosteroids

E. Panselinas, M.D. ($\boxtimes$)
Department of Pulmonary Medicine, 411 General Army Hospital, Tripoli, Greece
e-mail: spanselinas@yahoo.gr

M.A. Judson, M.D.
Division of Pulmonary and Critical Care Medicine, Department of Medicine,
Albany Medical College, Albany Medical Center, Albany, NY, USA

M.A. Judson (ed.), *Pulmonary Sarcoidosis: A Guide for the Practicing Clinician*,
Respiratory Medicine 17, DOI 10.1007/978-1-4614-8927-6_4,
© Springer Science+Business Media New York 2014

Abbreviations

APES   Acute pulmonary exacerbation of sarcoidosis
ART   Antiretroviral therapy
CT   Computed tomography
HIV   Human immunodeficiency virus
HLA   Human leukocyte antigen
INF   Interferon
SAPH   Sarcoidosis-associated pulmonary hypertension
TNF   Tumor necrosis factor

Introduction

Sarcoidosis is a multisystem granulomatous disease of unknown etiology. The histopathologic hallmark of the disease is the presence of noncaseating granulomas in various organs. The lung is the most common organ involved with sarcoidosis [1].

The clinical course of patients with pulmonary sarcoidosis is often problematic to predict. Some patients present with acute, self-limited disease that resolves in months to a few years after diagnosis. When anti-sarcoidosis treatment is tapered or withdrawn, granulomatous inflammation may recur and patients can experience acute pulmonary exacerbations of sarcoidosis (APES). APES may also develop spontaneously in patients diagnosed with sarcoidosis but not previously treated [2].

In this chapter we discuss a proposed definition, potential pathophysiologic mechanisms, risk factors, diagnostic criteria, and treatment of APES. It should be made clear that all of these issues are conjectural and have not been clearly resolved.

Definition and Diagnostic Criteria

Definition

There is no universally accepted definition of APES. Although several descriptions of sarcoidosis exacerbations have been reported, most have not focused specifically on lung involvement. We believe that APES should be defined as the development of new or worsening granulomatous inflammation from sarcoidosis that causes significant pulmonary symptoms.

Diagnostic Criteria

Several combinations of the following criteria have been used to diagnose APES and/or exacerbations of extrapulmonary sarcoidosis: (1) worsening of symptoms severe enough to warrant treatment [3]; (2) decline in pulmonary function[4–7]; (3) increase in biomarkers of disease activity [2, 7]; and (4) exclusion of other diagnosis responsible for symptoms and pulmonary dysfunction [5, 6].

We propose the following diagnostic criteria for APES: worsening of pulmonary symptoms in patients with known sarcoidosis that cannot be not explained by an alternative cause, combined with a decline in spirometry (≥ 10 % from previous baseline forced vital capacity (FVC) and/or forced expiratory volume in 1 s (FEV1)). The pulmonary symptoms should be present for at least 1 month. The 1-month timeframe, although arbitrary, is useful to differentiate APES from other common causes of pulmonary symptoms with an abrupt onset such as bronchitis or asthma. The specific decline in spirometry is also arbitrary, and we acknowledge that milder declines in spirometry could occur in patients experiencing pathophysiologic derangements identical to APES. We chose this specific spirometric cutoff in order to develop criteria with adequate specificity for the diagnosis, as lesser declines in spirometry could also commonly occur in patients experiencing infectious bronchitis, upper respiratory tract infections, and other pulmonary processes other than APES. Our diagnostic criteria are not contingent on whether or not the patient has been receiving anti-sarcoidosis therapy. In addition, it should be noted that our proposed diagnostic criteria are not synonymous with our definition of APES. We believe that our diagnostic criteria have a high sensitivity and specificity for APES. However, this remains to be determined.

Epidemiology/Risk Factors

The prevalence and incidence of APES have not specifically studied. Extrapolating from retrospective cohorts of sarcoidosis patients, the estimated frequency of APES is between 13 and 75 % [3, 4, 7, 8]. This wide variation is the result of differences in the diagnostic criteria of APES, treatment regimens, and length of the follow-up. In addition, these rates are not adjusted for sex, ethnicity, or race. Finally, these cohorts were reported from tertiary institutions, and, therefore, the above rates may not be representative of the general population of sarcoidosis patients.

Table 4.1 describes risk factors for APES. Most of these risk factors have been extrapolated from studies concerning relapses of sarcoidosis in general, irrespective of the organ involved. Blacks are thought to be at higher risk for exacerbations than Whites [3, 9]. Female sex and older age are also associated with relapses [3, 4]. Certain clinical manifestations of the disease influence the probability of exacerbations. Longer disease duration, extrapulmonary disease, and fibrocystic pulmonary disease have been identified as risk factors for APES [3, 4, 7, 8, 10].

Corticosteroid treatment has been implicated as a risk factor for APES. Retrospective studies have shown that sarcoidosis patients receiving corticosteroids are more likely to have relapses, including APES, when therapy has been tapered or withdrawn [3, 10]. In addition, patients who suffered sarcoidosis exacerbations including APES received statistically significant higher doses of corticosteroids compared to patients who did not have relapses [7]. Although this could be explained

Table 4.1 Risk factors for APES

Risk factors	Strength of association
Black race vs. white race [3, 9]	+++
Longer disease duration (median = 33 months vs. median = 12 months) [10]	+++
Female vs. male sex [3]	+
Older age [4]	+
Musculoskeletal sarcoidosis at presentation [3]	+
Calcium disorder, cardiac disease, or neurologic disease secondary to sarcoidosis [10]	+
Extrapulmonary sarcoidosis [7]	+
Fibrocystic pulmonary sarcoidosis [4, 8]	++
The presence or worsening of pulmonary symptoms [3, 10]	++
Treatment with corticosteroids [3, 10, 11]	+++
Treatment with anti-sarcoidosis medications other than corticosteroids [10]	+
Treatment with higher doses of corticosteroids (mean = 17 mg vs. mean 11 mg of daily prednisolone) [7]	+
Interferon-α therapy [12–14]	++
ART [15–17]	++
Post lung transplant[18–21]	+
Treatment with tumor necrosis factor alpha antagonists (usually etanercept) [22–24]	+

ART, antiretroviral therapy; +, some association; ++, moderate association; +++, strong association
Adapted with permission from Panselinas E, Judson MA. Acute pulmonary exacerbations of sarcoidosis. Chest. 2012;142(4):827–36

by the fact that patients treated with corticosteroids have more severe forms of disease which made them more prone to relapse, it is possible that treatment per se may be responsible for APES.

Interferon-α (INF-α) therapy has triggered APES in patients with sarcoidosis [12, 13]. This phenomenon is not surprising as INF-α stimulates T cells to produce interferon-γ that is known to promote granulomatous inflammation [25]. These cases usually occur between 1 and 9 months after the initiation of treatment, but have been described as far out as 2 years [26].

Sarcoidosis exacerbations and APES have been described following initiation of antiretroviral therapy (ART) for human immunodeficiency virus (HIV) infection [15, 27, 28]. In addition, new onset sarcoidosis has developed after initiation of ART [29, 30]. It is postulated that these phenomena represent a form of immune reconstitution syndrome where ART increases the population of CD4+ lymphocytes that heightens the granulomatous response [30].

Recurrence of pulmonary sarcoidosis may develop in the lung allograft after lung transplantation for end-stage pulmonary sarcoidosis [18–21, 31–38]. These episodes are usually asymptomatic and the diagnosis is typically confirmed via detection of granulomas on transbronchial biopsies performed as surveillance for lung rejection [21, 31, 38]. This condition often improves spontaneously or with escalation of immunosuppressive therapy in symptomatic patients [20, 21, 31, 34]. Recurrent sarcoidosis usually occurs within 15 months after lung transplantation [20], but it has been described within 100 days and as long as 56 months [31, 37].

Finally, APES has been described after treatment with tumor necrosis factor alpha (TNF-α) antagonists. Most reported cases have been associated with etanercept [22–24, 39] which, in contrast to infliximab, is not usually effective for the treatment of sarcoidosis [40]. However, new onset intrathoracic sarcoidosis has also been described after treatment with infliximab for rheumatoid, psoriatic arthritis, and ankylosing spondylitis [41–43]. It is presumed that TNF-α antagonists cause CD4+ Th1 cell proliferation in the peripheral blood and thereby stimulate interferon-γ production [23, 44].

Pathogenesis

Our definition of APES assumes that it is the result of recurrent or increased granulomatous inflammation within the lung. Granulomas in sarcoidosis are thought to result from the interaction of an antigen with the immune system [1]. It is postulated that the antigen(s), presently unknown, is engulfed by antigen-presenting cells and subsequently presented to CD4+ lymphocytes via human leukocyte antigen (HLA) class II molecules. The interplay of the antigen, HLA II molecules, and T-cell receptors leads to the polarization of naïve T lymphocytes to the Th1 phenotype, the production of cytokines, and the recruitment of inflammatory cells which result in granuloma formation [45]. It has been postulated that granulomatous inflammation in sarcoidosis is necessary to clear the antigen [46]. If this theory is correct, it is plausible that effective anti-sarcoidosis therapy may resolve granulomatous inflammation that may lead to failure of clearance of the putative sarcoidosis antigen(s). In this scenario, when treatment is withdrawn, the antigen may still present which may lead to recurrent granulomatous inflammation, and, therefore, relapse [47]. This schema is supported by the aforementioned data that relapse of sarcoidosis is more common in sarcoidosis patients previously treated for sarcoidosis [3] or with higher doses of corticosteroids [7]. In addition, this concept is consistent with the premise that anti-sarcoidosis treatment improves granulomatous inflammation but does not alter the natural course of the disease [11, 46, 48–52]. APES may occur by alternative mechanisms such as by exposure to the same or a different antigen after complete clearance of a previous antigen that triggered the initial granulomatous response.

In addition, APES could possibly occur by mechanisms only indirectly related to the granulomatous inflammation from sarcoidosis. Sarcoidosis patients have an increased prevalence of bronchial hyperresponsiveness, probably related to granulomatous inflammation in the airway [53, 54]. Therefore, a proportion of APES patients may develop symptoms because of bronchospasm [47]. We have observed sarcoidosis patients with APES who responded to an escalation of corticosteroid treatment within 48 h. This rapid response might be too rapid for the downregulation of the granulomatous inflammation, suggesting the possibility of bronchospasm or other non-granulomatous mechanisms as the cause of APES [47].

Diagnostic Algorithm

An algorithm for the diagnosis of APES is proposed in Table 4.2 and will be discussed in this section. As mentioned, the diagnostic criteria for APES have not been clearly established. Our proposed diagnostic criteria require worsening pulmonary symptoms, worsening of lung function, and the exclusion of other alternative causes for these findings. Of these three criteria, only the exclusion of alternative diagnoses is problematic for the clinician. This may be problematic because the symptoms and signs of APES are not specific and, therefore, it is problematic to differentiate APES from several alternative diseases. In some cases, the differentiation between APES and acute asthma or viral-induced bronchospasm is impossible on clinical grounds and both conditions may need to be treated concomitantly [55]. Fortunately, in many of these instances, the treatment of these conditions is similar. Table 4.3 describes several conditions that may mimic the clinical presentation of APES.

Cough is the most common symptom of APES, being present in 90 % of patients in one series [6]. In fact, the absence of cough raises suspicion that the patient is not experiencing APES. Other common symptoms of APES include dyspnea and wheeze, whereas constitutional symptoms such as fever and night sweats are less common [6]. APES may occur in patients who had only extrapulmonary manifestations of sarcoidosis previously [3].

Spirometry is mandatory for the diagnosis of APES based on our proposed diagnostic criteria. Patients may develop pulmonary symptoms suggestive of APES, have no evidence of an alternative cause for these findings but fail to meet our proposed spirometric diagnostic criteria for APES. Although such patients fail to fulfill our criteria for APES, they may have a disorder pathophysiologically identical (failure to meet the diagnostic criteria represents a "false negative") and, as such, could be considered for treatment of APES (scenario 8, Table 4.3).

The typical chest imaging findings of APES include parenchymal lung nodules 1–5 mm in diameter with perilymphatic distribution [55, 56]. It is important to note that these imaging findings are often not present with APES, especially if the chest radiography is performed. In fact, in a study of patients with APES, chest radiographs showed improvement or no change (51 %) in parenchymal infiltration in terms of ILO perfusion scores more frequently than they showed worsening (49 %) [5]. Nonetheless, chest radiographs should be performed routinely as part of an evaluation for APES, not to diagnose the condition but to exclude other alternative diagnoses (e.g., pneumonia, pulmonary edema).

Chest computed tomography (CT) is more sensitive than the chest radiograph to detect parenchymal abnormalities in patients with sarcoidosis. However, chest CT exposes patients to significant radiation, especially if it is performed serially [57]. Therefore, we do not recommend chest CT as a routine test in patients with APES. Chest CT may be useful when the chest radiograph is normal and APES is suspected in clinical grounds. Sarcoidosis has recently found to be associated with an increased risk of pulmonary embolism [58], and chest CT angiography may also be useful in selected patients.

Table 4.2 Diagnostic algorithm of APES

Scenario	1	2	3	4	5	6	7	8	9
Clinical feature									
New/worsening pulmonary symptoms	+	+	+	+	+	+	+	+	−
Receiving ≤10 mg/day of prednisone	+	+	+	+	+	+	−	+	
≥10 % decline in FVC and/or FEV1	+	+	+	+	+	+		−	
CXR typical for APES (see text)	+	+	−, CXR normal or not specific	−, CXR normal or not specific	+	−, CXR suggests alternative dx			
No alternative dx (see Table 4.3) likely	+	+	+	+	−	−			
Evidence of new/worsening extrapulmonary organ involvement	+	−	+	−					
Probability of APES	**Very high**	**High**	**High**	**Moderate to high**	**Low, unless alternative dx excluded**	**Very low**	**Very low**	**Nil**[a]	**Nil**
Empiric corticosteroid treatment for APES[b]	**Yes**	**Yes**	**Usually yes**	**Usually yes**	**No**[c] **unless alternative dx rigorously excluded**	**No**[c] **unless alternative dx rigorously excluded**	**No**[c]**, as dx of APES is unlikely. Consider other dx**	**N/A**	**No**[c]**, as dx of APES is unlikely. Consider other dx**

APES, acute pulmonary exacerbation of sarcoidosis; FVC, forced vital capacity; FEV1, forced expiratory volume in 1 s; CXR, chest radiograph; +, condition present; −, condition absent; dx, diagnosis; N/A, not applicable

Adapted with permission from Panselinas E, Judson MA. Acute pulmonary exacerbations of sarcoidosis. Chest. 2012;142(4):827–36

[a]Nil by spirometry criterion for APES. However this presentation may be pathophysiologically similar to APES. Therefore, if clinically indicated, would proceed in this table as if there was ≥10 % decline in FVC and/or FEV1

[b]A response in 2–3 weeks strongly supports the diagnosis. The diagnosis is questionable if there is no response in 2–3 weeks. In this case, an evaluation for alternative diagnosis may be required

[c]Empirical therapy may still be given with caution if the risks of such therapy, in terms of comorbidities and risks from potential alternative diagnosis (i.e., infection) are reasonable. A response to such therapy should be evident within 2–3 weeks. If there is an inadequate response, an evaluation for alternative diagnosis may be required

Table 4.3 Differential diagnosis of sarcoidosis

Alternative conditions
Pneumonia/bronchitis
Tuberculosis
Airway hyperresponsiveness/asthma
Acute decompensation of congestive heart failure
Pulmonary embolism
Ischemic heart disease
Cardiac sarcoidosis
Sarcoidosis-associated pulmonary hypertension
Psychogenic
Steroid myopathy
Sarcoidosis associated fatigue

Adapted with permission from Panselinas E, Judson MA. Acute pulmonary exacerbations of sarcoidosis. Chest. 2012;142(4):827–36

APES is a clinical diagnosis that usually does not require pathological confirmation. Therefore, bronchoscopy with bronchoalveolar lavage and/or transbronchial biopsy is not typically required to diagnose APES. These procedures may be indicated if the probability of APES is low or the risks of empiric corticosteroid therapy are significant (e.g., significant probability of infection, the patient has comorbid conditions such that empiric corticosteroid use would place the patient at a significant health risk).

Because sarcoidosis is a systemic disease, APES frequently occurs concomitantly with development or relapse of extrapulmonary sarcoidosis. APES is rare in patients currently treated with a prednisone equivalent >10 mg/day [6]. Therefore, an alternative diagnosis should be seriously considered when a patient is receiving such doses of corticosteroids.

The diagnostic algorithm underscores the fact that when there is a high probability of APES, empirical therapy should be started and the patient should be followed closely to detect a response (scenarios 1–3). Because APES usually responds to corticosteroids within 3 weeks [6], we recommend evaluating the patient after 1 month for a response in terms of symptoms and spirometry [47]. When the probability of APES is intermediate, the patient may still be treated, provided the risk of significant corticosteroid complications is low and alternative diagnoses (i.e., infection, heart disease) are unlikely. Otherwise, further testing to exclude alternative diagnoses may be appropriate. Patients who are empirically treated for APES and do not respond within 1 month may also need such additional procedures [47].

Treatment

Corticosteroids are the cornerstone of treatment for pulmonary sarcoidosis. The initial corticosteroid dose is controversial [59]. The American Thoracic Society/European Respiratory Society/World Association of Sarcoidosis and Other Granulomatous Diseases (WASOG) consensus statement recommends a starting dose of 20–40 mg/day prednisone equivalent for the treatment of pulmonary

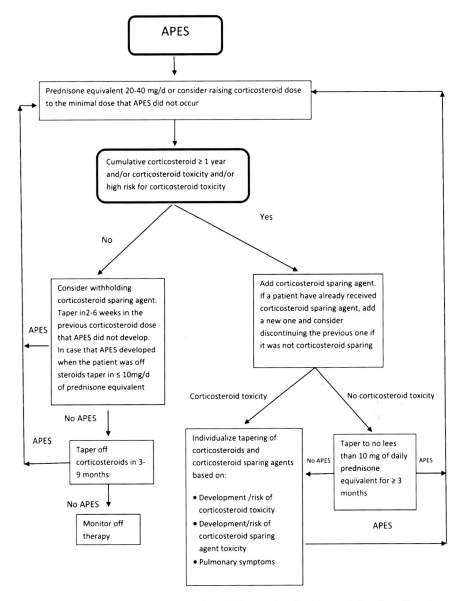

Fig. 4.1 A proposed treatment algorithm for APES (reproduced, with permission, from Panselinas E, Judson MA. Acute pulmonary exacerbations of sarcoidosis. Chest. 2012;142(4):827–36)

sarcoidosis [1]. Corticosteroids have also been recommended for the treatment of APES [5, 7, 60]. However, it is not known if APES is pathophysiologically similar to an initial presentation of sarcoidosis, and, therefore, the corticosteroid dose for APES remains to be determined. It has been suggested that 20 mg of prednisone daily equivalent can improve symptoms and spirometry in patients with APES [6]. Figure 4.1 proposes an algorithm for the treatment of APES. Corticosteroids should

Table 4.4 Corticosteroid-sparing drugs for the treatment of APES

Drug	Level of evidence	Standard dose	Reference
Methotrexate	1A	5–20 mg/week	[49, 60, 61]
Leflunomide	1B	10–20 mg/day	[62, 63]
Azathioprine	1B	50–200 mg/day	[64, 65]
Mycophenolate	1C	500–3,000 mg/day	[66, 67]
Infliximab	1A[a]	3–5 mg/kg intravenously, then 2 weeks later, then every 4–8 weeks	[68, 69]
Adalimumab	1C[a]	40 mg subcutaneously every 1–2 weeks	[70]
Pentoxifylline	2C	400–1,200 mg/day	[71, 72]
Chloroquine	2B	250–750 mg/day	[73, 74]
Thalidomide	2C	50–200 mg/day	[75, 76]

Level A: At least one double blind, placebo-controlled trial with positive results with one or more case series supporting the results. Level B: Majority of case series showing positive results. Level C: Case series with mixed reports of effectiveness, or only a small number of cases reported
1: Strong recommendation, 2: weak recommendation
Adapted with permission from Panselinas E, Judson MA. Acute pulmonary exacerbations of sarcoidosis. Chest. 2012;142(4):827–36
[a]Usually given after another strong recommended alternative medication has been ineffective/inadequate in terms of corticosteroid sparing

be tapered when the pulmonary symptoms and pulmonary function return near baseline. The proper weaning strategy in patients with APES remains to be determined; there are no evidence-based guidelines for any particular weaning strategy. Specific aspects of the tapering process depend on the initial dose of corticosteroids, the maintenance of corticosteroid dose to control the disease, the frequency of previous exacerbations, and the patient's risk for corticosteroid side effects. An attempt should be made to wean APES patients completely off corticosteroids. However, this may be problematic, especially in patients who develop APES while still receiving corticosteroids. In these cases, tapering to the previous lowest dose where APES did not develop is recommended.

Because many patients with APES cannot be successfully weaned off corticosteroids [8], the addition of a corticosteroid-sparing agent should be strongly considered to minimize corticosteroid side effects. These agents are recommended for patients who receive steroids for longer than 1 year or experience significant adverse effects from corticosteroids [47].

Table 4.4 summarizes the corticosteroid sparing agents used for the treatment of sarcoidosis. Methotrexate is the most studied corticosteroid-sparing agent for pulmonary sarcoidosis [49, 60] and has been recommended as the preferred initial corticosteroid-sparing agent [59]. Alternative agents to corticosteroids are rarely effective alone for the treatment of chronic sarcoidosis [71, 73]. Most of these agents require a period of 3–9 months to reach maximal efficacy [60]. An exception to this premise is infliximab which has been demonstrated to improve pulmonary function within 2 weeks [68].

The clinician must be cognizant that these corticosteroid-sparing agents have their own potential side effects that should be weighed against the adverse effects of steroids. If pulmonary sarcoidosis is controlled with ≤10 mg of prednisone per day without significant side effects, most sarcoidosis experts do not recommend the routine addition of a corticosteroid-sparing agent [59].

Prognosis

There is a paucity of data concerning the prognosis of APES. The short-term prognosis seems favorable since most patients respond to corticosteroid treatment [6]. The long-term prognosis of APES is unclear. In a retrospective cohort of patients with chronic sarcoidosis, many of whom had fibrotic disease, relapse occurred in three-quarters after the reduction or cessation of corticosteroid treatment; furthermore, most had recurrent episodes of APES with further attempts to taper corticosteroids. These data suggest that chronic, fibrotic pulmonary sarcoidosis patients who develop APES are likely to remain corticosteroid dependent and have additional episodes of APES when corticosteroids are again tapered [8]. However, it is unknown whether APES is a risk factor for the development of pulmonary fibrosis from sarcoidosis.

Unresolved Issues Concerning APES

Although APES is common in patients with chronic sarcoidosis, it is not well studied and, therefore, there are questions about this entity that remain unanswered. First, a consensus definition and diagnostic criteria for APES should be established that can be used in prospective and retrospective studies. Second, biomarkers need to be discovered that predict or confirm APES. Third, a standardized therapeutic regimen should be established and tailored according to the phenotypic expression of the disease. Finally, more information about impact of APES on the long-term prognosis of sarcoidosis is needed.

Conclusion

APES is a common clinical condition. The exact definition of APES has not been established, diagnostic criteria are unclear, and its prevalence and immunopathogenesis remain speculative. Several risk factors for APES have been identified. Although the chest radiograph is often not useful to diagnose APES, it should be performed when APES is suspected to exclude other alternative conditions. Patients may be treated empirically for APES if (a) the probability of this condition is high and potential alternative causes are unlikely and (b) the risk of corticosteroid side effects is not substantial. Corticosteroids are regarded the treatment of choice for APES.

References

1. Hunninghake GW, et al. ATS/ERS/WASOG statement on sarcoidosis. American Thoracic Society/European Respiratory Society/World Association of Sarcoidosis and other Granulomatous Disorders. Sarcoidosis Vasc Diffuse Lung Dis. 1999;16(2):149–73.
2. Mana J, et al. Recurrent sarcoidosis: a study of 17 patients with 24 episodes of recurrence. Sarcoidosis Vasc Diffuse Lung Dis. 2003;20(3):212–21.
3. Gottlieb JE, et al. Outcome in sarcoidosis. The relationship of relapse to corticosteroid therapy. Chest. 1997;111(3):623–31.
4. Hunninghake GW, et al. Outcome of the treatment for sarcoidosis. Am J Respir Crit Care Med. 1994;149(4 Pt 1):893–8.
5. Judson MA, et al. The utility of the chest radiograph in diagnosing exacerbations of pulmonary sarcoidosis. Respirology. 2008;13(1):97–102.
6. McKinzie BP, et al. Efficacy of short-course, low-dose corticosteroid therapy for acute pulmonary sarcoidosis exacerbations. Am J Med Sci. 2010;339(1):1–4.
7. Rizzato G, Montemurro L, Colombo P. The late follow-up of chronic sarcoid patients previously treated with corticosteroids. Sarcoidosis Vasc Diffuse Lung Dis. 1998;15(1):52–8.
8. Johns CJ, et al. Longitudinal study of chronic sarcoidosis with low-dose maintenance corticosteroid therapy. Outcome and complications. Ann N Y Acad Sci. 1986;465:702–12.
9. Israel HL, et al. Factors affecting outcome of sarcoidosis. Influence of race, extrathoracic involvement, and initial radiologic lung lesions. Ann N Y Acad Sci. 1986;465:609–18.
10. Rodrigues SC, et al. Factor analysis of sarcoidosis phenotypes at two referral centers in Brazil. Sarcoidosis Vasc Diffuse Lung Dis. 2011;28(1):34–43.
11. Eule H, et al. The possible influence of corticosteroid therapy on the natural course of pulmonary sarcoidosis. Late results of a continuing clinical study. Ann N Y Acad Sci. 1986;465:695–701.
12. Alazemi S, Campos MA. Interferon-induced sarcoidosis. Int J Clin Pract. 2006;60(2):201–11.
13. Li SD, et al. Reactivation of sarcoidosis during interferon therapy. J Gastroenterol. 2002;37(1):50–4.
14. Hurst EA, Mauro T. Sarcoidosis associated with pegylated interferon alfa and ribavirin treatment for chronic hepatitis C: a case report and review of the literature. Arch Dermatol. 2005;141(7):865–8.
15. Lenner R, et al. Recurrent pulmonary sarcoidosis in HIV-infected patients receiving highly active antiretroviral therapy. Chest. 2001;119(3):978–81.
16. Mirmirani P, et al. Sarcoidosis in a patient with AIDS: a manifestation of immune restoration syndrome. J Am Acad Dermatol. 1999;41(2 Pt 2):285–6.
17. Morris DG, et al. Sarcoidosis following HIV infection: evidence for CD4+ lymphocyte dependence. Chest. 2003;124(3):929–35.
18. Martinez FJ, et al. Recurrence of sarcoidosis following bilateral allogeneic lung transplantation. Chest. 1994;106(5):1597–9.
19. Barbers RG. Role of transplantation (lung, liver, and heart) in sarcoidosis. Clin Chest Med. 1997;18(4):865–74.
20. Walker S, et al. Medium term results of lung transplantation for end stage pulmonary sarcoidosis. Thorax. 1998;53(4):281–4.
21. Nunley DR, et al. Lung transplantation for end-stage pulmonary sarcoidosis. Sarcoidosis Vasc Diffuse Lung Dis. 1999;16(1):93–100.
22. Burns AM, Green PJ, Pasternak S. Etanercept-induced cutaneous and pulmonary sarcoid-like granulomas resolving with adalimumab. J Cutan Pathol. 2012;39(2):289–93.
23. Louie GH, Chitkara P, Ward MM. Relapse of sarcoidosis upon treatment with etanercept. Ann Rheum Dis. 2008;67(6):896–8.
24. Verschueren K, et al. Development of sarcoidosis in etanercept-treated rheumatoid arthritis patients. Clin Rheumatol. 2007;26(11):1969–71.
25. Parronchi P, et al. Effects of interferon-alpha on cytokine profile, T cell receptor repertoire and peptide reactivity of human allergen-specific T cells. Eur J Immunol. 1996;26(3):697–703.

26. Lopez V, et al. Cutaneous sarcoidosis developing after treatment with pegylated interferon and ribavirin: a new case and review of the literature. Int J Dermatol. 2011;50(3):287–91.
27. Foulon G, et al. Sarcoidosis in HIV-infected patients in the era of highly active antiretroviral therapy. Clin Infect Dis. 2004;38(3):418–25.
28. Haramati LB, et al. Newly diagnosed pulmonary sarcoidosis in HIV-infected patients. Radiology. 2001;218(1):242–6.
29. Naccache JM, et al. Sarcoid-like pulmonary disorder in human immunodeficiency virus-infected patients receiving antiretroviral therapy. Am J Respir Crit Care Med. 1999;159(6):2009–13.
30. Wittram C, Fogg J, Farber H. Immune restoration syndrome manifested by pulmonary sarcoidosis. AJR Am J Roentgenol. 2001;177(6):1427.
31. Johnson BA, et al. Recurrence of sarcoidosis in pulmonary allograft recipients. Am Rev Respir Dis. 1993;148(5):1373–7.
32. Bjortuft O, et al. Single lung transplantation as treatment for end-stage pulmonary sarcoidosis: recurrence of sarcoidosis in two different lung allografts in one patient. J Heart Lung Transplant. 1994;13(1 Pt 1):24–9.
33. Kazerooni EA, Jackson C, Cascade PN. Sarcoidosis: recurrence of primary disease in transplanted lungs. Radiology. 1994;192(2):461–4.
34. Carre P, et al. Recurrence of sarcoidosis in a human lung allograft. Transplant Proc. 1995;27(2):1686.
35. Kazerooni EA, Cascade PN. Recurrent miliary sarcoidosis after lung transplantation. Radiology. 1995;194(3):913.
36. Muller C, et al. Sarcoidosis recurrence following lung transplantation. Transplantation. 1996;61(7):1117–9.
37. Padilla ML, Schilero GJ, Teirstein AS. Sarcoidosis and transplantation. Sarcoidosis Vasc Diffuse Lung Dis. 1997;14(1):16–22.
38. Collins J, et al. Frequency and CT findings of recurrent disease after lung transplantation. Radiology. 2001;219(2):503–9.
39. van der Stoep D, et al. Sarcoidosis during anti-tumor necrosis factor-alpha therapy: no relapse after rechallenge. J Rheumatol. 2009;36(12):2847–8.
40. Utz JP, et al. Etanercept for the treatment of stage II and III progressive pulmonary sarcoidosis. Chest. 2003;124(1):177–85.
41. Clementine RR, et al. Tumor necrosis factor-alpha antagonist-induced sarcoidosis. J Clin Rheumatol. 2010;16(6):274–9.
42. O'Shea FD, Marras TK, Inman RD. Pulmonary sarcoidosis developing during infliximab therapy. Arthritis Rheum. 2006;55(6):978–81.
43. Toussirot E, et al. Sarcoidosis occurring during anti-TNF-alpha treatment for inflammatory rheumatic diseases: report of two cases. Clin Exp Rheumatol. 2008;26(3):471–5.
44. Maurice MM, et al. Treatment with monoclonal anti-tumor necrosis factor alpha antibody results in an accumulation of Th1 CD4+ T cells in the peripheral blood of patients with rheumatoid arthritis. Arthritis Rheum. 1999;42(10):2166–73.
45. Baughman RP, Culver DA, Judson MA. A concise review of pulmonary sarcoidosis. Am J Respir Crit Care Med. 2011;183(5):573–81.
46. Chen ES, et al. Serum amyloid A regulates granulomatous inflammation in sarcoidosis through Toll-like receptor-2. Am J Respir Crit Care Med. 2010;181(4):360–73.
47. Panselinas E, Judson MA. Acute pulmonary exacerbations of sarcoidosis. Chest. 2012;142(4):827–36.
48. Israel HL, Fouts DW, Beggs RA. A controlled trial of prednisone treatment of sarcoidosis. Am Rev Respir Dis. 1973;107(4):609–14.
49. Lower EE, Baughman RP. Prolonged use of methotrexate for sarcoidosis. Arch Intern Med. 1995;155(8):846–51.
50. Panselinas E, Rodgers JK, Judson MA. Clinical outcomes in sarcoidosis after cessation of infliximab treatment. Respirology. 2009;14(4):522–8.
51. Paramothayan NS, Lasserson TJ, Jones PW. Corticosteroids for pulmonary sarcoidosis. Cochrane Database Syst Rev. 2005;(2):CD001114.

52. Zaki MH, et al. Corticosteroid therapy in sarcoidosis. A five-year, controlled follow-up study. N Y State J Med. 1987;87(9):496–9.
53. Bechtel JJ, et al. Airway hyperreactivity in patients with sarcoidosis. Am Rev Respir Dis. 1981;124(6):759–61.
54. Shorr AF, Torrington KG, Hnatiuk OW. Endobronchial involvement and airway hyperreactivity in patients with sarcoidosis. Chest. 2001;120(3):881–6.
55. Lynch 3rd JP, et al. Pulmonary sarcoidosis. Semin Respir Crit Care Med. 2007;28(1):53–74.
56. Nunes H, et al. Imaging in sarcoidosis. Semin Respir Crit Care Med. 2007;28(1):102–20.
57. Smith-Bindman R, et al. Radiation dose associated with common computed tomography examinations and the associated lifetime attributable risk of cancer. Arch Intern Med. 2009;169(22):2078–86.
58. Swigris JJ, et al. Increased risk of pulmonary embolism among US decedents with sarcoidosis from 1988 to 2007. Chest. 2011;140(5):1261–6.
59. Schutt AC, Bullington WM, Judson MA. Pharmacotherapy for pulmonary sarcoidosis: a Delphi consensus study. Respir Med. 2010;104(5):717–23.
60. Baughman RP, Winget DB, Lower EE. Methotrexate is steroid sparing in acute sarcoidosis: results of a double blind, randomized trial. Sarcoidosis Vasc Diffuse Lung Dis. 2000;17(1):60–6.
61. Vucinic VM. What is the future of methotrexate in sarcoidosis? A study and review. Curr Opin Pulm Med. 2002;8(5):470–6.
62. Baughman RP, Lower EE. Leflunomide for chronic sarcoidosis. Sarcoidosis Vasc Diffuse Lung Dis. 2004;21(1):43–8.
63. Sahoo DH, et al. Effectiveness and safety of leflunomide for pulmonary and extrapulmonary sarcoidosis. Eur Respir J. 2011;38(5):1145–50.
64. Lewis SJ, Ainslie GM, Bateman ED. Efficacy of azathioprine as second-line treatment in pulmonary sarcoidosis. Sarcoidosis Vasc Diffuse Lung Dis. 1999;16(1):87–92.
65. Muller-Quernheim J, et al. Treatment of chronic sarcoidosis with an azathioprine/prednisolone regimen. Eur Respir J. 1999;14(5):1117–22.
66. Kouba DJ, et al. Mycophenolate mofetil may serve as a steroid-sparing agent for sarcoidosis. Br J Dermatol. 2003;148(1):147–8.
67. Moudgil A, Przygodzki RM, Kher KK. Successful steroid-sparing treatment of renal limited sarcoidosis with mycophenolate mofetil. Pediatr Nephrol. 2006;21(2):281–5.
68. Baughman RP, et al. Infliximab therapy in patients with chronic sarcoidosis and pulmonary involvement. Am J Respir Crit Care Med. 2006;174(7):795–802.
69. Rossman MD, et al. A double-blinded, randomized, placebo-controlled trial of infliximab in subjects with active pulmonary sarcoidosis. Sarcoidosis Vasc Diffuse Lung Dis. 2006;23(3):201–8.
70. Callejas-Rubio JL, et al. Treatment of therapy-resistant sarcoidosis with adalimumab. Clin Rheumatol. 2006;25(4):596–7.
71. Zabel P, et al. Pentoxifylline in treatment of sarcoidosis. Am J Respir Crit Care Med. 1997;155(5):1665–9.
72. Park MK, et al. Steroid-sparing effects of pentoxifylline in pulmonary sarcoidosis. Sarcoidosis Vasc Diffuse Lung Dis. 2009;26(2):121–31.
73. Baltzan M, et al. Randomized trial of prolonged chloroquine therapy in advanced pulmonary sarcoidosis. Am J Respir Crit Care Med. 1999;160(1):192–7.
74. Chloroquine in the treatment of sarcoidosis. A report from the Research Committee of the British Tuberculosis Association. Tubercle. 1967;48(4):257–72.
75. Carlesimo M, et al. Treatment of cutaneous and pulmonary sarcoidosis with thalidomide. J Am Acad Dermatol. 1995;32(5 Pt 2):866–9.
76. Judson MA, et al. The effect of thalidomide on corticosteroid-dependent pulmonary sarcoidosis. Sarcoidosis Vasc Diffuse Lung Dis. 2006;23(1):51–7.

Chapter 5
Advanced ("End-Stage") Pulmonary Sarcoidosis

Divya C. Patel, Marie Budev, and Daniel A. Culver

Abstract Sarcoidosis is rarely an "end-stage" disease—a concept that implies futility of further treatment. Instead, we suggest the use of the term advanced pulmonary sarcoidosis which encompasses the ideas that the disease has progressed to the point that there is substantial morbidity, there is relatively high risk of mortality, and less reversibility than usual pulmonary sarcoidosis. While it may be equated with chronic, progressive, or fibrotic disease, none of those phenotypes are synonymous with advanced pulmonary sarcoidosis, since all of them may be asymptomatic or do not require therapy.

Symptoms and functional impairment in advanced pulmonary sarcoidosis may be multifactorial. It is important to define the pathophysiologic mechanism for limitations to direct therapy appropriately. A substantial proportion of patients with advanced pulmonary sarcoidosis have related pathologies, including pulmonary hypertension, bronchiectasis, airways stenosis, and mycetoma. These issues should be sought out and treated specifically. Second, the concept that most advanced pulmonary sarcoidosis is irreversible may lead to under-treatment of fibrotic pulmonary disease. There are no biomarkers of disease activity that are adequate to predict futility of immunosuppressive therapy trials in advanced disease.

When immunosuppressive therapy is no longer effective, lung transplantation may be considered. Lung transplantation for sarcoidosis is as successful as for other indications. Although sarcoidosis may recur in the allograft, it is usually nonbothersome. This chapter will review the definition of advanced pulmonary sarcoidosis, risk factors for it, typical manifestations, and approach to nonspecific and specific therapy for it, including lung transplant as a last option.

D.C. Patel, D.O. (✉) • M. Budev, D.O. • D.A. Culver, D.O.
Respiratory Institute, Cleveland Clinic, 9500 Euclid Avenue, Mailcode A91,
Cleveland, OH 44195, USA
e-mail: Pateld4@ccf.org; divcpatel@gmail.com; BudevM@ccf.org; Culverd@ccf.org

M.A. Judson (ed.), *Pulmonary Sarcoidosis: A Guide for the Practicing Clinician,*
Respiratory Medicine 17, DOI 10.1007/978-1-4614-8927-6_5,
© Springer Science+Business Media New York 2014

Keywords End-stage sarcoidosis • Advanced pulmonary sarcoidosis • Pulmonary fibrosis • Stage 4 sarcoidosis • Lung transplantation • Mortality • Mycetoma

Abbreviations

ACCESS	A Case–Control Etiologic Sarcoidosis Study
ACE	Angiotensin-converting enzyme
BAE	Bronchial artery embolization
BAL	Bronchoalveolar lavage
BOS	Bronchiolitis obliterans syndrome
COPD	Chronic obstructive pulmonary disease
CT	Computed tomography
DLCO	Diffusing capacity of the lung for carbon monoxide
FDG	^{18}F-Fluorodeoxyglucose
FEV1	Forced expiratory volume in 1 s
FVC	Forced vital capacity
HLA	Human leukocyte antigen
IL	Interleukin
IPF	Idiopathic pulmonary fibrosis
ISHLT	International Society for Heart and Lung Transplantation
LAS	Lung Allocation Score
PET	Positron emission test
PFTs	Pulmonary function tests
PH	Pulmonary hypertension
SAPH	Sarcoidosis-associated pulmonary hypertension
TLC	Total lung capacity
UIP	Usual interstitial pneumonitis
VO2max	Maximal oxygen consumption
WASOG	World Association of Sarcoidosis and Other Granulomatous Disorders

Introduction

The term "end stage" colloquially refers to an organ that has irreversibly lost any meaningful function. For instance, in the case of chronic kidney disease, specific staging systems have been proposed to define when renal replacement therapy is necessary [1]. However, in patients with parenchymal lung disease, no such standardized or validated system exists and thus the term may be applied unequally.

For sarcoidosis, phenotypes that rely on clinical outcome status categorize patients based on persistence or resolution of disease, use of therapy, and symptoms at some time point after disease onset, but do not define which patients should be considered as having end-stage disease [2, 3]. Alternatively, a predominant fibrotic pattern on chest radiography such as Scadding stage 4 can be used to define severe disease

[4–7]. In a substantial proportion of patients, this radiographic presentation may correlate with a histopathologic pattern of "fibrotic granulomatous" disease without evidence of active inflammation [5]. However, some patients with pulmonary fibrosis are asymptomatic and have no functional impairment [8]. A third definition of "end stage" could be candidacy for lung transplantation when there are no other options for medical management [9]. However, this definition may have variable meanings depending on the access to health care, geographic variation, and practice patterns.

From a practical standpoint, physicians make the diagnosis of "end-stage" disease based on a subjective combination of symptom severity, response to treatment, pulmonary function tests (PFTs), and radiological findings. As an alternative, we propose the use of the term "advanced pulmonary sarcoidosis" to encompass the spectrum of physiologic impairments, radiographic abnormalities, histopathologic features, and secondary complications that are associated with substantial morbidity, that significantly increase the risk of mortality, and that are typically difficult to ameliorate.

In this chapter, our aim is to provide an overview of the manifestations of and risk factors for advanced pulmonary sarcoidosis and to convey that clinical judgment regarding the potential reversibility of sarcoidosis lung disease is not always accurate, implying that aggressive medical management and symptom control should be considered in all these patients. We will also review the indications, sarcoidosis-specific considerations, and outcomes of lung transplantation for sarcoidosis.

Risk Factors for Advanced Pulmonary Sarcoidosis

Advanced pulmonary sarcoidosis develops in no more than 5–6 % of all sarcoidosis patients, generally over one to two decades [10, 11]. Nonetheless, most of the known prognostic indicators of bothersome disease are apparent within 2 years of diagnosis [12–14]. While no specific risk factors for the development of advanced pulmonary disease have been identified, numerous factors for progressive and/or chronic disease have been defined (Table 5.1). Although sarcoidosis that is progressive or chronic does not always eventuate in "advanced disease," it is clear that these phenotypes are markers for those patients who will develop it [15]. Therefore, at this time, decisions about prognosis and management for advanced pulmonary sarcoidosis must necessarily rely in part on the surrogate phenotypes of chronic/progressive sarcoidosis.

Risk Factors for Persistent Disease

Obviously, non-resolution of sarcoidosis is a prerequisite for development of advanced disease. No study has comprehensively surveyed all the potential risk factors for persistence of sarcoidosis. Features that correlate with persistence of the disease include demographic characteristics, radiologic patterns, genetic polymorphisms, and the pattern of organ involvement.

Table 5.1 Risk factors for persistent pulmonary sarcoidosis and clinically bothersome pulmonary sarcoidosis

Persistent	Clinically bothersome
Black race	Black race
Older age	More dyspnea at time of diagnosis
Female gender	Need for treatment in the first 6 months after diagnosis
Multiple organ involvement	Multiple organ involvement
Ascending Scadding radiograph stage	Ascending Scadding radiograph stage
Scadding stage at presentation	Lower socioeconomic status
Architectural distortion of the airways or cystic changes	
Absence of lymphadenopathy	
Need for systemic therapy	
Splenomegaly	

Several radiologic studies suggested that non-resolution occurs in approximately one-third of all sarcoidosis patients [16, 17]. However, non-resolution alone does not indicate severe disease. For example, a survey conducted by the World Association of Sarcoidosis and Other Granulomatous Disorders (WASOG) at ten referral centers revealed that 36 % of patients with disease persistence at 5 years had no requirement for therapy [2].

Black race has been shown to be a risk factor for chronic disease and worse clinical outcomes [12, 18]. In one center, analysis of the 12-year clinical course of disease in 1,774 diverse patients at a university-based medical center showed that blacks were more likely to demonstrate advanced Scadding stages compared to whites [18]. Blacks are also more likely to develop severe disease at a younger age [19]. Ethnic risk factors for more advanced disease have also been reported [15]. For instance, one retrospective study from Great Britain showed that patients with English or West Indies ancestry had poor prognosis for disease resolution compared to those with Irish background [20]. Besides race, younger age, and male gender have repeatedly been associated with radiographic resolution of disease [10, 11, 14, 20].

The pattern of sarcoidosis onset dictates the likelihood of resolution, with more frequent persistence in those with indolent presentations [3]. More organ involvement also increases the likelihood for non-resolution of sarcoidosis [14, 20]. Specific organ involvement that associates with persistent disease includes cardiac, osseous, upper airways, lupus pernio, nephrocalcinosis, and splenic involvement [21]. Whether these all associate with non-resolution specifically of pulmonary sarcoidosis or increase the chances for development of pulmonary fibrosis is unknown.

The presenting chest radiographic pattern is one marker of the overall likelihood for resolution that has been repeatedly confirmed since its first description [13, 20, 22]. For example, a Spanish study of 193 patients demonstrated that the presence of parenchymal involvement or lack of lymphadenopathy at the time of diagnosis were independently associated with persistent disease at 2 years, even after adjustment for other possible prognostic variables such as gender and presence of respiratory symptoms [14]. Long-term studies evaluating the utility of computed tomography

(CT) of the chest to determine potentially reversible lesions have also been conducted. They showed that cystic spaces and architectural distortion of the airways are irreversible with or without treatment [17].

A variety of biologic markers are either associated with or causally implicated in non-resolving disease. The presence of elevated lymphocyte counts in bronchoalveolar lavage (BAL) fluid at the time of diagnosis correlates with higher chances for resolution [23]. Human leukocyte antigen (HLA) Class II molecule types that confer a higher chance for disease resolution include HLA-DRB1*0301 and HLA-DQB1*0201, whereas those with HLA-DRB1*15 and HLA-DQB1*0602 are more likely to have non-resolution [24]. Type I major histocompatibility complex genes are also associated with the course of the disease, though they have been less frequently studied [24]. Polymorphisms in a number of other genes, including transforming growth factor β1, tumor necrosis factor, and prostaglandin-endoperoxide synthase 2 correspond with prognosis in well-characterized sarcoidosis cohorts [25–27].

Risk Factors for Clinically Bothersome Disease

Clinically bothersome sarcoidosis can be defined as disease that is progressive, causes substantial symptoms, impairs the quality of life, or requires treatment. Most clinically bothersome sarcoidosis is also "persistent," but these categories are not synonymous. For example, only half of patients in A Case–Control Etiologic Study of Sarcoidosis Study (ACCESS) who required therapy in the first 6 months after diagnosis were still on treatment at 2 years [12]. In another series of predominantly white, US patients, 87 % of those treated for chronic sarcoidosis were able to stop all therapy [23]. These examples demonstrate that the development of advanced pulmonary sarcoidosis typically entails both persistence of disease and the presence of clinically bothersome disease.

In the ACCESS cohort, a population dominated by pulmonary sarcoidosis, the only two variables independently associated with a requirement for therapy at 2 years were the level of dyspnea and the requirement for systemic therapy at baseline [12]. Dyspnea at presentation may reflect more advanced impairment of ventilatory reserve and both have been related to more severe course of disease [28, 29]. Many of the other factors that predict persistent disease are also related to treatment requirement, and a review of those is beyond the scope of this chapter. These include radiologic, biochemical, genetic, socioeconomic, and demographic parameters.

Mortality and Prognostic Factors

The course of advanced pulmonary sarcoidosis is more variable than many other pulmonary conditions, such as idiopathic pulmonary fibrosis (IPF) or severe chronic obstructive pulmonary disease (COPD). As a result, the mortality that occurs with sarcoidosis is often overlooked. In addition, there are sparse data describing the morbidity due to advanced sarcoidosis or its therapies. Unlike IPF and COPD, sarcoidosis generally affects individuals in the prime years of life.

Historically, the mortality rate for sarcoidosis was thought to be 1–5 % [16]. These estimates were criticized on the basis of being influenced by referral bias [30]. However, recent population surveys have confirmed that sarcoidosis does significantly impact survival. For example, mortality rates in a British population survey from 1991 to 2003 were 5 % and 7 % at three and 5 years, respectively, compared to age- and gender-matched controls for whom mortality was 2 % and 4 % [31]. In a survey of all US death certificates from the National Center for Health Statistics, the age- and gender-adjusted mortality rate for sarcoidosis was 4.32 per 1,000,000 with a 3 % increase per year between 1988 and 2007 [19]. Sarcoidosis was selected as the "underlying cause of death" in 59 % of all patients with sarcoidosis; the mean age at death in this group of patients was 57 years. When the population is limited to those with radiographic stage 4 disease, the mortality is predictably higher [8]. For example, in a French cohort of 142 patients with radiographic stage 4 disease followed for an average for 7 years, the mortality rate was 11.8 % and the 15-year survival rate was 78.1 %, which was significantly worse than the general population [4]. The mean age of patients who died was 55, which was on average 12 years after the diagnosis of sarcoidosis was made.

Advanced lung disease and its complications have been implicated as the most common cause of death in US and European patients with sarcoidosis [4, 8, 32]. In Japan, however, cardiac involvement has historically been the leading cause of death [33]. Age adjusted risk for death is higher in non-Hispanic blacks than in non-Hispanic whites [19]. This finding may relate to differences in racial pathobiology or to differing socioeconomic status, including access to health care [34]. Females also have higher rates of death compared to males [19, 35]. In addition, the risk for death is increased with advancing age, which might be related to comorbid conditions, complications from chronic lung disease, and possibly the development of pulmonary fibrosis [19].

Other demographic factors are associated with mortality. Age-adjusted mortality among blacks in the USA was found to be higher in the Mid-Atlantic and Northern Midwestern States, whereas in whites, mortality was higher in the Northern States [35]. Disease-related factors such as the presence of symptoms at the time of diagnosis, radiographic stage 3 or 4 disease, lower ratio of forced expiratory volume in 1 s over the forced vital capacity (FEV1/FVC), lower FVC, lower FEV1, and lower total lung capacity (TLC) have also shown to confer increased risk of mortality [8, 29, 36]. In one center, almost all of the respiratory-related sarcoidosis deaths occurred in patients with FVC less than 1.5 l [8].

Complications of sarcoidosis, especially pulmonary hypertension (PH), are known to carry poor prognosis with a tenfold increase in mortality and a 5-year survival of 59 % [20, 37, 38]. In patients with radiographic stage 4 disease, only the presence of PH has been found to be an independent predictor of mortality [4].

Pulmonary Fibrosis

Approximately 5–10 % of patients with sarcoidosis will develop radiologically evident fibrotic lung disease [39, 40]. Most patients with pulmonary fibrosis will not experience a relentless progressive downhill course but rather stabilize without the need for indefinite medical therapy [13]. A minority of patients with fibrosis develop respiratory failure related to complications or infections. There are no autopsy series of unselected patients to answer the question of what proportion of persistent sarcoidosis has an element of fibrosis. However, some granulomas hyalinize with time (Fig. 5.1) so that it is probable that a high proportion of patients with chronic sarcoidosis harbor at least some scarred granulomas. For the overwhelming majority of patients, the fibrosis in sarcoidosis follows the same distribution as the granulomas, affecting predominantly the mid to upper lobes [41, 42]. When it is extensive, it characteristically leads to fibrocystic cavities and architectural distortion of the airways.

The fibrosis of sarcoidosis is probably an artifact of chronic granulomatous inflammation rather than an independent process. Evidence for the source of the fibrosis is observational only: the distribution of the fibrosis in autopsies and explants, as well as the presence of pro-fibrotic mediators in the granulomas. Studies of surgical lung biopsies show that interstitial pneumonitis is not common in fibrotic lungs [7, 43]. It is unclear why some granulomas in the same patient exhibit more exuberant fibrosis than others, but this observation may be related to the age of the granuloma.

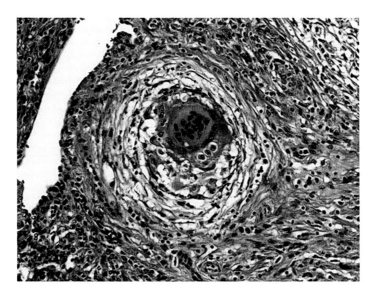

Fig. 5.1 Hyalinized granuloma in a patient with advanced pulmonary sarcoidosis; a multinucleate giant cell is visible in the center, but there is a paucity of the cellular constituents typically observed in inflammatory granulomas (courtesy of Carol Farver, MD)

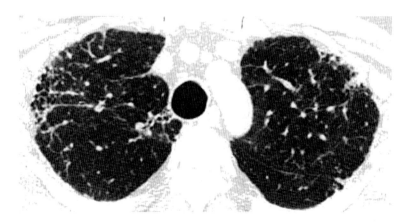

Fig. 5.2 Honeycombing and reticular opacities on computed tomography resembling usual interstitial pneumonitis in a patient with biopsy-proven sarcoidosis

There may be histologically and phenotypically distinct groups of patients with presumed fibrotic advanced pulmonary sarcoidosis. A recently published series of nine transplant patients evaluated the explanted lungs and chest CT scans for disease pattern [7]. Five of the nine patients had a predominant fibrotic scar pattern and four had evidence of active disease with granulomas around bronchovascular bundles in the periphery. Those with a predominant fibrotic pattern disease had relatively acellular septal, peribronchial, and pleural scarring with very few granulomas and central honeycombing. Fibroblastic foci may also be seen in association with the explants of fibrotic sarcoidosis lung [6]. Some patients with ground glass opacities on chest CT and active granulomatous inflammation have features of interstitial pneumonitis that resembles nonspecific interstitial pneumonitis [7].

A third radiologic–pathologic pattern in advanced pulmonary sarcoidosis bears striking resemblance to usual interstitial pneumonia (UIP) (Fig. 5.2). These patients may have honeycombing on radiography and fibroblastic foci on histopathology [5, 44–46]. In autopsy studies and radiologic studies of sarcoidosis patients with severe lung involvement, a "honeycomb" pattern with interstitial pulmonary fibrosis has also been reported [45, 47, 48]. It has been hypothesized that honeycombing may represent areas of prior intense inflammation in the early course of the disease [48].

The pathobiology of pulmonary fibrosis in sarcoidosis has not been well characterized. It has been hypothesized that a shift to a predominant T helper type-2 response, rather than a T helper type-1 response, leads to release of profibrotic cytokines such as interleukin (IL) 4 and IL-13 that may be involved in the fibrotic process [40]. Other mediators, such as transforming growth factor β and chemokine ligand 18, have reasonable biologic plausibility and have been associated with fibrotic sarcoidosis [49]. A transcriptome analysis from transbronchial biopsies comparing patients with bothersome sarcoidosis, including some with fibrosis, to those with self-resolving disease revealed that global gene expression patterns in severe sarcoidosis corresponded more closely to chronic hypersensitivity pneumonitis than to UIP [50]. The implication of that finding may be that a persistent cell-mediated immune system response rather than a separate fibrotic process may be responsible for fibrotic lung disease in patients with sarcoidosis. A variety of other pro-fibrotic growth factors and cytokines may be found in sarcoidosis [40, 51], but the absence of an accepted sarcoidosis animal model limits our ability to pinpoint which ones might be driving the fibrotic process.

Clinical Findings in Advanced Pulmonary Disease

Symptoms and Signs

Patients with advanced pulmonary sarcoidosis have nonspecific and variable clinical presentations, depending on where and how the pulmonary system is affected. For instance, patients with fibrocystic disease may have symptoms predominantly signifying the severe architectural distortion of the airways that usually occurs in this setting, such as wheezing and productive cough. Those with a predominance of honeycomb cystic changes or peripheral fibrosis may exhibit primarily dyspnea with or without nonproductive cough [52]. It should be recognized, however, that dyspnea is the common denominator with all phenotypes. The differential diagnosis of dyspnea is depicted schematically in Fig. 5.3.

Crackles or clubbing are extremely unusual except for two situations: diffuse lower lobe bronchiectasis [53] or a UIP-like pattern on chest imaging, respectively (see "Computed Tomography of the Chest" section, below). Although several

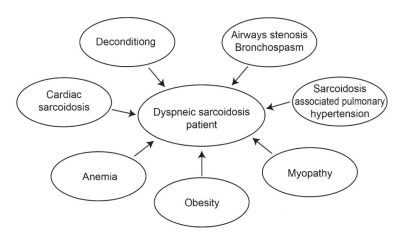

Fig. 5.3 Causes of dyspnea in sarcoidosis

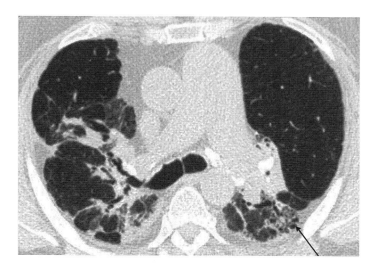

Fig. 5.4 Computed tomography of the chest demonstrating the fibrocystic pattern of advanced pulmonary sarcoidosis with predominantly mid and upper lung zone central fibrosis, architectural changes, dilated airways, and cysts (*arrow*)

review papers have suggested that crackles may occur in up to 20 % of advanced pulmonary sarcoidosis, the data are based on decades-old series where the diagnosis of sarcoidosis was established prior to modern criteria [42, 54]. More commonly, the presence of clubbing or crackles signifies that an alternate diagnosis or a super-imposed process is the cause of lung disease. In those situations, it is useful to search for evidence of extrapulmonary involvement to substantiate the diagnosis of sarcoidosis. Hemoptysis is rare but may be seen in patients with mycetomas or endobronchial involvement [55].

Computed Tomography of the Chest

It is probably not necessary to routinely obtain CT scans in all patients with Scadding stage 4 chest X-rays. Situations where CT of the chest may provide particular benefit include when there is clinical suspicion of mycetoma or complications unrelated to sarcoidosis such as infection or medication toxicity. There are little data to support a role for chest CT patterns in guiding therapy decisions [56].

Major CT findings suggesting fibrosis are fissure displacement, bronchial distortion, and fissure distortion [48]. The most common pattern is characterized by architectural distortion in a predominant central distribution (Fig. 5.4). It is frequently accompanied by micronodules and bronchovascular thickening. A CT pattern with substantial honeycomb cystic changes may occur as well, but it is less common (Fig. 5.4). The honeycombing typically involves the mid and upper lung zones. Patients with substantial honeycomb cystic changes have more impaired lung function [48, 56].

Pulmonary Function Tests

Advanced pulmonary sarcoidosis may manifest with any combination of restrictive or obstructive patterns on PFTs. The chest imaging pattern correlates poorly with physiologic findings and functional impairment [57–59]. Therefore, PFTs are useful tools to define the mechanism responsible for a patient's symptoms.

Obstruction is common in the setting of pulmonary fibrosis, occurring in up to 75 % of patients [52]. It generally occurs as part of a mixed obstructive–restrictive pattern and may relate to diminished elastic recoil and/or airway caliber [52]. Of interest, the presence of airways obstruction early in the disease is a predictor of worse long-term outcomes [36]. In a subset of patients, a bronchodilator response may be present, but the frequency of reversible obstruction in advanced sarcoidosis has not been systematically studied. The restrictive ventilatory impairment in advanced sarcoidosis reflects underlying reduction of static lung volumes and impairment of gas exchange [60]. The most sensitive of the standard PFT tests is the diffusing capacity of the lung for carbon monoxide (DLCO) [63]. For example, in a series of 607 patients with radiographic stage 2–4 disease, the prevalence of reduced TLC was only 7 %; in the same cohort, over 20 % of patients with normal TLC had low static compliance or low DLCO [60]. Compared to IPF, advanced sarcoidosis tends to exhibit less impairment of DLCO at the same lung volumes. This finding likely reflects the differences in the ventilation–perfusion relationships between the two disorders, especially the distribution of disease and the involvement of the airways.

Cardiopulmonary exercise testing can be useful in the setting of advanced pulmonary sarcoidosis. Impaired ventilatory reserve, widened alveolar–arterial gradient and reduced maximal oxygen consumption (VO2max) are seen more frequently in patients with fibrotic sarcoidosis than those with other radiographic patterns, even when FVC and DLCO are similar [61]. Elevated dead space fraction during exercise is the physiologic mechanism for nearly half of impaired VO2max [62]. Since the causes of dyspnea are multiple, cardiopulmonary exercise testing should be considered in all advanced pulmonary sarcoidosis when symptoms are substantial.

Other Presentations and Complications of Advanced Lung Disease

Pulmonary Hypertension

Pulmonary hypertension due to sarcoidosis is categorized by the World Health Organization in Group V (miscellaneous conditions) [38]. Up to 75 % of sarcoidosis patients listed for lung transplantation have pulmonary arterial hypertension associated with sarcoidosis (SAPH) based on right heart catheterization. The presence of SAPH is associated with a poor prognosis, compared to pulmonary venous hypertension in sarcoidosis patients [37].

Fig. 5.5 Explanted lung
with fibrotic sarcoidosis
with advanced bronchiectasis
(courtesy of Carol Farver, MD)

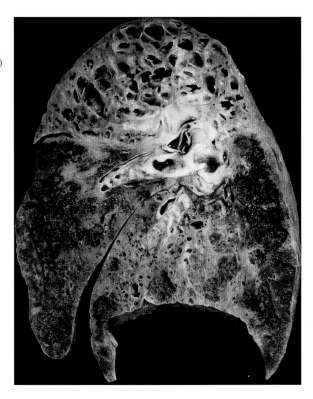

SAPH is most commonly found in patients with advanced fibrotic disease but may occur in those with minimal radiologic evidence of parenchymal disease For example, Sulica et al. found that 60 % of SAPH patients in one center had no significant fibrosis on chest radiography [63]. The extent of parenchymal involvement also may not correlate with the degree of PH and this suggests direct or indirect granulomatous involvement of the pulmonary arteries [64]. Screening for SAPH should be most avidly pursued in patients with fibrotic sarcoidosis, a disproportionate reduction of DLCO, reduced 6-min walk distance, or desaturation [63, 64]. SAPH is reviewed more extensively in Chap. 6.

Bronchiectasis

Bronchiectasis from sarcoidosis can be localized but it is usually diffuse. Diffuse cystic bronchiectasis is thought to originate from two mechanisms: traction-related fibrosis around the peribronchovascular bundles and direct damage to the airways from granulomatous inflammation (Fig. 5.5). In the less common scenario of localized or post-obstructive bronchiectasis, external compression from intrathoracic lymph nodes or long-standing endobronchial sarcoidosis is more often the cause [65].

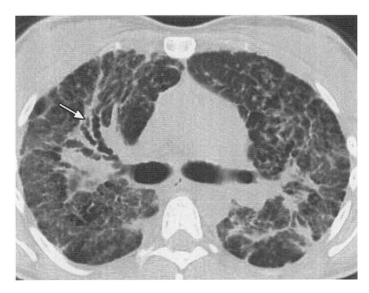

Fig. 5.6 Computed tomography of the chest with dilation of the large airways and segmental airways. The curvilinear distortion of the airway course is typical of the architectural distortion found in advanced pulmonary sarcoidosis (with permission from Culver DA. Immunol Allergy Clin North Am 2012;32(4):487)

The prevalence of bronchiectasis is related to the severity of lung involvement. Using CT of chest to make the diagnosis, bronchiectasis has been found on 18–40 % of patients (Fig. 5.6) with a stage 4 chest X-ray [48, 53]. The rate of bronchiectasis may approach 100 % in patients who require lung transplantation [7].

Most patients with traction bronchiectasis do not exhibit features typically seen with common causes of bronchiectasis, such as cystic fibrosis. However, in a minority of patients with bronchiectasis, the clinical course may be dominated by classical bronchiectasis features. In that situation, there may be a high rate of digital clubbing, lung rales on auscultation, hemoptysis, and recurrent exacerbations requiring hospitalization [53]. Management of recurrent infectious exacerbations may be more useful than escalating corticosteroid doses in that setting. In a small series of seven such patients acquired over 20 years, the mortality rate was 57 % [53].

In routine practice, it may be useful to consider a trial of corticosteroids or other immunosuppressive agents to assess the potential for reversible inflammation, since chest imaging is not reliable for this purpose. If no evidence of granulomatous inflammation is present or the patient has been adequately treated for sarcoidosis, the management of bronchiectasis should focus on the prevention and treatment of exacerbations rather than sarcoidosis itself. The foundation for management is non-pharmacologic airway clearance techniques such as routine chest physiotherapy [66]. Adjunctive pharmacotherapy may also be useful. Some suggested management techniques of chronic symptoms related to non-cystic fibrosis bronchiectasis are outlined in Table 5.2.

Table 5.2 Management strategies for stable bronchiectasis	Airway
	Clearance techniques
	Postural drainage
	Oscillating positive pressure device
	Forced expiration techniques
	Adjuncts for airway clearance
	Nebulized normal saline
	Nebulized hypertonic saline
	Inhaled Beta2 agonist
	Airway pharmacotherapy
	Inhaled Beta2 agnoist
	Inhaled anticholinergic bronchodilator
	Antibiotics
	Long-term oral antibiotics (azithromycin)
	Long-term inhaled antibiotics

Airway Stenosis

The classic anatomic distribution of sarcoidosis granulomas is along the bronchovascular bundles and lymphatics. Therefore sarcoidosis commonly involves the mucosa of the airways, most often the distal airways [67]. In advanced disease, endoluminal or extraluminal fibroproliferation, rather than inflammation, may be the dominant pathologic process [67, 68]. Airways compromise in advanced sarcoidosis may therefore result from a persistent endoluminal granulomatous inflammation, extrinsic compression from enlarged lymph nodes and conglomerate inflammatory masses, peribronchical fibrosis leading to bronchial architectural distortion, or focal bronchostenosis.

Bronchial stenosis may be isolated, involved multiple discrete sites of stenosis, or be diffuse [67, 68]. Severe stenosis is relatively uncommon, occurring in less than 1 % of all sarcoidosis patients [68]. However, the prevalence is higher in those with radiographic stage 4 chest X-rays [68]. Some patients with diffuse endoluminal stenosis disease may have concomitant bronchiectasis, which is unique to sarcoidosis [65].

Common symptoms of airway stenosis include dyspnea, wheezing, and stridor. Worsening airflow obstruction is common [65]. Central airway obstruction may be suspected in patients with FVC/FVC ratio less than 70 %, flattening of the flow-volume loop, or focal wheezing on chest exam. Bronchoscopy for airway examination is a useful tool to diagnose, determine location, extent, and etiology of proximal stenosis in the airways (Fig. 5.7) [68, 69]. Bronchial abnormalities can also be detected on CT, but the specificity of CT findings for diagnosis of clinically important airways stenosis is suspect. In a series of 60 consecutive patients who had both bronchoscopy and CT scan within 15 days, only eight of 39 patients with bronchial abnormalities on CT scan were found to have clinically important endoluminal abnormalities during direct visualization [70].

Fig. 5.7 Bronchoscopic image demonstrating almost complete web-like airway stenosis of the left lower lobe (*bottom*) and relatively spared left upper lobe (*top*)

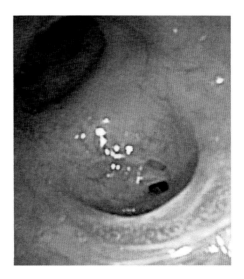

Early treatment with corticosteroids or cytotoxic agents such as methotrexate at the time of initial presentation is important since delay in treatment greater than 3 months may lead to irreversible endoluminal stenosis [67]. Adjunctive broncho-scopic modalities may be helpful for those with primarily discrete endoluminal ste-noses. These may include combinations of balloon bronchoplasty, mitomycin C application, cryoablation, laser photoresection, electrocautery, and brachytherapy [71–73]. Commonly, more than one therapeutic session is necessary, since manipu-lation of the airways frequently induces granulation tissue but with repeated therapy this reaction tends to be less exuberant. In our center, we most often use a combina-tion of balloon bronchoplasty, cryotherapy, corticosteroid injections, and topical application of mitomycin C. Given the propensity of sarcoidosis to react to manipu-lation and foreign bodies, endoluminal stents should be avoided unless all other options are exhausted.

Cavitary Lung Disease and Mycetomas

True cavitation due to dense granulomatous inflammation invading the intra-alveolar septa and leading to ischemic necrosis has been reported, but it is distinctly unusual [74]. Instead, "cavitary" disease in sarcoidosis almost always occurs in the setting of fibrotic lung disease and represents pseudocavities comprised of ectatic bronchi that are lined by fibrotic lung in the upper lobes [75]. When the pseudocavities of advanced pulmonary sarcoidosis are secondarily infected by bacteria, they may resemble pyogenic abscess. However, the most common infectious complication of pseudocavities is the mycetoma [76].

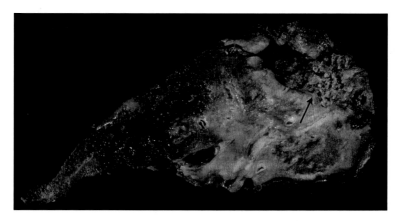

Fig. 5.8 Explanted lung with large upper lobe mycetoma (*arrow*) (courtesy of Carol Farver, MD)

Mycetomas represent a conglomeration of fungal mycelia colonizing the fibrocystic cavities, most commonly by *Aspergillus fumigatus* [77]. They communicate with the airways and are composed of saprophytic fungal elements, fibrin, mucus, and host cellular debris. Two types have been defined: simple and complex. Simple aspergillomas occur in cysts lined by epithelium with no peri-cavitary fibrosis. In distinction, the walls of complex aspergillomas are thick and are surrounded by diseased lung parenchyma [78]. A higher incidence of the complex type has been reported; the distinction in type may have implications for surgical management [79].

Mycetomas occur in less than 5 % of all patients with sarcoidosis when case ascertainment is by routine means such as radiography and longitudinal follow-up [18]. However, the true incidence of aspergillomas may be higher. For example, 10 % of patients in a cohort of 100 consecutive patients screened with serial aspergillus precipitins eventually developed aspergillomas over a decade follow-up. Among patients with stage 4 chest X-rays, aspergillomas developed in 11.3 % of a series of 142 French sarcoidosis patients [4]. At the time of diagnosis of cavitary sarcoidosis, up to 44 % of patients already have radiologic evidence of mycetomas [10, 80].

Mycetomas affect both the right and left lungs equally, but occur most commonly in the upper lobes (Fig. 5.8) [55]. They may be single or multiple. The classic radiographic appearance is that of a round, mobile mass topped by a clear crescent that separates the mass from the wall of the cavity (Fig. 5.9). It has the same density as water. The so-called crescent sign or Monod's sign is considered diagnostic [75]. Most patients with *Aspergillus fumigatus* infection will have positive serum precipitins against *Aspergillus* [77, 81]. Diagnosis can be established in the setting of the classic radiographic presentation and positive serum precipitins [81]. In patients with significant risk factors for tuberculosis, it is important to perform confirmatory tests when considering the diagnosis of aspergillosis, since the presentation may be similar [82]. Invasive fungal infection or dissemination of the infection even in the setting of immune-modulating therapy is thought to be rare [83], but the true incidence of semi-invasive fungal disease is unknown [84].

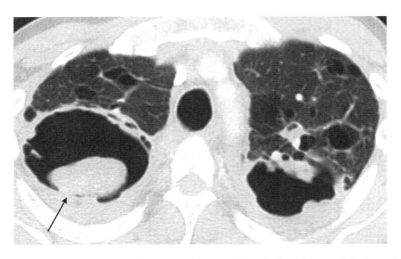

Fig. 5.9 Computed tomography of the chest with aspergilloma in the right upper lobe (*arrow*) and an obvious "crescent sign"

Most patients are asymptomatic. Hemoptysis may occur when there is invasion of local blood vessels in the cavity wall by fungal hyphae. In a retrospective study of 85 patients admitted to the hospital with aspergillomas due to various underlying lung disease, hemoptysis occurred in 83 % of the cases [55]. Similar rates have been reported in more recent series [85]. The size of the aspergilloma is unrelated to the risk of hemoptysis [55]. When hemoptysis occurs, the mortality rate from the acute episode varies from 5 to 26 % [10, 55, 81].

Due to the lack of robust evidence, there are no specific consensus recommendations for the management of aspergillomas. Fortunately, given the quiescent nature of the disease, not all patients require therapy. Surgical resection is the only definitive therapy [81], usually for the indication of hemoptysis [86]. However, resection for patients with mild or isolated hemoptysis is not recommended due to high operative morbidity and mortality which may be due to the coexistence of impaired pulmonary function and widespread vascular adhesions [55, 79]. Operative morality has been reported to be as high as 33 % in patients with complex aspergillomas [79] and approximately 2–5 % in all patients [55, 85, 86]. The rate of complications such as secondary hemorrhage, bronchopulmonary fistulas, empyema, respiratory failure, and death are higher in complex (78 %) than in simple (33 %) mycetomas [83]. When the mycetoma is complex, there is a 2.5-fold higher rate of surgical complications [83]. As a result, surgical resection is generally reserved for patients with clinically significant hemoptysis who fail less invasive treatment options. A rarely used surgical option is a cavernostomy, where a flap of pectoralis, rhomboid, trapezius, or serratus muscles is permanently placed through the chest wall into the cavity, obliterating it and providing good vascular supply for antimicrobial delivery. Historically, caveronstomies are associated with high mortality rates [55] but newer series show relatively good outcomes [85].

A common approach to the management of hemoptysis from mycetomas is bronchial artery embolization (BAE) with polyvinyl alcohol particles or gelatin sponge. It should be noted that that the procedure is usually only a temporizing measure and may be ineffective in the long term due to the formation of collateral circulation [87]. The immediate success rate of BAE ranges from 75 to 90 %, but with aspergillomas the recurrence rate may be as high as 100 % [88, 89].

Treatment of aspergillomas with systemic antifungal agents is attractive but the success rate is low, perhaps due to inability of the antimicrobial to penetrate into the cavity [90]. For example, in one retrospective study, none of the 18 patients treated with intravenous amphotericin B demonstrated any radiographic improvement [55]. There is some evidence supporting the use of azoles for treatment of mycetomas but these studies are limited by lack of standardization, sample size, or poor study design [91, 92]. Their use received only a Grade BIII recommendation from the Infectious Disease Society of America [81].

A novel approach is to deliver antifungal agents more effectively to the cavity itself. Direct CT-guided intracavitary amphotericin installation may effectively stop bleeding [93–95]. In one institution, daily installation of amphotericin via an indwelling percutaneous catheter was highly effective, with cessation of bleeding in 17 of 23 (74 %) of bleeding episodes and prolonged remission in more than 50 % of patients [95].

Risk factors for recurrent hemoptysis included radiologic evidence of active aspergilloma growth, bleeding diathesis, and lack of bronchial artery embolization [95]. Spontaneous resolution of aspergillomas has been reported and occurs in approximately 5–10 % patients over 1–5 years from the time of diagnosis [55, 96, 97].

Management

Symptom Control

There are no specific guidelines or statements that address the management of respiratory symptoms due to advanced pulmonary sarcoidosis. A combined non-pharmacologic and pharmacologic strategy for symptom control should be considered similar to other chronic lung diseases such as COPD and IPF. For instance, patients with airflow obstruction or bronchiectasis should have treatment targeted specifically to these aspects of the clinical presentation. In formulating the treatment strategy, it may be helpful to consider the mechanism for the particular symptom, which can vary considerably among sarcoidosis patients. In the example of airflow obstruction, for example, there may be bronchospasm, bronchiectasis, airways involvement by granulomatous inflammation, fixed or reversible laryngeal sarcoidosis, vocal cord dysfunction, extrinsic compression of airways from conglomerate lymph node masses, or bronchostenosis. Obviously, the approach to each of these situations must be individualized.

Dyspnea is another symptom that may be multifactorial. There are no studies addressing the role of oxygen supplementation or pulmonary rehabilitation for the management of dyspnea in sarcoidosis. However, there is a high prevalence of respiratory muscle and appendicular muscle weakness in sarcoidosis patients that is only partly explained by corticosteroid use [98, 99]. The impaired muscle strength correlates with reduced 6-min walk distance, lower quality of life, depression and fatigue, so pulmonary rehabilitation that includes resistance training may theoretically be very helpful in advanced pulmonary sarcoidosis [100].

Disease Activity and Medical Therapy

Two competing priorities must be balanced when considering medical therapy in advanced lung disease: risk for under-treatment of granulomatous inflammation versus risk of medication toxicities. There is a temptation to equate "advanced or fibrotic sarcoidosis" with "irremediable" sarcoidosis, a viewpoint that is based more on opinion than on evidence. A closely related aspect of treatment decisions is the goal of reducing the burden of granulomatous inflammation with an intention to modify symptoms and decrease functional impairment, just as in acute disease. Given the morbidity associated with advanced disease and the dangers inherent to lung transplantation, as well as the substantial likelihood that a transplant may not materialize, it may be useful to aggressively search for evidence of treatable (i.e., "active") disease.

A widely held viewpoint is that sarcoidosis "activity" must be documented by some testing prior to treatment of advanced disease. There have been a variety of attempts to define "active sarcoidosis." For example, the 1983 WASOG conference participants defined active sarcoidosis as the presence of (1) ongoing T-cell and macrophage-driven inflammation, (2) persistence of granuloma formation, or (3) active progression to fibrosis [101]. In the current era, all of the available tests to assess can still be described by the 1983 rubric. However, the tools to assess activity such as angiotensin-converting enzyme (ACE) level, BAL fluid analysis, and CT suffer from inadequate sensitivity and specificity. For example, in a series of 96 French patients with Scadding stage 4 chest X-rays who had escalation of therapy, 84 (88 %) exhibited objective improvement [4]. Interestingly age, sex, ethnicity, baseline FVC and DLCO, honeycombing pattern on CT, high serum ACE level, and alveolar lymphocytosis did not predict response to therapy. Only a shorter duration of diagnosis prior to initiation of treatment was useful to differentiate patients who improved or worsened. Other studies have confirmed the lack of association between radiograph stage and the quantity of inflammatory cells in tissue biopsies or BAL fluid [102].

Further support of the poor utility of conventional testing to define whether active granulomatous inflammation is present comes from the lung transplant experience. Four of seven consecutive explants from a single US center exhibited persistent granulomatous inflammation despite radiologic evidence of "end-stage" lung disease with extensive honeycomb cystic changes [5]. Anecdotally, the experience at our institution is similar, where roughly half of explants harbor substantial active

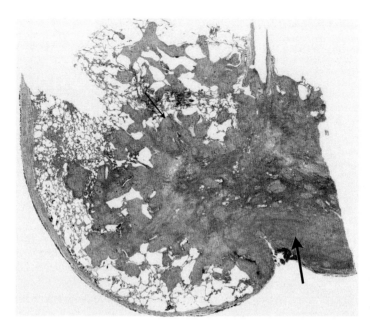

Fig. 5.10 Explant from a patient with "end-stage" lung disease who underwent lung transplantation. There is substantial fibrosis (*thick arrow*), but in the areas adjacent to more normal lung, there are multiple inflammatory (non-fibrotic) granulomas (*thin arrows*) (courtesy Carol Farver, MD)

granulomatous inflammation after clinical and radiologic diagnosis of irreversible sarcoidosis (personal communication, Carol Farver, MD) (Fig. 5.10). These observations imply that conventional assessment of "end stage" is flawed, that there is a role for empiric trials of escalated treatment when faced with advanced pulmonary sarcoidosis, and possibly also point out that none of the currently available immunosuppressive medications are 100 % effective for granuloma dissolution. In our practice, we administer a trial of prednisone (30–40 mg daily) for approximately 4 weeks to assess reversibility in advanced pulmonary sarcoidosis. In selected patients, we also may consider a trial of infliximab, since responses to it are generally evident within three to four infusions [103].

Lung imaging using positron emission tomography (PET) with ^{18}F-Fluorodeoxyglucose (FDG) is a promising tool to help guide the intensity of treatment trials, but there are insufficient data available about the predictive values of PET scan to advocate its routine use at this juncture. Even in individuals with stage 0 or 4 chest radiographs, PET scan may demonstrate uptake in the lung parenchyma [6, 104]. In early sarcoidosis and in refractory sarcoidosis, increased FDG uptake in the lung has been able to define individuals with potential to improve after treatment, as well as serve as a marker of treatment response [105, 106]. Besides PET, serum markers of disease activity such as ACE, soluble interleukin 2 receptor, chitotriosidase, vascular endothelial growth factor, and IL-6 may also be considered, although the data supporting their usefulness are sparse and many are available only in a research setting [107–109].

Lung Transplantation

Sarcoidosis patients comprise 3.5 % of the total population listed for transplantation [110]. According to the International Society for Heart and Lung Transplantation (ISHLT) 2012 report, sarcoidosis accounts for 2.5 % of lung and 1.6 % of heart–lung transplants [111]. As a result, sarcoidosis is currently the seventh leading cause for lung transplantation. Compared to the overall lung transplant population in the USA, those with sarcoidosis are younger (45.8 ± 8.8 years versus 48.9 ± 12.3 years; $p < 0.001$), and more likely to be female and African American [112]. These characteristics mirror the population that is affected by sarcoidosis in the USA.

Transplant Window

The median survival time after lung transplantation is 5½ years. The survival after sarcoidosis is no different than for transplant as a whole [111]. Given the limited number of studies, it is unclear if transplantation in patients with advanced pulmonary sarcoidosis leads to improved survival [113]. Thus, it is advisable to list patients at the point in time when the risk for death from advanced disease clearly exceeds the risks from transplantation. A second consideration, analogous to that for COPD, would be to consider transplantation in an individual with such severely symptomatic disease that the risks of transplantation are outweighed by its potential for improved quality of life.

In general, orthotopic lung transplantation should be considered when the 2-year mortality for patients with chronic pulmonary disease is 50 % [114]. This determination can be challenging in patients with sarcoidosis since the disease course is often long and variable. Despite the longer time-to-death, the risk of death for patients with sarcoidosis on the lung transplant list is high. Prior to adoption of the Lung Allocation Score (LAS) in 2005, the mortality rate for those on the transplant list was estimated to be 30–58 %, a figure that higher than for IPF [115–117]. In that era, risk factors for death while waiting for lung transplantation included black race, higher oxygen requirements, elevated pulmonary artery pressures, and right atrial pressure greater than 15 mmHg [115, 116]. Using these data, the ISHLT derived guidelines for referral for transplantation which are summarized below [117]:

- New York Heart Association functional classification III or IV

  and
  Any of the following:

- Hypoxemia at rest
- Pulmonary hypertension
- Right atrial pressure greater than 15 mmHg

However, the ISHLT parameters can be criticized on the basis of referral and ascertainment bias, and they have never been validated. As a rule, a decision to proceed with evaluation for lung transplantation should include a careful

Table 5.3 Suggested work-up and testing prior to lung transplantation for patients with advanced pulmonary sarcoidosis	Physical exam
	Chest wall and axial skeleton for mobility
	Diaphragm movement
	Evidence for systemic involvement: skin, liver, spleen, neurologic, and cardiac
	Imaging studies
	Computed tomography scan of the chest
	Quantitative nuclear medicine ventilation and perfusion scan
	Functional evaluation
	Spirometry
	Lung volumes
	Diffusing capacity of the lung for carbon monoxide
	Six-minute walk distance
	Oximetry at rest and with exercise
	Cardiac evaluation
	Echocardiogram with bubble study
	Right heart catheterization
	Left heart catheterization
	Studies specific for sarcoidosis
	Sputum culture for *Aspergillus*
	Aspergillus serum precipitins
	Electrocardiogram or 24–72-h ambulatory electrocardiography

assessment about the course and pace of the disease, the degree of physiologic impairment, potential for reversibility or stabilization, absence of data about the survival benefit, and the risk factors listed above.

Candidacy

Besides severity of pulmonary involvement, predicted mortality, and comorbid conditions, pre-transplant evaluation in patients with sarcoidosis should include a review of any extrapulmonary disease burden that could complicate post-transplant management or represent contraindications for lung transplantation (Table 5.3). Extrapulmonary sarcoidosis was present in 47 % of patients listed for transplant at one US center [116]. Cardiac involvement is especially important since it may carry a high risk of mortality [9]. Individuals with impaired left ventricular ejection fraction or sustained ventricular dysrhythmias are at higher risk of death and may be appropriately considered for heart and lung transplantation [118]. On the other hand, severe right ventricular impairment due to PH may regress after bilateral lung transplantation and does not necessarily indicate a need for a combined procedure [119].

Severe liver involvement leading to end-stage liver disease or severe skin involvement with secondary infections are also important issues to consider. At the same time, it may be important to emphasize that liver involvement usually follows a benign course and would be unlikely to impact the long-term outcome or limit medication options in most cases. The intensity of screening for extrapulmonary disease ideally should focus on manifestations likely to cause morbidity or mortality, and therefore screening for occult organ involvement (e.g., by whole body PET scan) is generally unnecessary. A thorough history and review of systems, as well as some basic screening for cardiac sarcoidosis with echocardiogram and ambulatory electrocardiography are generally the only tools necessary to determine the extent of disease involvement and plan for post-transplant management.

As mentioned previously, mycetomas are common in advanced pulmonary sarcoidosis. Among all explanted lungs with mycetomas, sarcoidosis is the most common underlying lung disease [120]. In a series of 303 consecutive explants, the presence of a mycetoma was associated with a median survival rate of 16 months (versus 57 months for those without mycetomas) and a 2-year survival rate of 14.3 % [106]. However, the accelerated mortality in those with mycetomas cannot be definitively attributed to their presence, since other covariates were not analyzed. Antifungal therapy may have a role in the prevention of poor outcomes in this setting [106].

Type of Transplantation

The decision to list a patient for a single lung, double lung, or heart–lung transplantation involves consideration of the underlying physiology, extrapulmonary involvement, complications of the lung involvement, comorbid conditions, and the probability of organ procurement given a patient's size and ABO blood group. The importance of a thorough evaluation and thoughtful consideration should not be underestimated since the type of transplantation impacts peri- and post-op care and outcomes [111, 117, 121]. Survival after lung transplant for sarcoidosis is similar to the transplant population as a whole, even for those receiving single lung transplants [122, 123]. The development of post-transplant chronic rejection, bronchiolitis obliterans syndrome (BOS), is similar in sarcoidosis and IPF [108]. However, due to the higher prevalence of PH and other factors, sarcoidosis patients are more likely to receive a double lung transplant (51 % vs. 40 %) or a heart–lung transplant (5.3 % vs. 1.4 %) compared to those transplanted for other reasons [112].

Patients with significant SAPH should be considered for double lung transplantation. It has been theorized that single lung transplantation may risk primary graft failure as a result of persistently high vascular resistance in the native lung, leading to a disproportionate fraction of the cardiac output flowing through the donor lung [121]. If there is evidence of significant cardiac sarcoidosis [124], a combined en bloc heart and lung transplantation may be the appropriate choice.

It has not been definitively demonstrated, but seems theoretically plausible, that patients with unilateral mycetomas in the explanted lung may be at increased risk for development of de novo fungal infection in the native lung. Therefore, some authors have advocated that all patients with mycetomas should receive a double lung transplant [116]. In our center, we routinely prefer to list patients for double lung transplantation when possible if there is a history of a mycetoma.

Table 5.4 Summary of survival rates in patients with sarcoidosis undergoing lung transplantation from six series

	30 Days	3 Months	1 Year	2 Years	3 Years	5 Years	10 Years
Arcasoy (n = 12)	–	–	62 %	62 %	50 %	50 %	–
Milman (n = 7)	–	–	100 %	85 %	85 %	85 %	85 %
Nunley (n = 9)	100 %	–	67 %	56 %	56 %	–	–
Shorr (n = 133)	83 %	–	–	–	–	–	–
Walker (n = 12)	75 %	–	75 %	–	70 %	56 %	–
Wille (n = 15)	–	86.7 %	80 %	66.7 %	66.7 %	46.7 %	–

Outcomes

Overall intermediate and long-term survival is similar to that for transplant in general [112, 116, 122, 125]. Unadjusted survival rates for the entire lung transplant population are 88 % at 3 months, 79 % 1 year, 64 % at 3 years, 53 % at 5 years, and 30 % at 10 years [111]. Survival rates based on the ISHLT registry and six retrospective studies are summarized in Table 5.4.

In contrast to long-term survival, short-term outcomes in sarcoidosis are worse than average [111]. The risk of death within the first year is fourth highest for sarcoidosis (after re-transplantation, pulmonary arterial hypertension, and miscellaneous unusual indications) among all the indications for transplant; the relative risk for death compared to the overall transplant population is 1.66 (95 % CI 1.25–2.19, $p = 0.0004$) [111]. In analysis conducted prior to adoption of the LAS, black race was found to be a risk factor for worse 30-day survival, but it is unclear whether that finding reflects intrinsic biologic factors or the effects of delayed access to transplant centers due to socioeconomic factors [112]. A similar analysis has not been published since the LAS was adopted in 2005.

BOS is the main cause of mortality after the first year after lung transplant. The frequency and severity of episodes of acute rejection is one the most important factors associated with the development of BOS [126]. Rates of BOS in sarcoidosis reportedly range from 25 to 57 % [123, 125]. In a single center study comparing outcomes in sarcoidosis and IPF transplant groups, there was no difference in the development of BOS (33.3 % for sarcoidosis vs. 31.2 % for IPF, OR 0.91, 95 % CI 0.23–4.01, $p = 1.0$) when adjusted for age, race, and gender [123].

Disease Recurrence

Sarcoidosis is the most common underlying disease to recur in patients who undergo allogenic lung transplantation. Recurrence has been defined by the presence of non-caseating granulomas in the donor lung tissue not attributable to infection or foreign bodies [127, 128]. Recurrence of non-caseating granulomas has been reported in kidney, liver, heart, and lung transplant recipients. Interestingly transmission of sarcoidosis with dissemination to the lungs has occurred after bone marrow transplantation from a donor with sarcoidosis [129].

Sarcoidosis is estimated to recur in approximately half to two-third of lung allografts as early as 14 days after transplantation [130]. The estimated average time to recurrence is 15 months [128]. However, recurrent sarcoidosis is usually not clinically bothersome [122, 131–133]. One multicenter study published as an abstract suggested a slight survival advantage in patients with disease recurrence, which was attributed to more careful detection and treatment of subclinical rejection [134]. However, there has been at least one reported case where re-transplant was required after failure of intensified immunosuppression [135].

Evidence of recurrence has been reported to precede radiographic evidence of disease, and hilar adenopathy is surprisingly absent from descriptions [122, 128, 131, 135]. Frequently, the only evidence of the disease is an isolated pathologic finding at the time of surveillance bronchoscopy [122, 125, 130]. Thus the rate of recurrence at any given center is likely dependent on surveillance practices. The benign course of recurrent sarcoidosis may be related to the fact that patients are on immunosuppressive agents to prevent allograft rejection [127].

Recurrence of sarcoidosis has provided an opportunity to study granuloma formation. Milman et al. performed fluorescent in situ hybridization to probe for X- and Y-chromosomes on lung tissue from transbronchial biopsies obtained from a single lung, graft–sex mismatch patient with recurrent sarcoidosis [133]. The granulomas in that patient were comprised of immune cells from the recipient rather than the donor. In another study Ionescu et al. analyzed histiocyte microchimerism to identity the origin of the epithelioid cells comprising recurrent granulomas in donor lung [127]. They also concluded that the presence of granulomas in the donor lung signifies repopulation of the donor lung by recipient monocytes. These observations accord with the hypothesis that sarcoidosis is caused by a transmissible, poorly degraded antigen, first popularized by the Norwegian pathologist, Morten Ansgar Kveim [136].

Our Experience

The lung transplantation program at our institution was started in 1990 and in that time we have preformed lung transplantation in over 1,155 patients. Of these, 38 (3.4 %) were in patients with sarcoidosis and 40 % were transplanted after the 2005 adoption of the LAS. The average age of our cohort is 50 years, 79 % have either sequential or en bloc double lung transplantation, and unlike what is reported in the lung transplantation literature, 52 % are men [115, 137]. The overall mortality rate for this group of patients is 52 % over 20 years.

Conclusion

Determining when a patient with sarcoidosis has reached the point of irreversible loss of lung function ("end stage") is difficult, and it implies futility of further treatment. Instead, there are often specific and nonspecific therapies that can be beneficial for how a patient feels, functions, or survives. Thus the term "end stage" may not be appropriate in patients with advanced pulmonary sarcoidosis. Not only is clinical presentation heterogenous, but functional implications may also vary. Prior to referral to lung transplantation, strong consideration for aggressive medical therapy should be considered. Patients should also be monitored for related complications of advanced lung disease, such as SAPH or mycetoma. However, once a referral for transplantation is made, sarcoidosis-specific considerations regarding candidacy and type of transplantation must be borne in mind. While advanced pulmonary sarcoidosis may be considered more difficult to treat than less severe disease, a number of interventions can benefit these patients.

References

1. Bellomo R, Ronco C, Kellum JA, Mehta RL, Palevsky P. Acute renal failure – definition, outcome measures, animal models, fluid therapy and information technology needs: the Second International Consensus Conference of the Acute Dialysis Quality Initiative (ADQI) Group. Crit Care. 2004;8(4):R204–12.
2. Baughman RP, Nagai S, Balter M, Costabel U, Drent M, du Bois R, et al. Defining the clinical outcome status (COS) in sarcoidosis: results of WASOG Task Force. Sarcoidosis Vasc Diffuse Lung Dis. 2011;28(1):56–64.
3. Prasse A, Katic C, Germann M, Buchwald A, Zissel G, Muller-Quernheim J. Phenotyping sarcoidosis from a pulmonary perspective. Am J Respir Crit Care Med. 2008;177(3): 330–6.
4. Nardi A, Brillet PY, Letoumelin P, Girard F, Brauner M, Uzunhan Y, et al. Stage IV sarcoidosis: comparison of survival with the general population and causes of death. Eur Respir J. 2011;38(6):1368–73.
5. Shigemitsu H, Oblad JM, Sharma OP, Koss MN. Chronic interstitial pneumonitis in end-stage sarcoidosis. Eur Respir J. 2010;35(3):695–7.
6. Teirstein AT, Morgenthau AS. "End-stage" pulmonary fibrosis in sarcoidosis. Mt Sinai J Med. 2009;76(1):30–6.
7. Xu L, Kligerman S, Burke A. End-stage sarcoid lung disease is distinct from usual interstitial pneumonia. Am J Surg Pathol. 2013;37(4):593–600.
8. Baughman RP, Winget DB, Bowen EH, Lower EE. Predicting respiratory failure in sarcoidosis patients. Sarcoidosis Vasc Diffuse Lung Dis. 1997;14(2):154–8.
9. Judson MA. Lung transplantation for pulmonary sarcoidosis. Eur Respir J. 1998;11(3): 738–44.
10. Johns CJ, Michele TM. The clinical management of sarcoidosis. A 50-year experience at the Johns Hopkins Hospital. Medicine (Baltimore). 1999;78(2):65–111.
11. Nagai S, Shigematsu M, Hamada K, Izumi T. Clinical courses and prognoses of pulmonary sarcoidosis. Curr Opin Pulm Med. 1999;5(5):293–8.
12. Judson MA, Baughman RP, Thompson BW, Teirstein AS, Terrin ML, Rossman MD, et al. Two year prognosis of sarcoidosis: the ACCESS experience. Sarcoidosis Vasc Diffuse Lung Dis. 2003;20(3):204–11.
13. Chappell AG, Cheung WY, Hutchings HA. Sarcoidosis: a long-term follow up study. Sarcoidosis Vasc Diffuse Lung Dis. 2000;17(2):167–73.
14. Mana J, Salazar A, Manresa F. Clinical factors predicting persistence of activity in sarcoidosis: a multivariate analysis of 193 cases. Respiration. 1994;61(4):219–25.
15. Mana J, Badrinas F. Prognosis of sarcoidosis. An unresolved issue. Sarcoidosis. 1992;9(1): 15–20.

16. Costabel U, Hunninghake GW. ATS/ERS/WASOG statement on sarcoidosis. Sarcoidosis Statement Committee. American Thoracic Society. European Respiratory Society. World Association for Sarcoidosis and Other Granulomatous Disorders. Eur Respir J. 1999;14(4):735–7.
17. Akira M, Kozuka T, Inoue Y, Sakatani M. Long-term follow-up CT scan evaluation in patients with pulmonary sarcoidosis. Chest. 2005;127(1):185–91.
18. Judson MA, Boan AD, Lackland DT. The clinical course of sarcoidosis: presentation, diagnosis, and treatment in a large white and black cohort in the United States. Sarcoidosis Vasc Diffuse Lung Dis. 2012;29(2):119–27.
19. Swigris JJ, Olson AL, Huie TJ, Fernandez-Perez ER, Solomon J, Sprunger D, et al. Sarcoidosis-related mortality in the United States from 1988 to 2007. Am J Respir Crit Care Med. 2011;183(11):1524–30.
20. Neville E, Walker AN, James DG. Prognostic factors predicting the outcome of sarcoidosis: an analysis of 818 patients. Q J Med. 1983;52(208):525–33.
21. Lazar CA, Culver DA. Treatment of sarcoidosis. Semin Respir Crit Care Med. 2010;31(4):501–18.
22. Scadding JG. Prognosis of intrathoracic sarcoidosis in England. A review of 136 cases after five years' observation. Br Med J. 1961;2(5261):1165–72.
23. Hunninghake GW, Gilbert S, Pueringer R, Dayton C, Floerchinger C, Helmers R, et al. Outcome of the treatment for sarcoidosis. Am J Respir Crit Care Med. 1994;149(4 Pt 1):893–8.
24. Grunewald J. Review: role of genetics in susceptibility and outcome of sarcoidosis. Semin Respir Crit Care Med. 2010;31(4):380–9.
25. Hill MR, Papafili A, Booth H, Lawson P, Hubner M, Beynon H, et al. Functional prostaglandin-endoperoxide synthase 2 polymorphism predicts poor outcome in sarcoidosis. Am J Respir Crit Care Med. 2006;174(8):915–22.
26. Kruit A, Grutters JC, Ruven HJ, van Moorsel CH, Weiskirchen R, Mengsteab S, et al. Transforming growth factor-beta gene polymorphisms in sarcoidosis patients with and without fibrosis. Chest. 2006;129(6):1584–91.
27. Yamaguchi E, Itoh A, Hizawa N, Kawakami Y. The gene polymorphism of tumor necrosis factor-beta, but not that of tumor necrosis factor-alpha, is associated with the prognosis of sarcoidosis. Chest. 2001;119(3):753–61.
28. Lopes AJ, Menezes SL, Dias CM, Oliveira JF, Mainenti MR, Guimaraes FS. Cardiopulmonary exercise testing variables as predictors of long-term outcome in thoracic sarcoidosis. Braz J Med Biol Res. 2012;45(3):256–63.
29. Vestbo J, Viskum K. Respiratory symptoms at presentation and long-term vital prognosis in patients with pulmonary sarcoidosis. Sarcoidosis. 1994;11(2):123–5.
30. Reich JM. Mortality of intrathoracic sarcoidosis in referral vs population-based settings: influence of stage, ethnicity, and corticosteroid therapy. Chest. 2002;121(1):32–9.
31. Gribbin J, Hubbard RB, Le Jeune I, Smith CJ, West J, Tata LJ. Incidence and mortality of idiopathic pulmonary fibrosis and sarcoidosis in the UK. Thorax. 2006;61(11):980–5.
32. Huang CT, Heurich AE, Sutton AL, Lyons HA. Mortality in sarcoidosis. A changing pattern of the causes of death. Eur J Respir Dis. 1981;62(4):231–8.
33. Iwai K, Tachibana T, Hosoda Y, Matsui Y. Sarcoidosis autopsies in Japan. Frequency and trend in the last 28 years. Sarcoidosis. 1988;5(1):60–5.
34. Rabin DL, Thompson B, Brown KM, Judson MA, Huang X, Lackland DT, et al. Sarcoidosis: social predictors of severity at presentation. Eur Respir J. 2004;24(4):601–8.
35. Gideon NM, Mannino DM. Sarcoidosis mortality in the United States 1979-1991: an analysis of multiple-cause mortality data. Am J Med. 1996;100(4):423–7.
36. Viskum K, Vestbo J. Vital prognosis in intrathoracic sarcoidosis with special reference to pulmonary function and radiological stage. Eur Respir J. 1993;6(3):349–53.
37. Baughman RP, Engel PJ, Taylor L, Lower EE. Survival in sarcoidosis-associated pulmonary hypertension: the importance of hemodynamic evaluation. Chest. 2010;138(5):1078–85.

38. Shlobin OA, Nathan SD. Management of end-stage sarcoidosis: pulmonary hypertension and lung transplantation. Eur Respir J. 2012;39(6):1520–33.
39. Baughman RP, Teirstein AS, Judson MA, Rossman MD, Yeager Jr H, Bresnitz EA, et al. Clinical characteristics of patients in a case control study of sarcoidosis. Am J Respir Crit Care Med. 2001;164(10 Pt 1):1885–9.
40. Moller DR. Pulmonary fibrosis of sarcoidosis. New approaches, old ideas. Am J Respir Cell Mol Biol. 2003;29(3 Suppl):S37–41.
41. Rosen Y. Pathology of sarcoidosis. Semin Respir Crit Care Med. 2007;28(1):36–52.
42. Cavazza A, Harari S, Caminati A, Barbareschi M, Carbonelli C, Spaggiari L, et al. The histology of pulmonary sarcoidosis: a review with particular emphasis on unusual and underrecognized features. Int J Surg Pathol. 2009;17(3):219–30.
43. Rosen Y, Athanassiades TJ, Moon S, Lyons HA. Nongranulomatous interstitial pneumonitis in sarcoidosis. Relationship to development of epithelioid granulomas. Chest. 1978;74(2):122–5.
44. El-Husseini A, Mahmood MA, Sabry A. Pulmonary sarcoidosis developing fatal interstitial pneumonia-like lesions: a case report and literature review. Intern Emerg Med. 2011;6(5): 479–81.
45. Nobata K, Kasai T, Fujimura M, Mizuguchi M, Nishi K, Ishiura Y, et al. Pulmonary sarcoidosis with usual interstitial pneumonia distributed predominantly in the lower lung fields. Intern Med. 2006;45(6):359–62.
46. Shigemitsu H, Azuma A. Sarcoidosis and interstitial pulmonary fibrosis; two distinct disorders or two ends of the same spectrum. Curr Opin Pulm Med. 2011;17(5):303–7.
47. Perry A, Vuitch F. Causes of death in patients with sarcoidosis. A morphologic study of 38 autopsies with clinicopathologic correlations. Arch Pathol Lab Med. 1995;119(2):167–72.
48. Abehsera M, Valeyre D, Grenier P, Jaillet H, Battesti JP, Brauner MW. Sarcoidosis with pulmonary fibrosis: CT patterns and correlation with pulmonary function. AJR Am J Roentgenol. 2000;174(6):1751–7.
49. Prasse A, Pechkovsky DV, Toews GB, Jungraithmayr W, Kollert F, Goldmann T, et al. A vicious circle of alveolar macrophages and fibroblasts perpetuates pulmonary fibrosis via CCL18. Am J Respir Crit Care Med. 2006;173(7):781–92.
50. Lockstone HE, Sanderson S, Kulakova N, Baban D, Leonard A, Kok WL, et al. Gene set analysis of lung samples provides insight into pathogenesis of progressive, fibrotic pulmonary sarcoidosis. Am J Respir Crit Care Med. 2010;181(12):1367–75.
51. Chen ES, Greenlee BM, Wills-Karp M, Moller DR. Attenuation of lung inflammation and fibrosis in interferon-gamma-deficient mice after intratracheal bleomycin. Am J Respir Cell Mol Biol. 2001;24(5):545–55.
52. Miller A, Teirstein AS, Jackler I, Chuang M, Siltzbach LE. Airway function in chronic pulmonary sarcoidosis with fibrosis. Am Rev Respir Dis. 1974;109(2):179–89.
53. Lewis MM, Mortelliti MP, Yeager Jr H, Tsou E. Clinical bronchiectasis complicating pulmonary sarcoidosis: case series of seven patients. Sarcoidosis Vasc Diffuse Lung Dis. 2002;19(2): 154–9.
54. Lynch 3rd JP, Kazerooni EA, Gay SE. Pulmonary sarcoidosis. Clin Chest Med. 1997;18(4): 755–85.
55. Jewkes J, Kay PH, Paneth M, Citron KM. Pulmonary aspergilloma: analysis of prognosis in relation to haemoptysis and survey of treatment. Thorax. 1983;38(8):572–8.
56. Remy-Jardin M, Giraud F, Remy J, Wattinne L, Wallaert B, Duhamel A. Pulmonary sarcoidosis: role of CT in the evaluation of disease activity and functional impairment and in prognosis assessment. Radiology. 1994;191(3):675–80.
57. Sharma OP, Johnson R. Airway obstruction in sarcoidosis. A study of 123 nonsmoking black American patients with sarcoidosis. Chest. 1988;94(2):343–6.
58. Medinger AE, Khouri S, Rohatgi PK. Sarcoidosis: the value of exercise testing. Chest. 2001;120(1):93–101.
59. Keogh BA, Hunninghake GW, Line BR, Crystal RG. The alveolitis of pulmonary sarcoidosis. Evaluation of natural history and alveolitis-dependent changes in lung function. Am Rev Respir Dis. 1983;128(2):256–65.

60. Boros PW, Enright PL, Quanjer PH, Borsboom GJ, Wesolowski SP, Hyatt RE. Impaired lung compliance and DL, CO but no restrictive ventilatory defect in sarcoidosis. Eur Respir J. 2010;36(6):1315–22.

61. Lopes AJ, de Menezes SL, Dias CM, de Oliveira JF, Mainenti MR, Guimaraes FS. Comparison between cardiopulmonary exercise testing parameters and computed tomography findings in patients with thoracic sarcoidosis. Lung. 2011;189(5):425–31.

62. Wallaert B, Talleu C, Wemeau-Stervinou L, Duhamel A, Robin S, Aguilaniu B. Reduction of maximal oxygen uptake in sarcoidosis: relationship with disease severity. Respiration. 2011;82(6):501–8.

63. Sulica R, Teirstein AS, Kakarla S, Nemani N, Behnegar A, Padilla ML. Distinctive clinical, radiographic, and functional characteristics of patients with sarcoidosis-related pulmonary hypertension. Chest. 2005;128(3):1483–9.

64. Nunes H, Humbert M, Capron F, Brauner M, Sitbon O, Battesti JP, et al. Pulmonary hypertension associated with sarcoidosis: mechanisms, haemodynamics and prognosis. Thorax. 2006;61(1):68–74.

65. Udwadia ZF, Pilling JR, Jenkins PF, Harrison BD. Bronchoscopic and bronchographic findings in 12 patients with sarcoidosis and severe or progressive airways obstruction. Thorax. 1990;45(4):272–5.

66. Pasteur MC, Bilton D, Hill AT. British Thoracic Society guideline for non-CF bronchiectasis. Thorax. 2010;65 Suppl 1:i1–58.

67. Chambellan A, Turbie P, Nunes H, Brauner M, Battesti JP, Valeyre D. Endoluminal stenosis of proximal bronchi in sarcoidosis: bronchoscopy, function, and evolution. Chest. 2005;127(2):472–81.

68. Olsson T, Bjornstad-Pettersen H, Stjernberg NL. Bronchostenosis due to sarcoidosis: a cause of atelectasis and airway obstruction simulating pulmonary neoplasm and chronic obstructive pulmonary disease. Chest. 1979;75(6):663–6.

69. Lavergne F, Clerici C, Sadoun D, Brauner M, Battesti JP, Valeyre D. Airway obstruction in bronchial sarcoidosis: outcome with treatment. Chest. 1999;116(5):1194–9.

70. Lenique F, Brauner MW, Grenier P, Battesti JP, Loiseau A, Valeyre D. CT assessment of bronchi in sarcoidosis: endoscopic and pathologic correlations. Radiology. 1995;194(2):419–23.

71. Mayse ML, Greenheck J, Friedman M, Kovitz KL. Successful bronchoscopic balloon dilation of nonmalignant tracheobronchial obstruction without fluoroscopy. Chest. 2004;126(2):634–7.

72. Teo F, Anantham D, Feller-Kopman D, Ernst A. Bronchoscopic management of sarcoidosis related bronchial stenosis with adjunctive topical mitomycin C. Ann Thorac Surg. 2010;89(6):2005–7.

73. Fouty BW, Pomeranz M, Thigpen TP, Martin RJ. Dilatation of bronchial stenoses due to sarcoidosis using a flexible fiberoptic bronchoscope. Chest. 1994;106(3):677–80.

74. Rohatgi PK, Schwab LE. Primary acute pulmonary cavitation in sarcoidosis. AJR Am J Roentgenol. 1980;134(6):1199–203.

75. Rockoff SD, Rohatgi PK. Unusual manifestations of thoracic sarcoidosis. AJR Am J Roentgenol. 1985;144(3):513–28.

76. Winterbauer RH, Kraemer KG. The infectious complications of sarcoidosis: a current perspective. Arch Intern Med. 1976;136(12):1356–62.

77. Israel HL, Ostrow A. Sarcoidosis and aspergilloma. Am J Med. 1969;47(2):243–50.

78. Battaglini JW, Murray GF, Keagy BA, Starek PJ, Wilcox BR. Surgical management of symptomatic pulmonary aspergilloma. Ann Thorac Surg. 1985;39(6):512–6.

79. Daly RC, Pairolero PC, Piehler JM, Trastek VF, Payne WS, Bernatz PE. Pulmonary aspergilloma. Results of surgical treatment. J Thorac Cardiovasc Surg. 1986;92(6):981–8.

80. Hours S, Nunes H, Kambouchner M, Uzunhan Y, Brauner MW, Valeyre D, et al. Pulmonary cavitary sarcoidosis: clinico-radiologic characteristics and natural history of a rare form of sarcoidosis. Medicine (Baltimore). 2008;87(3):142–51.

81. Stevens DA, Kan VL, Judson MA, Morrison VA, Dummer S, Denning DW, et al. Practice guidelines for diseases caused by Aspergillus. Infectious Diseases Society of America. Clin Infect Dis. 2000;30(4):696–709.

82. Gorske KJ, Fleming RJ. Mycetoma formation in cavitary pulmonary sarcoidosis. Radiology. 1970;95(2):279–85.
83. Rubinstein I, Baum GL, Rosenthal T. Fungal infections complicating pulmonary sarcoidosis. J Infect Dis. 1985;152(6):1360.
84. Waldhorn RE, Tsou E, Kerwin DM. Invasive pulmonary aspergillosis associated with aspergilloma in sarcoidosis. South Med J. 1983;76(2):251–3.
85. Regnard JF, Icard P, Nicolosi M, Spagiarri L, Magdeleinat P, Jauffret B, et al. Aspergilloma: a series of 89 surgical cases. Ann Thorac Surg. 2000;69(3):898–903.
86. Khan MA, Dar AM, Kawoosa NU, Ahangar AG, Lone GN, Bashir G, et al. Clinical profile and surgical outcome for pulmonary aspergilloma: nine year retrospective observational study in a tertiary care hospital. Int J Surg. 2011;9(3):267–71.
87. Uflacker R, Kaemmerer A, Neves C, Picon PD. Management of massive hemoptysis by bronchial artery embolization. Radiology. 1983;146(3):627–34.
88. Kalva SP. Bronchial artery embolization. Tech Vasc Interv Radiol. 2009;12(2):130–8.
89. Mossi F, Maroldi R, Battaglia G, Pinotti G, Tassi G. Indicators predictive of success of embolisation: analysis of 88 patients with haemoptysis. Radiol Med. 2003;105(1–2):48–55.
90. Hammerman KJ, Sarosi GA, Tosh FE. Amphotericin B in the treatment of saprophytic forms of pulmonary aspergillosis. Am Rev Respir Dis. 1974;109(1):57–62.
91. Campbell JH, Winter JH, Richardson MD, Shankland GS, Banham SW. Treatment of pulmonary aspergilloma with itraconazole. Thorax. 1991;46(11):839–41.
92. De Beule K, De Doncker P, Cauwenbergh G, Koster M, Legendre R, Blatchford N, et al. The treatment of aspergillosis and aspergilloma with itraconazole, clinical results of an open international study (1982-1987). Mycoses. 1988;31(9):476–85.
93. Dar MA, Ahmad M, Weinstein AJ, Mehta AC, Golish JA. Thoracic aspergillosis (Part I). Overview and aspergilloma. Cleve Clin Q. 1984;51(4):615–30.
94. Jackson M, Flower CD, Shneerson JM. Treatment of symptomatic pulmonary aspergillomas with intracavitary instillation of amphotericin B through an indwelling catheter. Thorax. 1993;48(9):928–30.
95. Kravitz JN, Steed LL, Judson MA. Intracavitary voriconazole for the treatment of hemoptysis complicating Pseudallescheria angusta pulmonary mycetomas in fibrocystic sarcoidosis. Med Mycol. 2011;49(2):198–201.
96. Wollschlager C, Khan F. Aspergillomas complicating sarcoidosis. A prospective study in 100 patients. Chest. 1984;86(4):585–8.
97. Hammerman KJ, Christianson CS, Huntington I, Hurst GA, Zelman M, Tosh FE. Spontaneous lysis of aspergillomata. Chest. 1973;64(6):677–9.
98. Marcellis RG, Lenssen AF, Elfferich MD, De Vries J, Kassim S, Foerster K, et al. Exercise capacity, muscle strength and fatigue in sarcoidosis. Eur Respir J. 2011;38(3):628–34.
99. Spruit MA, Thomeer MJ, Gosselink R, Troosters T, Kasran A, Debrock AJ, et al. Skeletal muscle weakness in patients with sarcoidosis and its relationship with exercise intolerance and reduced health status. Thorax. 2005;60(1):32–8.
100. Phillips WT, Benton MJ, Wagner CL, Riley C. The effect of single set resistance training on strength and functional fitness in pulmonary rehabilitation patients. J Cardiopulm Rehabil. 2006;26(5):330–7.
101. Consensus conference: activity of sarcoidosis. Third WASOG meeting, Los Angeles, USA, September 8-11, 1993. Eur Respir J. 1994;7(3):624–7.
102. Hunninghake GW, Crystal RG. Pulmonary sarcoidosis: a disorder mediated by excess helper T-lymphocyte activity at sites of disease activity. N Engl J Med. 1981;305(8):429–34.
103. Rossman MD, Newman LS, Baughman RP, Teirstein A, Weinberger SE, Miller Jr W, et al. A double-blinded, randomized, placebo-controlled trial of infliximab in subjects with active pulmonary sarcoidosis. Sarcoidosis Vasc Diffuse Lung Dis. 2006;23(3):201–8.
104. Mostard RL, Voo S, van Kroonenburgh MJ, Verschakelen JA, Wijnen PA, Nelemans PJ, et al. Inflammatory activity assessment by F18 FDG-PET/CT in persistent symptomatic sarcoidosis. Respir Med. 2011;105(12):1917–24.

105. Keijsers RG, Grutters JC, Thomeer M, Du Bois RM, Van Buul MM, Lavalaye J, et al. Imaging the inflammatory activity of sarcoidosis: sensitivity and inter observer agreement of (67)Ga imaging and (18)F-FDG PET. Q J Nucl Med Mol Imaging. 2011;55(1):66–71.
106. Keijsers RG, Verzijlbergen JF, van Diepen DM, van den Bosch JM, Grutters JC. 18F-FDG PET in sarcoidosis: an observational study in 12 patients treated with infliximab. Sarcoidosis Vasc Diffuse Lung Dis. 2008;25(2):143–9.
107. Sekiya M, Ohwada A, Miura K, Takahashi S, Fukuchi Y. Serum vascular endothelial growth factor as a possible prognostic indicator in sarcoidosis. Lung. 2003;181(5):259–65.
108. Kobayashi J, Kitamura S. Serum KL-6 for the evaluation of active pneumonitis in pulmonary sarcoidosis. Chest. 1996;109(5):1276–82.
109. Ziegenhagen MW, Rothe ME, Schlaak M, Muller-Quernheim J. Bronchoalveolar and serological parameters reflecting the severity of sarcoidosis. Eur Respir J. 2003;21(3):407–13.
110. Nathan SD. Lung transplantation: disease-specific considerations for referral. Chest. 2005;127(3):1006–16.
111. Christie JD, Edwards LB, Kucheryavaya AY, Benden C, Dipchand AI, Dobbels F, et al. The Registry of the International Society for Heart and Lung Transplantation: 29th adult lung and heart-lung transplant report-2012. J Heart Lung Transplant. 2012;31(10):1073–86.
112. Shorr AF, Helman DL, Davies DB, Nathan SD. Sarcoidosis, race, and short-term outcomes following lung transplantation. Chest. 2004;125(3):990–6.
113. De Meester J, Smits JM, Persijn GG, Haverich A. Listing for lung transplantation: life expectancy and transplant effect, stratified by type of end-stage lung disease, the Eurotransplant experience. J Heart Lung Transplant. 2001;20(5):518–24.
114. Kreider M, Kotloff RM. Selection of candidates for lung transplantation. Proc Am Thorac Soc. 2009;6(1):20–7.
115. Shorr AF, Davies DB, Nathan SD. Predicting mortality in patients with sarcoidosis awaiting lung transplantation. Chest. 2003;124(3):922–8.
116. Arcasoy SM, Christie JD, Pochettino A, Rosengard BR, Blumenthal NP, Bavaria JE, et al. Characteristics and outcomes of patients with sarcoidosis listed for lung transplantation. Chest. 2001;120(3):873–80.
117. Orens JB, Estenne M, Arcasoy S, Conte JV, Corris P, Egan JJ, et al. International guidelines for the selection of lung transplant candidates: 2006 update – a consensus report from the Pulmonary Scientific Council of the International Society for Heart and Lung Transplantation. J Heart Lung Transplant. 2006;25(7):745–55.
118. Yazaki Y, Isobe M, Hiroe M, Morimoto S, Hiramitsu S, Nakano T, et al. Prognostic determinants of long-term survival in Japanese patients with cardiac sarcoidosis treated with prednisone. Am J Cardiol. 2001;88(9):1006–10.
119. Kasimir MT, Seebacher G, Jaksch P, Winkler G, Schmid K, Marta GM, et al. Reverse cardiac remodelling in patients with primary pulmonary hypertension after isolated lung transplantation. Eur J Cardiothorac Surg. 2004;26(4):776–81.
120. Hadjiliadis D, Sporn TA, Perfect JR, Tapson VF, Davis RD, Palmer SM. Outcome of lung transplantation in patients with mycetomas. Chest. 2002;121(1):128–34.
121. Shah L. Lung transplantation in sarcoidosis. Semin Respir Crit Care Med. 2007;28(1):134–40.
122. Nunley DR, Hattler B, Keenan RJ, Iacono AT, Yousem S, Ohori NP, et al. Lung transplantation for end-stage pulmonary sarcoidosis. Sarcoidosis Vasc Diffuse Lung Dis. 1999;16(1):93–100.
123. Wille KM, Gaggar A, Hajari AS, Leon KJ, Barney JB, Smith KH, et al. Bronchiolitis obliterans syndrome and survival following lung transplantation for patients with sarcoidosis. Sarcoidosis Vasc Diffuse Lung Dis. 2008;25(2):117–24.
124. Scott J, Higenbottam T. Transplantation of the lungs and heart and lung for patients with severe pulmonary complications from sarcoidosis. Sarcoidosis. 1990;7(1):9–11.
125. Milman N, Burton C, Andersen CB, Carlsen J, Iversen M. Lung transplantation for end-stage pulmonary sarcoidosis: outcome in a series of seven consecutive patients. Sarcoidosis Vasc Diffuse Lung Dis. 2005;22(3):222–8.

126. Girgis RE, Tu I, Berry GJ, Reichenspurner H, Valentine VG, Conte JV, et al. Risk factors for the development of obliterative bronchiolitis after lung transplantation. J Heart Lung Transplant. 1996;15(12):1200–8.
127. Ionescu DN, Hunt JL, Lomago D, Yousem SA. Recurrent sarcoidosis in lung transplant allografts: granulomas are of recipient origin. Diagn Mol Pathol. 2005;14(3):140–5.
128. Padilla ML, Schilero GJ, Teirstein AS. Sarcoidosis and transplantation. Sarcoidosis Vasc Diffuse Lung Dis. 1997;14(1):16–22.
129. Heyll A, Meckenstock G, Aul C, Sohngen D, Borchard F, Hadding U, et al. Possible transmission of sarcoidosis via allogeneic bone marrow transplantation. Bone Marrow Transplant. 1994;14(1):161–4.
130. Johnson BA, Duncan SR, Ohori NP, Paradis IL, Yousem SA, Grgurich WF, et al. Recurrence of sarcoidosis in pulmonary allograft recipients. Am Rev Respir Dis. 1993;148(5):1373–7.
131. Kazerooni EA, Jackson C, Cascade PN. Sarcoidosis: recurrence of primary disease in transplanted lungs. Radiology. 1994;192(2):461–4.
132. Kiatboonsri C, Resnick SC, Chan KM, Barbers RG, Marboe CC, Khonsary A, et al. The detection of recurrent sarcoidosis by FDG-PET in a lung transplant recipient. West J Med. 1998;168(2):130–2.
133. Milman N, Andersen CB, Burton CM, Iversen M. Recurrent sarcoid granulomas in a transplanted lung derive from recipient immune cells. Eur Respir J. 2005;26(3):549–52.
134. Burke M, Stewart S, Ashcroft T, Corbishley C, Bishop P, Kjellstrom C. Biopsy diagnosis of disease recurrence after transplantation (TX) for pulmonary sarcoidosis: a multicentre study. J Heart Lung Transplant. 2001;20(2):154–5.
135. Walker S, Mikhail G, Banner N, Partridge J, Khaghani A, Burke M, et al. Medium term results of lung transplantation for end stage pulmonary sarcoidosis. Thorax. 1998;53(4):281–4.
136. Sharma OP. Sarcoidosis: a historical perspective. Clin Dermatol. 2007;25(3):232–41.
137. Shorr AF, Davies DB, Nathan SD. Outcomes for patients with sarcoidosis awaiting lung transplantation. Chest. 2002;122(1):233–8.

Chapter 6
Sarcoidosis-Associated Pulmonary Hypertension

Oksana A. Shlobin and Steven D. Nathan

Abstract There is growing appreciation for the prevalence and impact of pulmonary hypertension in patients with sarcoidosis (SAPH). This chapter will focus on the pathophysiology of this complication and its association with patients' outcomes, including functional ability and survival. When to suspect complicating SAPH will be addressed with a suggested work-up algorithm presented. The potential role and data supporting the use of pulmonary vasoactive agents in SAPH will be addressed. However, there is a paucity of data in this area and the need for further investigation in the form of multicenter, double-blind, randomized controlled studies will be underscored.

Keywords 6-min walk • Mean pulmonary artery pressure • Pulmonary hypertension • Right heart catherization • Sarcoid associated pulmonary hypertension

Abbreviations

6MWT	6-min walk
BAL	Bronchoalveolar lavage
DL_{CO}	Diffusing capacity for carbon monoxide
ET-1	Endothelin 1
ERA	Endothelin receptor antagonist
ILD	Interstitial lung disease
mPAP	Mean pulmonary artery pressure

O.A. Shlobin, M.D. • S.D. Nathan, M.D. (✉)
Advanced Lung Disease and Transplant Program, Department of Medicine, Inova Fairfax Hospital, 3300 Gallows Road, Falls Church, VA 22024, USA
e-mail: Steven.Nathan@inova.org

M.A. Judson (ed.), *Pulmonary Sarcoidosis: A Guide for the Practicing Clinician*, Respiratory Medicine 17, DOI 10.1007/978-1-4614-8927-6_6, © Springer Science+Business Media New York 2014

NO	Nitric oxide
PAH	Pulmonary arterial hypertension
PCWP	Pulmonary capillary wedge pressure
PDE-5	Phosphodiesterase 5
PFTs	Pulmonary function tests
PH	Pulmonary hypertension
PVR	Pulmonary vascular resistance
RAP	Right atrial pressure
RHC	Right heart catheterization
RVSP	Right ventricular systolic pressure
SAPH	Sarcoid-associated pulmonary hypertension
TTE	Transthoracic echocardiogram

Introduction

Sarcoidosis is a multinational disease that is prevalent throughout the world including in Europe, the USA, and Japan [1, 2]. In Europe, especially in the Scandinavian countries and Ireland, it affects the Caucasian population, while in the USA it tends to occur in African Americans more commonly. It has a reported incidence in females of 21.6 and in males 15.3 cases per 100,000 population per year [2].

Sarcoidosis is a multisystem disorder of unknown etiology characterized by the formation of non-caseating granulomas in affected tissues, particularly in the lung and the lymphatic system. Multiple phenotypes may be found based on the clinical presentation, involved organs, disease course, and severity of disease [3]. However, lung involvement is seemingly invariable with up to 95 % of patients manifesting some form of pulmonary disease during the course of their lifetime [1].

The natural history of sarcoidosis in the lung is quite variable and spans the spectrum from spontaneous resolution to advanced fibrocystic disease. Fortunately, in most cases, there is more of a propensity for the former and hence a more benign clinical course, with spontaneous resolution in half of the cases within 2 years from disease onset [3]. However, in about 5 % of cases permanent severe pulmonary dysfunction in the form of fibrosis occurs, accounting for most of the morbidity and mortality associated with the disease (Fig. 6.1) [1]. Indeed, respiratory failure is the most common cause of death from sarcoidosis in the USA and Europe [3]. As with all forms of advanced parenchymal lung disease, there is a growing appreciation for the prevalence and impact of pulmonary hypertension (PH) toward the later stages of disease. However, sarcoidosis-related pulmonary hypertension (SAPH) may also occur in the context of earlier disease stages. As opposed to other forms of fibrotic lung disease, where supervening PH tends to be milder, in many cases SAPH is on the severe side of the spectrum. The ready availability and use of echocardiography has resulted in increased discovery of SAPH which, as an increasingly recognized complication of sarcoidosis, will be the focus of this chapter.

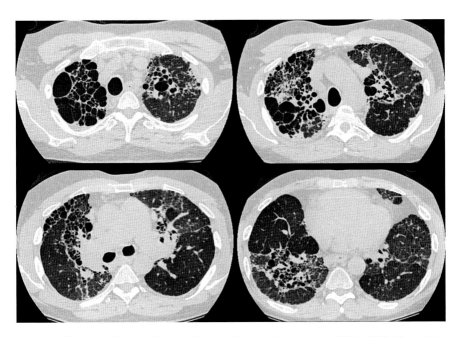

Fig. 6.1 CT scan of chest of stage IV sarcoidosis with associated PH (mPAP 49 mmHg). Reproduced with permission of the European Respiratory Society. Eur Respir J. 2012;39:1520–33; published ahead of print January 12, 2012, doi:10.1183/09031936.00175511

Overview

Pulmonary hypertension is defined hemodynamically as an increased mean pulmonary arterial pressure (mPAP) greater than or equal to 25 mmHg at rest on right heart catheterization (RHC) [4]. The reported prevalence of PH in the wide spectrum of sarcoidosis patients is between 1 and 28 % at rest and up to 43 % with exercise [5–7]. PH most commonly occurs in association with advanced stage IV disease, but can also occur in the context of relatively normal lung function and preserved parenchymal architecture. Patients with recalcitrant dyspnea and normal left ventricular function have a higher reported PH prevalence of approximately 53 % [8]. Sarcoidosis patients who are listed for lung transplantation have an even higher rate of PH at ~74 % [9]. In our own clinic, we have found a similar prevalence of PH (~75 %) based on right heart catheterization of 104 transplant and non-transplant candidates with advanced sarcoidosis evaluated over a 14-year period (Fig. 6.2).

Over the last decade, there has been a surge of interest in sarcoidosis-associated PH (SAPH). As a result, there is now a greater understanding of its pathogenesis and better characterization of the associated prognosis. Specifically, there is a growing appreciation for the substantial morbidity and mortality that accompanies the development of SAPH. What remains somewhat uncertain is whether the PH is a

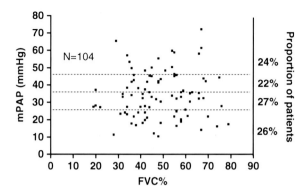

Fig. 6.2 Distribution of mean pulmonary artery pressures in relation to the FVC% predicted in a cohort of 104 patients with sarcoidosis. The *horizontal dashed lines* and right *y* axis stratify the patients by severity of PH (Inova Fairfax Hospital data). Abbreviations: *FVC* forced vital capacity, *mPAP* mean pulmonary artery pressure. Reproduced with permission of the European Respiratory Society. Eur Respir J. 2012;39:1520–33; published ahead of print January 12, 2012, doi:10.1183/09031936.00175511

surrogate for the extent of disease that determines these outcomes or whether it is the PH itself that is the primary driver. It is conceivable that both notions are true in different patients with "disproportionate" PH playing a larger role in determining outcomes in the latter group. This ill-defined concept variably termed "disproportionate" or "out of proportion" PH has led to a growing interest and an emerging literature on the potential role of therapies directed at SAPH.

Pathophysiology of SAPH

The most recent World Health Organization (WHO) conference (Nice, France 2013) reaffirmed the categorization of PH into five groups. Group I (Pulmonary Arterial Hypertension (PAH)) includes the prototypical entity of idiopathic disease and other forms of associated PAH, while group II is PH related to left-sided heart disease, group III is associated with underlying parenchymal lung disease, group IV is due to chronic thromboembolic disease, and group V is comprised of miscellaneous conditions [10]. SAPH remains categorized within the last group since its pathogenesis is complex and multifactorial with variable characteristics of the other four groups (Fig. 6.3) [11].

Sarcoidosis might be accompanied by a primary vasculopathic process due to the bronchovascular, or more specifically perivascular, distribution of the non-caseating granulomas. Additionally, there are accompanying fibrotic and fibrocavitary changes that typify stage IV disease and result in architectural distortion which invariably favors a more central and upper lobe distribution. Parenchymal remodeling may also result in vessel tortuosity, turbulent flow, and shear stresses which may perpetuate the development and progression of PH [12]. The heterogenous distribution of

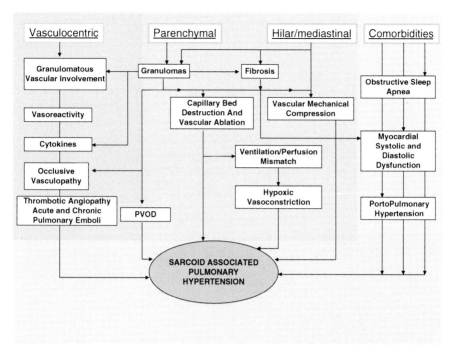

Fig. 6.3 Schematic representation of the interplaying factors contributing to the pathogenesis of PH in sarcoidosis. Abbreviation: *PVOD* pulmonary veno-occlusive disease. Reproduced with permission of the European Respiratory Society. Eur Respir J. 2012;39:1520–33; published ahead of print January 12, 2012, doi:10.1183/09031936.00175511

disease might contribute to the apparent dissociation between the degree of restrictive physiology, a surrogate for the parenchymal disease burden, and the prevalence and severity of PH. The central predilection specifically may involve the proximal lobar vessels with a greater propensity for the subsequent development of PH. Fibrosis in proximity to the pulmonary arterial circulation may also adversely affect the vascular capacitance, a surrogate of vessel stiffness. A low vascular capacitance has been demonstrated to portend a worse prognosis in patients with PAH [13]. If the same holds true for the SAPH, this might help explain the significant morbidity and mortality implications of even mild elevations in PA pressures.

In most parenchymal lung diseases (ILD), it is commonly regarded that mild to moderate PH is due to vascular destruction that occurs as the result of fibrosis and regional hypoxemia. Until recently the term cor pulmonale was used to describe the ensuing development of right heart failure. The concept alluded to previously of "out of proportion" or "disproportionate" PH has also been used in reference to PH, where the degree of elevation of pressures cannot be explained solely by the hypoxia and magnitude of the parenchymal process [14]. An arbitrary mPAP value of 35 mmHg or greater has been proposed to identify this category of patients [15]. However, there is as yet a paucity of data to support this concept and this proposed level to define it.

Mechanical Destruction of the Distal Capillary Bed

The majority of sarcoidosis patients with PH have stage IV radiographic disease and associated impaired pulmonary function testing (PFTs) (Fig. 6.2) [16]. PH is therefore usually attributed to destruction of the capillary bed by the fibrotic process and regional hypoxemic vasoconstriction. However, the severity of PH does not always correlate with the degree of parenchymal lung disease and blood gas abnormalities, suggesting that other mechanisms may be playing a role [5, 9, 16]. Moreover, the degree of PH is often apparently disproportionate to functional abnormalities [9, 16, 17]. This attests to other contributors, either directly related to the pulmonary vasculature or extrapulmonary in nature, playing important roles in the pathogenesis of SAPH.

Granulomatous Vasculopathy

Granulomatous involvement of the pulmonary vessels is common in sarcoidosis-associated PH and has been described in 69–100 % of patients with PH [18]. The granulomatous inflammation tends to involve the lung in a lymphatic distribution, thus neighboring the granulomas with the pulmonary arteries and veins in the bronchovascular bundles and interlobular septae. The granulomas may be found in all layers of the vessel wall, while other pathologic findings commonly seen include inflammation, necrosis, destruction of the musculoelastic media of the small and medium-sized vessels, endothelial proliferation, and disruption of the basal lamina. As a result, an occlusive vasculopathy may develop, especially in the small arterioles and venules [18, 19]. When the granulomatous infiltration involves the pulmonary veins preferentially, this may result in a clinical picture that mimics pulmonary veno-occlusive disease (PVOD) [20–22]. In situ thrombosis (thrombotic angiopathy) is yet another intravascular mechanism described and that may play a role in the pathogenesis of SAPH [19].

Local Vasoreactivity

There may also be increased pulmonary vasoreactivity in sarcoidosis, as suggested by the favorable acute response to vasodilators, including nitric oxide (NO) and prostacyclin. The mechanism for this is not clear, but may be partially explained by endothelial damage from sarcoidosis granulomas, with a subsequent decrease in synthesis and release of NO and prostaglandins. This may have long-term sequela with chronic, pulmonary vasoconstriction and associated remodeling [23, 24].

Cytokine Derangement

There are a number of cytokines that have been found to be upregulated in sarcoidosis that could perpetuate the development of PH. One such example is endothelin-1

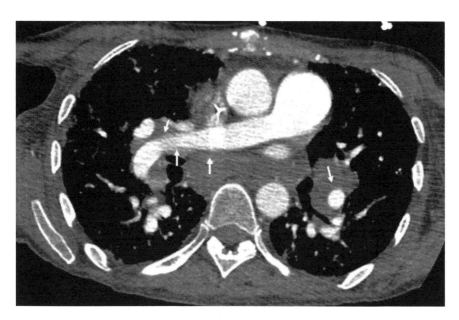

Fig. 6.4 CT scan of the chest of a SAPH patient with lymphadenopathy (*white arrows*) surrounding the right pulmonary artery. Reproduced with permission of the European Respiratory Society. Eur RespirJ.2012;39:1520–33;publishedaheadofprintJanuary12,2012,doi:10.1183/09031936.00175511

(ET-1), which has been implicated in the pathogenesis of both idiopathic PAH and various interstitial lung diseases [25–27]. One study examining ET-1 concentrations in bronchoalveolar lavage (BAL) specimens from patients with various pulmonary disorders and healthy controls demonstrated raised ET-1 levels in sarcoidosis patients, in comparison to scleroderma and idiopathic pulmonary fibrosis patients [28]. ET-1 is produced primarily by endothelial cells, smooth muscle and airway epithelial cells, with production induced by hypoxia, shear stress, and various growth factors and cytokines. It is a potent vasoconstrictor which is also thought to have long-term vascular remodeling properties [27].

Tumor necrosis factor alpha which is thought to play a central role in the pathogenesis of sarcoidosis has also recently been implicated in the inflammatory pathway of PAH [29, 30]. Conceptually therefore, the upregulation of these and perhaps other cytokines may contribute to the development of PH. The prospect of cytokine "cross talk" may therefore provide an additional explanation for the disproportionate PH seen in the context of well-preserved lung volumes.

Extrinsic Compression of Pulmonary Vessels

Mediastinal or hilar adenopathy and/or interstitial fibrosis can result in mechanical extrinsic compression of the large pulmonary arteries and an increased pulmonary vascular resistance (Figs. 6.1 and 6.4) [16, 31–33]. Although occasionally described in early stages of sarcoidosis, pulmonary artery compression is much more frequent in patients with longstanding disease when lymph nodes become fibrotic and calcify. This mechanism has been demonstrated in 21.4 % of patients with PH and radiographic stage IV in one study [16].

Extrapulmonary Manifestations

In some cases, extra-pulmonary manifestations of sarcoidosis may also contribute to the development of PH. Not infrequently, direct myocardial involvement by granulomas and myocardial fibrosis may lead to left ventricular systolic and diastolic dysfunction [34]. In one study, 30 % of sarcoidosis patients with evidence of PH demonstrated elevated pulmonary capillary wedge pressures (PCWP). This underscores the need to rule out left-sided heart disease in the comprehensive evaluation of PH related to sarcoidosis [17]. As with all forms of PH, right heart catheterization is therefore mandatory in establishing the diagnosis.

Hepatic granulomatous infiltration and subsequent cirrhosis may be seen as a complication of the disease and therefore portopulmonary hypertension should be considered in patients with stigmata of liver dysfunction [35]. Other common comorbidities, which are not necessarily sarcoidosis specific, should not be overlooked if patients are thus predisposed. For example, the prevalence of obstructive sleep apnea (OSA) in sarcoidosis has been reported to be 17 %, which is much higher than what might be expected in a healthy patient population [36].

A potential link between sarcoidosis and thromboembolic events has been emphasized in two epidemiological studies both in the USA and Europe [37, 38]. However, whether or not sarcoidosis patients are more predisposed to chronic thromboembolic disease (CTEPH) remains to be determined.

Impact and Outcomes of PH in Sarcoidosis

The presence of PH has been shown to be associated with greater supplemental oxygen requirements and reduced exercise capacity [39]. Additionally, its burden on functional and employment status is substantial [9], with greater caregiver dependency resulting [39]. The mortality implications of any PH in the context of sarcoidosis are also profound with a >10-fold increase in mortality and an associated estimated 5-year survival of only 59 % [16, 17]. SAPH patients are more likely to be listed for lung transplantation and not surprisingly, based on the data prior to inception of lung allocation score (LAS), also had a greater likelihood of succumbing while on the wait list [9, 40].

One of the issues in sarcoidosis, as with all forms of parenchymal lung disease associated PH, is whether patients are succumbing because of PH or in the presence of PH. With regards to the latter scenario, it might be that PH is a surrogate for other disease-related processes that are driving mortality. In any event, the occurrence of

SAPH has been shown to confer an up to 8.1-fold increase risk of mortality with intractable right heart failure as a significant mortality contributor [41]. Indeed, in one study demonstrating the association of PH with mortality, the only hemodynamic factor that remained predictive of outcomes after multivariable analysis was the right atrial pressure (RAP) [40]. Moreover, this analysis also demonstrated hemodynamic progression of PH in the patient cohort. This evidence of right-sided heart failure suggests that patients with SAPH are indeed dying from their PH once it progresses, rather than the PH being an epiphenomenon.

Clinical Presentation and Diagnostic Testing

The most common symptom of SAPH is worsening dyspnea on exertion. This makes the diagnosis of PH in sarcoidosis difficult, as the symptom is frequently attributed to the underlying parenchymal lung disease [42]. Moreover, one study reported no difference in the presenting symptoms in patients with and without SAPH [5]. The clinical signs of right heart failure also have a low sensitivity, manifesting in as few as 21 % of patients with SAPH [5]. Nevertheless, a high index of suspicion should be maintained and PH should be suspected in any patient with symptoms that appear to be out of proportion to the degree of their underlying parenchymal disease. A heightened index of suspicion for PH in the context of other common symptoms including lower extremity swelling, dizziness, chest pain, syncope, or even palpitations, is prudent.

One prospective study of a large cohort of sarcoidosis patients with the hemodynamic diagnosis of SAPH demonstrated that prolonged disease duration, advanced parenchymal disease, and a single breath diffusing capacity for carbon monoxide (DL_{CO}) less than 50 % of predicted were all associated with the development of PH [43].

A number of retrospective studies have sought to examine the association of radiographic, physiological, and laboratory factors with the presence of SAPH. Although PH is more common in patients with advanced fibrosis, there are no specific radiographic findings that predict the presence or absence of PH [6, 16]. Patients often have hilar fullness on chest roentgenography, however, this may be due to either adenopathy or pulmonary artery enlargement. Computed tomography (CT) chest scans can be very helpful in providing the structural detail necessary to differentiate these. The presence of enlarged PA segments (diameter greater than 29 mm or diameter larger than that of the ascending aorta) on CT scanning should raise the suspicion for underlying PH, although the predictive accuracy of these findings does require further study in sarcoidosis patients. There are additional CT findings that should raise the suspicion for PH including evidence of extrinsic compression of large pulmonary arteries by lymphadenopathy or fibrosis (Fig. 6.4). One study demonstrated that patients with SAPH had a significantly higher frequency of ground-glass attenuation and septal lines as compared to sarcoidosis controls without PH [16].

Blood tests that have been shown to correlate with the presence or severity of PH include brain natriuretic peptide (BNP) and N-terminal fragment-proBNP (NT-proBNP) levels. There are data to suggest that an elevated BNP is a marker of a poor prognosis in patients with chronic lung diseases [44]. In one study of patients with interstitial lung disease, an elevated BNP was the strongest predictor of overall mortality, independent of the severity of the underlying fibrosis [45]. However, the BNP might be a global biomarker of cardiac dysfunction, rather than being specific for PH. Indeed, in a recently published echocardiography-based prospective study of 150 Japanese patients with sarcoidosis, NT-proBNP was found to be a useful biomarker in identifying cardiac sarcoidosis, but not PH [46].

A study of 212 ILD patients, 10 % of whom had sarcoidosis, examined the relation of NT-proBNP, fibrin, D-dimer, troponin-T, uric acid and exhaled nitric oxide (NO) to the presence of PH and mortality. The analysis suggested that a NT-proBNP value <95 ng/l may be used to accurately rule-out the presence of PH in ILD, while an abnormally high uric acid indicates the possibility of PH. NT-proBNP, troponin-T, uric acid and fibrin D-dimer, but not exhaled levels of NO, were all demonstrated to have prognostic value in predicting PH or mortality [47].

Pulmonary function data may provide helpful information. Specifically, there is some indication that the lower the DL_{CO}, the greater the likelihood of underlying PH. A $DL_{CO} < 60$ % of predicted has been reported to be associated with a sevenfold increase in prevalence of underlying PH [48]. Although SAPH patients tend to have more restrictive disease, the correlation between PH and measures of lung volumes is poor, since PH can develop at any stage of the underlying disease (Fig. 6.2). Although the ability of the forced vital capacity (FVC) %/DL_{CO} % ratio in screening for PH has never been tested in sarcoidosis, several authors have postulated that a high ratio (>1.4–1.5), reflecting a disproportionately reduced DL_{CO}, alone or together with the oxygen saturation (SpO_2), may be a better screening tool for PH in ILDs than any other pulmonary function test parameter [49, 50].

SAPH patients have greater supplemental oxygen needs, shorter 6-min walk test distances (6MWT) and lower oxygen saturations (SpO_2) with exercise than sarcoidosis patients without complicating PH [5, 9]. Patients who desaturate below 90 % are 12-fold more likely to have associated PH [48, 51]. Conversely, the absence of desaturation below 90 % with exercise implies a low likelihood of significant PH [48, 51]. In a cohort of sarcoidosis transplant candidates, the amount of supplemental oxygen requirements was associated with the presence and severity of PH after adjusting for multiple covariates including age, gender, race, FVC, FEV_1, and 6-min walk (6MWT) distance [9]. The association of PH with a lower SpO_2 raises the pathophysiologic conundrum of whether the PH causes the desaturation or if hypoxemia perpetuates the PH. It is likely that both scenarios are true with each pathologic element perpetuating the other. Therefore, any hypoxemia should warrant institution of supplemental oxygen, especially in the presence of documented PH [51].

PH can affect both the distance attained as well as the oxygen saturation (SpO_2) nadir during the course of a 6MWT. The multisystem nature of sarcoidosis invokes other reasons for a lower distance attained during the 6MWT. Therefore it is possible that the distance component is more useful to evaluate response to therapy, rather than as a screening tool for PH [33, 51, 52]. In an attempt to account for the impact of both the distance and SpO_2 components on the 6MWT, the composite distance saturation product (DSP) has been examined in sarcoidosis. Indeed, in comparison to the 6MWT distance, a lower DSP correlated with a greater number of factors associated with decreased functional status in sarcoidosis patients [53].

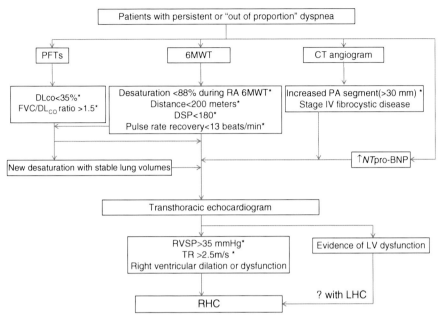

Fig. 6.5 Screening and work up algorithm in sarcoidosis patients with suspected PH

Continuous Doppler flow transthoracic echocardiogram (TTE) is the most reliable noninvasive test to screen for the presence of PH in the absence of concomitant lung disease. TTE allows calculation of the right ventricular systolic pressures (RVSP) from the maximal velocity of the tricuspid regurgitation jet together with an estimation of the right atrial pressure. However, there are inherent variables that can affect the accuracy of this calculation, which may be further compromised in the presence of chronic lung diseases [54]. For example, in a study of 374 subjects with various forms of advanced lung disease including sarcoidosis, the RVSP could only be estimated in 44 % of the patients. Additionally, in approximately one half of these cases, pressure estimations were inaccurate when compared to right heart catheterization measurements. TTE tends to overestimate but can also underestimate the true RVSP, and therefore does not have sufficient predictive properties to be solely relied on to diagnose or rule out PH [54]. However, TTE is very useful in assessing for other cardiac abnormalities, such as left ventricular systolic or diastolic dysfunction, valvular abnormalities, the presence of shunts, and pericardial effusions [52]. In the absence of tricuspid regurgitation, the diagnosis of PH should still be suspected when there are signs of right ventricular (RV) dysfunction, including dilatation, hypertrophy, decreased systolic function as well as flattening or bowing of the interventricular septum [52]. The presence of any of these should prompt RHC to further characterize the pulmonary hemodynamics [42] (Fig. 6.5).

As with all forms of PH, RHC remains the gold standard for the diagnosis of PH in sarcoidosis. In addition to allowing the direct measurement of the pulmonary artery pressures (PAPs), the right atrial pressure and cardiac output are also obtained, all of which impart additional important prognostic information [39, 40]. Measurement of the PCWP is also essential in differentiating between arterial and venous pulmonary hypertension [17], as the results dictate a different management approach. Once PH is diagnosed, even in the presence of a cause, a comprehensive workup is still recommended to rule out other contributory factors, such as OSA, CTEPH, portopulmonary hypertension, HIV, and concomitant connective tissue disease.

Management of PH in Sarcoidosis

The optimal management approach to SAPH is unknown and based on limited evidence. Modifiable risk factors and comorbidities should be sought and treated where indicated. Hypoxemia correlates to some extent with the severity of PH, and supplemental oxygen is thus recommended to reverse resting, nocturnal and exertional hypoxemia. The presence of any contributory co-morbidities, including OSA, cardiac dysfunction or thromboembolic disease, warrants standard therapeutic interventions [33]. The treatment of sarcoidosis with anti-inflammatory and other immunomodulating therapies has a theoretic role if the predominant pathologic potentiator of the PH is active sarcoidosis. However, such an approach has not demonstrated consistent benefits with response rates of only 20–30 % reported in small series [16, 55–57]. Moreover, no studies with Stage IV disease patients, which is the most common stage associated with PH, showed a significant hemodynamic response to corticosteroids. Thus, steroids ought to be considered only for patients with evidence of active disease and/or compression of central vascular structures by bulky lymphadenopathy [56, 57].

The use of currently available pulmonary vasoactive agents is controversial since there have been no randomized, placebo-controlled studies to demonstrate their efficacy in sarcoidosis patients. According to the ERS Task Force guidelines, the use of PAH targeted therapy is discouraged in Group 3 or 5 PH when the mPAP is less than 40 mmHg. It may be considered in patients with "out of proportion" PH and should be offered by PH referral centers, ideally in the context of randomized controlled trials with judicious monitoring [58]. There is a theoretical possibility to do more harm than good in patients with significant parenchymal lung disease due to potential ventilation/perfusion mismatching resulting in worsening hypoxemia. In addition, it is also possible that a pulmonary edema pattern might be precipitated in patients with pre-existing PVOD-like lesions [33, 42, 52]. Despite these cautionary caveats, there are a number of small case series attesting to the potential utility of PAH-specific therapies in patients with sarcoidosis (Table 6.1). A recently initiated registry of SAPH patients (RESAPH) will hopefully provide a wealth of data on both the clinical course and impact of available therapies in this patient population [59].

The currently available approved therapies for WHO group 1 PAH target one of three pathways, which include the endothelin, nitric oxide, and prostacyclin pathways. If any one of these pathways plays more of a role in SAPH remains to be determined as are the effects of therapies that target these.

Table 6.1 Summary of SAPH treatment studies

	Type of study/subject number treated	Therapy	Outcomes
Preston et al. [23]	Prospective observational (8)	Inhaled NO (5), inhaled NO with IV EPO (1), CCBs (2)	Short term 20 % decrease in PVR and mPAP; Long term ↑ in 6MWT
Baughman et al. [66]	Prospective open-label 16-week trial (22)	Inhaled iloprost (15)	6/15 patients showed ↓ mPAP/PVR, 3/15 improvement in 6MWT
Fisher et al. [65]	Retrospective case series (7)	IV EPO (6), SQ treprostinil (1)	Improved NYHA Class
Barnett et al. [61]	Retrospective case series (22)	Initial: IV EPO (1), bosentan (12), sildenafil (9) Subsequent: S/B (3), S/I (2), S/B/I (2), Epo/B (1)	Improved 6MWT, NYHA Class Reduction in mPAP and PVR in 12 patients with f/u RHC data
Milman et al. [64]	Retrospective chart review (12)	Sildenafil (12)	↓ mPAP/PVR, ↑ cardiac output, no change in 6MWT
Culver et al. [60]	Retrospective chart review (7)	Bosentan (3), bosentan and IV EPO (4)	Reduction in mPAP at 6–18 months in half of the patients
Baughman et al. [17]	Retrospective chart review (5)	Bosentan (5)	Reduction in mPAP from 50 to 35 mmHg in 3/5 patients at 4 months
Judson et al. [62]	Prospective placebo-controlled 12-week study (20)	Ambrisentan (17 patients at 4 weeks, 12 patients at 8 weeks and 7 patients at 12 weeks)	No change in 6MWT 9 patients discontinued drug

Reproduced with permission of the European Respiratory Society. Eur Respir J. 2012;39:1520–33; published ahead of print January 12, 2012, doi:10.1183/09031936.00175511

The Endothelin Pathway

The finding of increased endothelin-1 levels in patients with sarcoidosis and con-comitant PH provides a rationale for the use of endothelin receptor antagonists (ERAs) in these patients. Experience in SAPH, however, is mostly limited to a few retrospective case series, where ERAs have been used either alone or in combina-tion with other medications. Baughman and colleagues reported five patients in whom there was a decrease in the mPAP from an average of 50 to 35 mmHg after at least 4 months of treatment [8]. Another study described seven patients treated either with bosentan alone ($n=3$) or in combination with prostanoids ($n=4$), in whom ~50 % responded to therapy after 6–18 months of follow-up [60]. A two-center retrospective study by Barnett et al. reported outcomes in 22 SAPH who received a variety of vasoactive therapies, including bosentan ($n=12$) and sildenafil ($n=9$) [61]. An overall improvement in the mPAP, pulmonary vascular resistance (PVR) and 6MWT distance was demonstrated, especially in those patients with limited fibrosis. Despite this apparent salutary response, the overall prognosis remained quite poor, with a 3-year survival of only 74 %.

There has been one open-label study of ambrisentan, a selective endothelin receptor A blocker, in 21 patients with SAPH. Unfortunately this drug was not well tolerated by a significant proportion of these subjects, and the 6-min walk distance (the study's primary endpoint) did not improve. In subjects who did tolerate ambris-entan, there was a large improvement in WHO functional class and health related quality of life, although it failed to reach statistical significance [62]. A large pro-spective randomized 16-week study of bosentan in this patient population is cur-rently underway, with an anticipated completion date of early 2013 [63].

Nitric Oxide and Phosphodiesterase Inhibitors

Nitric oxide is potent vasodilator with a very short half-life that may be delivered via the inhaled route. There is one report describing the use of ambulatory inhaled NO in eight patients with sarcoidosis, of whom five had improvements in their 6MWT distance [23]. This may become a feasible therapeutic option as several ambulatory delivery systems are currently under development. The NO pathway may be targeted by selective phosphodiesterase type 5 inhibitors (PDE-5). This blockade increases local NO levels in the arterial smooth muscle cells, thereby pro-moting short and long-term vasodilation and possibly long-term antiproliferation of vascular smooth muscle cells [33, 42]. Aside from the nine patients reported in the Barnett paper, there is one additional retrospective study of 12 patients treated with sildenafil for a range of 1–12 months [61, 64]. Although no significant change in the 6MWT distance was observed, the study did demonstrate an improvement in the pulmonary hemodynamic profile with a reduction in the mPAP and PVR accompa-nied by an increase in the cardiac index. Although these findings are encouraging, the ultimate role of phosphodiesterase 5 (PDE-5) inhibitors in SAPH remains to be determined by further prospective studies.

The Prostacyclin Pathway

This pathway is targeted by prostanoid analogues that may be administered intravenously, subcutaneously, or via the inhaled route. These agents are potent vasodilators which may also inhibit platelet aggregation [30, 33]. There is very limited data on use of IV epoprostenol in SAPH. In one study of six patients with advanced fibrotic disease there was an improvement in functional class in all but one of the patients [65]. Improvements in functional class and pulmonary hemodynamics have also been demonstrated in another study that included the use of either inhaled nitric oxide (iNO) or iNO in combination with epoprostenol [30]. Finally, an open-label study of inhaled iloprost in 22 patients demonstrated hemodynamic improvement in six patients, with a >20 % decrease in the PVR [66]. Additionally, there were downstream clinical correlates noted with an overall increase in the 6MWT distance (~30 m) and improvements in patients' quality of life.

Conclusion

The cumulative evidence from the growing body of literature suggests a potential benefit of PAH-specific agents in select patients with SAPH. However, before these therapies can be universally endorsed and adopted, it is essential for the appropriate prospective, randomized, double-blind clinical trials to be undertaken and completed. Such studies are mandatory to validate that such a therapeutic approach is of benefit as well as to best define the patient phenotypes most likely to respond and least likely to deteriorate from therapy. In the absence of such trials, if any such therapy is contemplated, it should be implemented with caution and with the full consent of the patient. Each case should be treated as an "N of one" study with close serial follow-up. Monitoring of patients should include an assessment of their symptoms, the impact on their quality of life and an objective functional study, such as the 6MWT. Consideration should be given to discontinuing the medication in the absence of any improvement or in the presence of any untoward side-effects.

References

1. Baughman RP, Teirstein AS, Judson MA, et al. Clinical characteristics of patients in a case control study of sarcoidosis. Am J Respir Crit Care Med. 2001;164:1885–9.
2. Rybicki BA, Major M, Popovich Jr J, Maliarik MJ, Iannuzzi MC. Racial differences in sarcoidosis incidence: a five year study in a health maintenance organization. Am J Epidemiol. 1997;145:234–41.
3. Iannuzzi MC, Rybicki BA, Teirstein AS. Sarcoidosis. N Engl J Med. 2007;357:2153–62.
4. Simonneau G, Robbins I, Beghetti M, et al. Updated clinical classification of pulmonary hypertension. J Am Coll Cardiol. 2009;54(1):S43–54.
5. Sulica R, Teirstein AS, Kakarla S, Nemani N, Behnegar A, Padilla ML. Distinctive clinical, radiographic and functional characteristics of patients with sarcoidosis-related pulmonary hypertension. Chest. 2005;128:1483–9.

6. Handa T, Nagai S, Miki S, et al. Incidence of pulmonary hypertension and its clinical relevance in patients with sarcoidosis. Chest. 2006;129:1246–52.

7. Gluskowski J, Hawrylkiewicz I, Zych D, Wojtczak A, Zielinski J. Pulmonary haemodynamics at rest and during exercise in patients with sarcoidosis. Respiration. 1984;46(1):26–32.

8. Baughman RP, Engel PJ, Meyer CA, Barrett AB, Lower EE. Pulmonary hypertension in sarcoidosis. Sarcoidosis Vasc Diffuse Lung Dis. 2006;23:108–16.

9. Shorr AF, Helman DL, Davies DB, Nathan SD. Pulmonary hypertension in advanced sarcoidosis: epidemiology and clinical characteristics. Eur Respir J. 2005;25(5):783–8.

10. http://www.wsph2013.com/pdf/final_program.pdf

11. Baughman RP. Pulmonary hypertension associated with sarcoidosis. Arthritis Res Ther. 2007;9 Suppl 2:S8.

12. Thannickal VJ, Toews GB, White ES, Lynch III JP, Martinez FJ. Mechanisms of pulmonary fibrosis. Annu Rev Med. 2004;55:395–417.

13. Mahapatra S, Nishimura RA, Sorajja P, Cha S, McGoon MD. Relationship of pulmonary arterial capacitance and mortality in idiopathic pulmonary arterial hypertension. J Am Coll Cardiol. 2006;47(4):799–803.

14. Hoeper MM, Andreas S, Bastian A, et al. PH due to chronic lung diseases: updated recommendations of the Cologne Consensus Conference 2011. Int J Cardiol. 2011;1545S:S45–53.

15. Harari S. Out-of-proportion pulmonary hypertension: a paradigm for rare diseases. Chest. 2012;142(5):1087–8.

16. Nunes H, Humbert M, Capron F, et al. Pulmonary hypertension associated with sarcoidosis: mechanisms, haemodynamics and prognosis. Thorax. 2006;61:68–74.

17. Baughman RP, Engel PJ, Taylor L, et al. Survival in sarcoidosis associated pulmonary hypertension: the importance of hemodynamic evaluation. Chest. 2010;138(5):1078–85.

18. Takemura T, Matsui Y, Saiki S, et al. Pulmonary vascular involvement in sarcoidosis: a report of 40 autopsy cases. Hum Pathol. 1992;23:1216–23.

19. Corte T, Wells AU, Nicholson AG, et al. Pulmonary hypertension in sarcoidosis: a review. Respirology. 2011;16:69–77.

20. Damuth TE, Biwer JS, Cho K, et al. Major pulmonary artery stenosis causing pulmonary hypertension in sarcoidosis. Chest. 1980;78:888–91.

21. Hiffstein V, Ranganathan N, Mullen JBM. Sarcoidosis stimulating pulmonary veno-occlusive disease. Am Rev Respir Dis. 1986;134:809–11.

22. Portier F, Lerebourg-Pigeonnaiere G, Thiberville L, et al. Sarcoidosis simulating pulmonary veno-occlusive disease. Rev Mal Respir. 1991;8:101–2.

23. Preston IR, Klinger JR, Landzberg MJ, et al. Vasoresponsiveness of sarcoid-associated pulmonary hypertension. Chest. 2001;120:866–72.

24. Barst RJ, Ratner SJ. Sarcoidosis and reactive pulmonary hypertension. Arch Intern Med. 1985;145(11):2112–4.

25. Galie N, Manes A, Branzi A. The endothelin system in pulmonary arterial hypertension. Cardiovasc Res. 2004;61:227–37.

26. Terashita K, Kato S, Sata M, et al. Increased endothelin-1 levels of BAL fluid in patients with pulmonary sarcoidosis. Respirology. 2006;11:145–51.

27. Letizia C, Danese A, Reale MG, et al. Plasma levels of endothelin-1 increase in patients with sarcoidosis and fall after disease remission. Panminerva Med. 2001;43:257–61.

28. Reichenberger F, Schauer J, Kellner K, Sack U, Stiehl P, Winkler J. Different expression of endothelin in the bronchoalveolar lavage in patients with pulmonary diseases. Lung. 2001;179:163–74.

29. Sutendra G, Dromparis P, Bonnet S, et al. Pyruvate dehydrogenase inhibition by the inflammatory cytokine TNF alpha contributes to the pathogenesis of pulmonary aterial hypertension. J Mol Med. 2011;89:771–83.

30. Chen ES, Moller DR. Sarcoidosis – scientific progress and clinical challenges. Nat Rev Rheumatol. 2011;7:457–67.

31. Toonkel RL, Borczuk AC, Pearson GD, et al. Sarcoidosis-associated fibrosing mediastinitis with resultant pulmonary hypertension: a case report and review of literature. Respiration. 2009;79:341–5.

32. Smith LJ, Lawrence JB, Katzenstein AL. Vascular sarcoidosis: a rare case report of pulmonary hypertension. Am J Med Sci. 1983;285:38–44.
33. Rosen Y, Moon S, Huang CT, et al. Granulomatous pulmonary angiitis in sarcoidosis. Arch Pathol Lab Med. 1977;101:170–4.
34. Bargout R, Kelly RF. Sarcoid heart disease: clinical course and treatment. Int J Cardiol. 2004;97:173–82.
35. Salazaar A, Mana J, Sala J, et al. Combined portal and pulmonary hypertension in sarcoidosis. Respiration. 1994;61:517–20.
36. Turner GA, Lower EE, Corser BC, et al. Sleep apnea in sarcoidosis. Sarcoidosis Vasc Diffuse Lung Dis. 1997;14:61–4.
37. Crawshaw AP, Wotton CJ, Yeates DG, Goldacre MJ, Ho LP. Evidence for association between sarcoidosis and pulmonary embolism from 35-year record linkage study. Thorax. 2011;66:447–8.
38. Swigris JJ, Olson AL, Huie TJ, et al. Increased risk of pulmonary embolism among US decedents with sarcoidosis from 1988 to 2007. Chest. 2011;140:1261–6.
39. Shorr AF, Davies DB, Nathan SD. Predicting mortality in patients with sarcoidosis awaiting lung transplantation. Chest. 2003;124:922–8.
40. Arcasoy SM, Christie JD, Pochettino A, et al. Characteristics and outcomes of patients with sarcoidosis listed for lung transplantation. Chest. 2001;120:873–80.
41. Nardi A, Brillet PY, Letoumelin P, et al. Stage IV sarcoidosis: comparison of survival with the general population and causes of death. Eur Respir J. 2011;38:1368–73.
42. Diaz-Guzman E, Farver C, Parambil J, Culver D. Pulmonary hypertension caused by sarcoidosis. Clin Chest Med. 2008;29(3):549–66.
43. Pabst S, Hammerstingl C, Grau N, et al. Pulmonary arterial hypertension in patients with sarcoidosis: the Pulsar single experience. In: Pokorski M, editor. Respiratory regulation – clinical advances, Advances in experimental medicine and biology. Dordrecht: Springer; 2013. p. 299–304.
44. Leuchte HH, Baumgartner RA, Nounou ME, et al. Brain natriuretic peptide is a prognostic parameter in chronic lung diseases. Am J Respir Crit Care Med. 2006;173:744–50.
45. Corte TJ, Wort SJ, Gatzoulis MA, et al. Elevated brain natriuretic peptide predicts mortality in interstitial lung disease. Eur Respir J. 2010;36:819–25.
46. Handa T, Nagai S, Ueda S, et al. Significance of plasma NT-preBNP levels as a biomarker in the assessment of cardiac involvement and pulmonary hypertension in patients with sarcoidosis. Sarcoidosis Vasc Diffuse Lung Dis. 2010;27(1):27–35.
47. Andersen C, Mellemkjær S, Nielsen-Kudsk JE, et al. Diagnostic and prognostic role of biomarkers for pulmonary hypertension in interstitial lung disease. Respir Med. 2012;106: 1749–55.
48. Bourbonnais JM, Samavati L. Clinical predictors of pulmonary hypertension in sarcoidosis. Eur Respir J. 2008;32:296–302.
49. Steen VD, Graham G, Conte C, Owens G, Medsger Jr TA. Isolated diffusing capacity reduction in systemic sclerosis. Arthritis Rheum. 1992;35:765–70.
50. Nathan SD, Shlobin OA, Ahmad S, Urbanek S, Barnett SD. Pulmonary hypertension and pulmonary function testing in idiopathic pulmonary fibrosis. Chest. 2007;131:657–63.
51. Baughman RP, Sparkman BK, Lower EE. Six minute walk test and health status assessment in sarcoidosis. Chest. 2007;132:207–13.
52. Palmero V, Sulica R. Sarcoidosis-associated pulmonary hypertension: assessment and management. Semin Respir Crit Care Med. 2010;31(4):494–500.
53. Alhamad EH, Ahmad Shaik S, Idrees MM, Alanezi MO, Isnani AC. Outcome measures of the 6 minute walk test: relationships with physiologic and computed tomography findings in patients with sarcoidosis. BMC Pulm Med. 2010;10:42–9.
54. Arcasoy SM, Christie JD, Ferrari VA, et al. Echocardiographic assessment of pulmonary hypertension in patients with advanced lung disease. Am J Respir Crit Care Med. 2003;167:735–40.
55. Rodman DM, Lindenfeld J. Successful treatment of sarcoidosis-associated pulmonary hypertension with corticosteroids. Chest. 1990;97:500–2.

56. Davies J, Nellen M, Goodwin JF. Reversible pulmonary hypertension in sarcoidosis. Postgrad Med J. 1982;58(679):282–5.

57. Gluskowski J, Hawrylkiewicz I, Zych D, Zielinski J. Effects of corticosteroid treatment on pulmonary hemodynamics in patients with sarcoidosis. Eur Respir J. 1990;3:403–7.

58. Galie N, Hoeper MM, Humbert M, et al. Guidelines for the diagnosis and treatment of pulmonary hypertension. Eur Respir J. 2009;34:1219–63.

59. http://www.clinicaltrials.gov/ct2/show/NCT01467791?term=sarcoid+registry&rank=1 (last accessed 3/5/2013)

60. Culver DA, Minai OA, Chapman JT, et al. Treatment of pulmonary hypertension in sarcoidosis. Proc Am Thorac Soc. 2005;2:A862.

61. Barnett CF, Bonura EJ, Nathan SD, et al. Treatment of sarcoidosis-associated pulmonary hypertension. A two-center experience. Chest. 2009;135:1455–61.

62. Judson MA, Highland KB, Kwon S, et al. Ambrisentan for sarcoidosis associated pulmonary hypertension. Sarcoidosis Vasc Diffuse Lung Dis. 2011;28(2):139–45.

63. http://clinicaltrials.gov/ct2/show/NCT00581607 (last accessed on 3/5/2013)

64. Milman N, Burton CM, Iversen M, Videbaek R, Jensen CV, Carlsen J. Pulmonary hypertension in end-stage pulmonary sarcoidosis: therapeutic effect of sildenafil? J Heart Lung Transplant. 2008;75:329–34.

65. Fisher KA, Serlin DM, Wilson KC, Walter RE, Berman JS, Farber HW. Sarcoidosis-associated pulmonary hypertension: outcome with long-term epoprostenol treatment. Chest. 2006;130(5): 1481–8.

66. Baughman RP, Judson MA, Lower EE, et al. Inhaled iloprost for sarcoidosis associated pulmonary hypertension. Sarcoidosis Vasc Diffuse Lung Dis. 2009;26:110–20.

Chapter 7
Monitoring Pulmonary Sarcoidosis

Athol U. Wells

Abstract The monitoring of serial changes in disease severity is an essential part of the clinical management of pulmonary sarcoidosis. Historically, symptomatic change, pulmonary function trends, and changes on serial imaging have all been evaluated in routine practice. However, each of these three domains has significant limitations when used in isolation. Symptomatic change is confounded by the long list of causes, other than change in the severity of interstitial lung disease, for serial reductions in exercise tolerance. The interpretation of pulmonary function trends is complicated by (a) the major heterogeneity in pulmonary function patterns in sarcoidosis; (b) the limitations of thresholds for "significant" change; and (c) the fact that pulmonary function trends do not always represent changes in the severity of pulmonary sarcoidosis. Serial chest radiography is somewhat insensitive in the detection of change and uncertainties exist on the optimal method of quantifying radiographic change. Given these limitations, a multidisciplinary approach is required in the routine monitoring of pulmonary sarcoidosis, with the reconciliation of symptomatic change, radiographic change, and pulmonary function trends, although no guidance on this process exists in current guidelines. This principle applies equally to defining responses to treatment, detecting changes in disease severity in other contexts and the identification of increasing pulmonary vascular disease.

Keywords Monitoring • Pulmonary sarcoidosis • Pulmonary function tends • Chest radiography • Symptomatic change

A.U. Wells, M.D. (✉)
Interstitial Lung Disease Unit, Royal Brompton Hospital, C/O Emmanuel Kaye Building, Manresa Rd, Chelsea, London, SW3 6LR, UK
e-mail: Athol.Wells@rbht.nhs.uk

M.A. Judson (ed.), *Pulmonary Sarcoidosis: A Guide for the Practicing Clinician*, Respiratory Medicine 17, DOI 10.1007/978-1-4614-8927-6_7,
© Springer Science+Business Media New York 2014

Introduction

In the most recent international consensus document on the management of sarcoidosis states, it was recommended that serial chest radiography and spirometry should be used to identify changes in disease severity [1]. This deceptively simple statement summarises routine clinical practice during previous decades but does not capture the major limitations in the application of these tests to routine monitoring in individual cases. In the absence of a reference standard for the identification of change in disease severity, accumulated clinical experience has taught clinicians that in interstitial lung disease, "objective" evaluation of change in severity is more reliable than subjective symptomatic change [2]. Tellingly, in the 1999 recommendations, symptomatic change was not given the same weight as serial radiography and spirometry in routine monitoring [1].

This point of view is based on the view that the primary goals in monitoring pulmonary sarcoidosis are to identify regression of disease with treatment and to detect clinically important disease progression with a view to therapeutic intervention, in order to prevent increasing respiratory disability. However, in reality, when pulmonary disease severity is mild to moderate, as judged by "objective" measures, therapeutic intervention is often directed primarily towards addressing disabling loss of quality of life which may result from unrelenting cough or wheeze due to bronchial hyper-reactivity, even in the absence of severe pulmonary involvement, as judged by imaging and pulmonary function tests. It follows logically that the first step in routine monitoring is to focus on changes in symptoms: often, changes in therapy are warranted for symptomatic reasons, even when disease appears to be stable, judging from serial chest radiography and pulmonary function tests. Accurate monitoring requires multidisciplinary evaluation, amounting to the reconciliation of overall disease severity and symptomatic chest radiographic and pulmonary function change. Only by integrating all these considerations can a clear judgement be made as to whether treatment changes are needed to address unacceptable loss in quality of life in isolation or whether there is overt pulmonary disease progression, signalling a risk of future disability due to loss of pulmonary reserve. It should be stressed that when the full range of pulmonary disease severity is taken into account, accumulated experience has taught us that intervention is required solely for symptomatic reasons as often it is for major ("dangerous") disease progression.

A glossary of abbreviations for routine PFT is given in Table 7.1.

Table 7.1 A glossary of abbreviations for routine pulmonary function variables

DLco	Carbon monoxide diffusing capacity
FEV1	Forced expiratory volume in 1 s
FVC	Forced vital capacity
Kco	Carbon monoxide transfer coefficient
RV	Residual volume
TLC	Total lung capacity
VA	Alveolar volume

Symptomatic Change in Monitoring

However, if the importance of evaluating symptomatic change in monitoring pulmonary disease is sometimes understated, the difficulties that may arise in interpreting symptomatic change cannot be overemphasised. Pulmonary involvement is often accompanied by systemic manifestations which may have a profound effect on the level of exercise tolerance, both at a single point in time and with regard to serial change. Fatigue is common in sarcoidosis and often disabling [3]. When severe fatigue is present in sarcoidosis, it can be difficult for the patient to deconstruct the relative contributions of fatigue and loss of pulmonary reserve to changes in exercise tolerance, with the two symptoms often amalgamated as "breathlessness". Musculoskeletal involvement (whether of joints or muscles) is also a major confounding factor. Arthralgia and myalgia may result in major increases in the work of locomotion, giving rise to severe exertional dyspnoea, even in the absence of pulmonary involvement. Limitation due to systemic or stable pulmonary disease may also lead to significant reductions in exercise tolerance due to inactivity with consequent weight gain and loss of fitness. As discussed later, exercise testing has no routine role in the monitoring of pulmonary sarcoidosis. However, when increasing exercise intolerance is associated with systemic morbidity, the 6-min walk test may provide invaluable information. It is sometimes obvious from observation of the patient that exercise limitation is primarily due to non-pulmonary factors, especially when oxygen saturation is normal when dyspnoea causes early cessation of the test.

However, difficulties in interpreting symptomatic change are not confined to extra-pulmonary confounding factors. Progressive reductions in exercise tolerance in the setting of stable interstitial lung disease may result from cardiac involvement, pulmonary vascular disease, or infection. Increasing cardiac or pulmonary vascular limitation, in particular, may simulate progression of pulmonary sarcoidosis as worsening exertional dyspnoea is often the sole clinical manifestation of advancing disease. Whenever progressive exercise limitation appears disproportionate to the severity of pulmonary disease, cardiac evaluation is appropriate.

Acute or subacute infection is an occasional cause of apparent progression of pulmonary sarcoidosis but is often disclosed by sputum production or systemic symptoms. However, the extra-pulmonary symptoms of infection may be suppressed by immunosuppression and, when present, may be difficult to distinguish from symptoms due to systemic sarcoidosis. Moreover, in treated patients with advanced fibrotic disease, the clearance of infected secretions may be compromised due to a combination of structural damage and the inhibition of host defence mechanisms by immunosuppressive therapy. Supervening chronic lung suppuration may result in insidiously increasing exercise intolerance which is difficult to distinguish from worsening pulmonary sarcoidosis. Chronic *Aspergillus* infection with aspergillomas or, less frequently, semi-invasive aspergillosis is a notorious complication of advanced fibro-bullous pulmonary sarcoidosis [4] and is often associated with low-grade systemic symptoms which may be suggestive of systemic sarcoidosis disease activity.

Table 7.2 Possible reasons for increased exertional dyspnoea, with causes due to sarcoidosis disease activity emboldened

Pulmonary causes	**Progression of interstitial lung disease**
	Bronchial hyperactivity due to airway involvement
	Acute or subacute infection
	Chronic infection (especially *Aspergillus* infection)
Cardiac causes	**Pulmonary hypertension**
	Cardiac sarcoidosis
	Coexistent cardiac disease, unrelated to sarcoidosis
Musculoskeletal causes	**Arthritis**
	Myositis
	Chest wall discomfort
	Coexistent arthritis, unrelated to sarcoidosis
Other systemic causes	**Fatigue**
	Anaemia
Iatrogenic causes	Corticosteroids (weight gain, myopathy)
	Methotrexate (interstitial lung disease)
Other causes	Weight gain
	Loss of fitness
	Psychogenic factors

Finally, in sarcoidosis patients with a predominantly obstructive ventilatory defect, bronchial hyper-reactivity due to endobronchial inflammation may give rise to cough, wheeze, and variable exercise intolerance, without necessarily being indicative of progressive interstitial lung disease [5]. The clinical difficulty in this context usually lies in discriminating between this presentation and concurrent asthma. The distinction is less problematic when bronchocentric symptoms develop only after the onset of sarcoidosis and are associated with increasing chronic airflow obstruction. However, in patients with low-grade cough and wheeze, and in those with long-standing asthma, it is often difficult to ascribe symptoms to pulmonary sarcoidosis.

In summary, the interpretation of symptomatic change in pulmonary sarcoidosis requires the consideration of all the confounding factors discussed above. It might be supposed that studies of symptomatic change in sarcoidosis (whether centred on exercise tolerance or quality of life) might provide useful guidance to the clinician. However, in reality, the validation of dyspnoea and quality of life scales, although providing a means of evaluation of cohort change in therapeutic trials, add little or nothing to routine clinical monitoring in individual patients. The use of semi-quantitative scales may allow symptomatic change to be described with greater precision but do not distinguish between progression of pulmonary disease and the many confounders that may confuse the clinical picture. It should also be stressed that in insidiously progressive pulmonary sarcoidosis, significant progression of interstitial lung disease may occur without symptomatic worsening, especially in patients with mild to moderate disease and a good pulmonary reserve. For all these reasons, symptomatic change, although a key consideration in routine monitoring, cannot be used in isolation. The many causes of declining exercise tolerance are listed in Table 7.2. The objective evaluation of change in disease severity is required, using pulmonary function tests and chest radiography.

Pulmonary Function Tests in Monitoring

In routine monitoring, serial pulmonary function tests have consistently had a central role. In interstitial lung disease, pulmonary function variables have long been regarded as a more accurate reflection of the underlying histologic severity of disease than symptoms and chest radiography [2]. However, it should be stressed that in pulmonary sarcoidosis, the prognostic accuracy of pulmonary function trends has not been "validated" against subsequent mortality. It is likely that standard monitoring in sarcoidosis has been influenced by studies of idiopathic pulmonary fibrosis (IPF), which have consistently shown that serial declines in FVC are predictive of increased mortality [6–8]. In sarcoidosis, there is no reference standard for change in pulmonary disease severity. In particular, the relatively low mortality and greater efficacy of treatment in sarcoidosis (compared to IPF) have undermined the use of mortality as an "anchor" against which to evaluate the prognostic value of pulmonary function trends. By default, clinical experience in monitoring change in IPF and other progressive forms of pulmonary fibrosis has been adapted to the serial evaluation of sarcoidosis. The current recommendations in IPF [9] that FVC and DLco levels should be monitored at three to six monthly intervals have largely captured routine practice in pulmonary sarcoidosis early in the course of disease, when the primary clinical question is whether disease has stabilised, with or without treatment. Similarly, in both sarcoidosis and IPF, responses to higher dose therapy have been largely defined by short-term pulmonary function trends, usually at 4–6 weeks.

The central role of serial FVC in monitoring is based on ease of performance and reproducibility. Pulmonary function trends are stated as percentage changes from absolute baseline values. Calculations of change are made from absolute values, rather than from percentages of predicted normal values, because the latter are influenced by patient age and are modified if the birthday of the patient occurs within the time interval of monitoring. Thus, a change in FVC from 2.0 to 1.8 l represents a 10 % decline, but a change from 60 to 54 % of predicted cannot be interpreted with quite the same precision. This is an important consideration because a 10 % change in FVC has been considered to denote "significant change" and this threshold has been widely used by clinicians to identify a response to treatment or, in the event of a 10 % decline, progression of disease.

It should be stressed that the designation of threshold values to define "significant change" comes from studies of the variability of individual variables in normal subjects and, to a lesser extent, in patients with pulmonary disease. In reproducibility studies, FVC values have differed by less than 10 % at repeat measurement in approximately 95 % of cases (and thus the threshold of 10 % represents two standard deviations of FVC change).

In pulmonary function laboratories with rigorous quality assurance and regular evaluation of normal biological control subjects (e.g. healthy staff members), it is possible to achieve greater FVC reproducibility [10], but the threshold of 10 % is broadly applicable to routine pulmonary function estimation. Crucially, based on this threshold, spurious change in FVC values of 10 % or more due to measurement variation can be expected on repeat testing in 5 % of normal subjects and sarcoidosis patients. A 10 % threshold to identify change that is likely to exceed measurement variation is also appropriate for FEV1.

By contrast, the estimation of DLco is less reproducible and a 15 % threshold for change is needed to minimise the confounding effect of measurement variation. In part, this reflects the fact that the quantification of DLco is relatively complex, with a number of technical variations in measurement protocols that differ between pulmonary function laboratories. For this reason, DLco trends defined by measurements made at different laboratories are notoriously inaccurate, an important consideration in patients who are referred to a regional centre or change their city of residence. However, even when patients are evaluated in the same pulmonary function laboratory, a 15 % threshold for "significant change" is appropriate. Variability in DLco estimation is significantly reduced with daily calibration of lung function equipment against normal biological controls, but this is seldom practicable. It should not be overlooked that DLco levels are a composite of *two* measurements, each with its own inherent variability. Carbon monoxide uptake is measured per unit volume (corresponding to the gas transfer coefficient or Kco) and is adjusted by the alveolar volume, which is derived from helium dilution in the same measurement manoeuvre. Much confusion has arisen from the term "DLco/VA" as a widely used synonym for Kco, implying incorrectly that DLco and VA are the cardinal measurements and that Kco is a derived ratio [11].

It should be recognised that no formal comparison exists in pulmonary sarcoidosis between change in FVC as described above, expressed as percentage change of absolute baseline values, and a number of alternative approaches. In some treatment trials in IPF, change in predicted normal values has been used with a 10 % threshold for decline representing a fall in FVC values from, for example, 60–50 % of predicted normal. This higher threshold has also been used in routine monitoring by some clinicians but suffers from the disadvantage that in severe disease, major change (e.g. a fall from 40 to 30 %) is required before it is designated as "significant". In any case, as measurement variation is quantified as variation from *measured* values, the designation of thresholds for "significant" change based on predicted normal values appears illogical. The use of FVC, rather than other lung volumes such as TLC and VA, reflects the ready availability and ease of performance of simple spirometry and the view that FVC trends and trends in other volumes provide essentially the same information.

Based on these considerations, can FVC change, evaluated in isolation, be viewed as a robust means of identifying clinically significant changes in the severity of pulmonary sarcoidosis? Despite the attractiveness of this proposition, accumulated clinical experience has taught us that this is emphatically not the case, due to three important confounding factors that apply to other interstitial lung disease but are more problematic in sarcoidosis (Table 7.3).

Table 7.3 Problems in the interpretation of pulmonary function trends and the optimal clinical approach to address these difficulties

Problem	Optimal clinical approach
Heterogeneity of patterns of pulmonary function impairment	Establish which cardinal PFT variable (FEV1, FVC, DLco) provides the most abnormal signal Focus on this variable during serial monitoring, although continue to monitor other variables
The limitations of thresholds for "significant" change	When the pretest probability of decline is low, always view isolated changes in a single PFT variable with scepticism Evaluate concurrent trends in other PFT variables Integrate PFT trends with serial symptoms and chest radiographic data
Pulmonary function trends do not always represent changes in the severity of pulmonary sarcoidosis	Consider the following confounding factors – Bronchial hyperactivity – Pulmonary infection (acute, subacute, or chronic) – Extrapulmonary restriction (myopathy, weight gain, chest wall pain, sub-maximal effort) – Pulmonary hypertension (selectively affecting DLco and Kco levels) – Left heart failure – Iatrogenic (methotrexate lung, weight gain due to corticosteroid therapy)

The Heterogeneity of Patterns of Pulmonary Function Impairment

The heterogeneity of pulmonary function patterns in sarcoidosis is well recognised. Although pulmonary sarcoidosis is widely regarded as a restrictive interstitial lung disease, non-caseating granulomas may be located in the alveolar walls, small lymphatics, perivascular and peribronchiolar regions, larger airways, and, less frequently, in the respiratory muscles. Lung function abnormalities in sarcoidosis may arise from any of these compartments, with variable patterns of airflow obstruction, lung restriction, a mixed obstructive/restrictive ventilatory effect, and disproportionate reduction in gas transfer. In severe parenchymal lung disease, a restrictive ventilatory defect is often evident, especially in patients with chest radiographic stages III and IV [12–14], but also in association with any chest radiographic stage, including radiological stage 0 disease [14, 15]. In this context, changes in disease severity may be best captured by FVC trends.

However, airflow obstruction has been more prevalent than lung restriction in some sarcoidosis cohorts. Airflow obstruction has been viewed as an early feature of sarcoidosis, representing a granulomatous bronchiolitis that precedes the development of fibrotic disease. However, airflow obstruction is encountered at all radiographic stages of disease and, in one longitudinal study, increased in prevalence with increasing chest radiographic stage [15]. In two HRCT studies, morphologic abnormalities associated with airflow obstruction have included fibrotic reticular abnormalities, peribronchial thickening, and mosaic attenuation [16, 17].

These observations are likely to reflect the histological finding of peribronchiolar fibrosis in pulmonary sarcoidosis [18], but airflow obstruction may also result from fibrotic stenoses of large airways [19] or, rarely, airway compression by enlarged lymph nodes.

A disproportionate impairment in gas transfer is a less frequent pattern of impairment than obstruction or restriction. DLco reductions occur in up to 50 % of patients with sarcoidosis, but these are more commonly at a level that is compatible with interstitial lung disease and are usually less severe than in patients with IPF [20]. However, in an important patient subgroup, DLco levels are disproportionately reduced, as shown by major reductions in Kco. It is likely, although not proven, that this reflects pulmonary vascular limitation, although, in most cases, this is not sufficiently severe to result in pulmonary hypertension at rest.

Thus, the inflexible use of FVC trends to monitor pulmonary disease does not take into account the spectrum of patterns of pulmonary function impairment in pulmonary sarcoidosis. In one study, FEV1 levels better reflected global morphologic abnormalities on HRCT than FVC or DLco levels [17], probably because FEV1 levels are reduced in both obstructive and restrictive disease, whereas FVC levels are less impaired in mild to moderate airflow obstruction. The inescapable conclusion is that no single pulmonary function variable is equal to the accurate monitoring of pulmonary disease in all cases. It can be argued, although not proven, that in individual patients, pulmonary function variables that are most impaired at baseline are the most likely to signal disease progression on serial evaluation. In a patient with predominant airflow obstruction, changes in disease severity may be most likely to manifest as a "significant" change in FEV1. By contrast, it appears most logical to expect a higher prevalence of change in DLco in patients with a disproportionate reduction in DLco at baseline.

Essentially, no single pulmonary function variable can be regarded as the primary arbiter of changes in disease severity in all sarcoidosis patients. This constraint creates obvious difficulties in pharmaceutical studies in pulmonary sarcoidosis, in which a single primary end-point is required. The idea that the primary end-point should be chosen individually in each patient, based on the pattern of pulmonary function impairment, is unlikely to appeal to regulatory authorities. In routine practice, accurate pulmonary function monitoring requires that FEV1, FVC, and DLco trends are evaluated in combination and reconciled with the baseline pulmonary function profile. This, in turn, underlines the need for detailed pulmonary function evaluation at baseline, including spirometric volumes and the measurement of gas transfer. Only by this means will the pattern of pulmonary function impairment be disclosed in individual patients as an aid to accurate monitoring. Ideally, plethysmographic volumes should also be evaluated at baseline as knowledge of a mixture of airflow obstruction and lung restriction (not reliably identified by simple spirometry) may also have important implications for subsequent pulmonary function monitoring. Importantly, baseline plethysmography also allows monitoring of TLC or RV levels as a substitute for FVC in patients who develop contraindications to forced spirometric manoeuvres such as chest wall pain and glaucoma.

The Limitations of Thresholds for "Significant" Change

Thresholds for "significant" change reduce the likelihood that pulmonary function trends represent measurement variability but do not indicate that the amplitude of change is *clinically significant*. It should not be forgotten that measurement variation results equally frequently in the overstatement and understatement of change. Given the known variability in FVC estimation, an observed change of 10 % represents, in reality, a change that lies somewhere between 1 and 19 %. In other words, variability thresholds establish merely that change in an individual pulmonary function parameter is likely to be real but do not discriminate reliably between trivial and major change [21].

A related problem is that the accurate use of variability thresholds to identify genuine trends is influenced by the pretest probability of change, which varies greatly between interstitial lung diseases. As discussed earlier, measurement variation will result in a spurious change in FVC of at least 10 % in approximately 5 %, and thus a spurious decline in 2.5 % of patients. In a rapidly progressive disease such as IPF, this matters little. True declines in FVC, exceeding 10 % of baseline values, can be expected in up to 50 % of patients at a time interval of 12 months. In a cohort of 40 IPF patients, a spurious decline of at least 10 % will occur, on average, in only one case whereas a true decline of over 10 % can be expected in approximately 20 cases: the likelihood that an observed decline of 10 % is real is approximately 95 % (20/21). However, in pulmonary sarcoidosis, a less progressive disease, a very different picture emerges with the application of Bayesian principles. If, for example, the prevalence of pulmonary function decline of greater than 10 % in a cohort of 40 sarcoidosis patients approximates 10–15 %, the likelihood that decline to this threshold represents disease progression in an individual patient will be only 80–85 %. The use of standardised thresholds for change across all interstitial lung diseases takes no account of the pretest probability of disease progression and is likely to mislead the clinician in less progressive disorders, in which observed change is relatively less likely to denote disease progression and relatively more likely to result from measurement variation.

Both these problems can be addressed by the consideration of pulmonary function trends measured using separate techniques (i.e. spirometry and estimation of gas transfer). Although isolated changes in gas transfer can represent increasing pulmonary vascular limitation, progression of interstitial lung disease generally results in parallel declines in DLco and spirometric variables. A compatible DLco trend increases the likelihood that an observed change in FEV1 or FVC is genuine, even if thresholds for "significant change" are not reached for all variables. Similarly, it is essential that FVC and FEV1 trends are integrated with symptomatic and chest radiographic change. In the absence of symptomatic and radiographic support, an isolated increase or fall in a single pulmonary function variable should be viewed with suspicion, especially if the increase exceeds variability thresholds by only a small amount.

Pulmonary Function Trends Do Not Always Represent Changes in Disease Severity

The use of variability thresholds to define "significant" pulmonary function change does not, in itself, distinguish between change due to the progression or regression of interstitial lung disease and change for other reasons. In interstitial lung disease at large, acute or subacute infection is a common cause of apparent disease progression, as judged by increased symptoms and pulmonary function decline. In pulmonary sarcoidosis, symptoms due to viral infection such as fevers and myalgia may be difficult to distinguish from the systemic symptoms of sarcoidosis. Moreover, in patients treated with immunosuppressive therapies, which, in themselves, predispose to pulmonary infection, the systemic symptoms of infection may be attenuated due to the effects of immunomodulation.

In pulmonary sarcoidosis, a number of other complications may result in pulmonary function trends that simulate progression of interstitial lung disease. Bronchial hyper-reactivity is commonly associated with bronchocentric inflammation and may give rise to a clinical picture similar to asthma with variable wheeze and transient reductions in spirometric variables. Reductions in FEV1 and FVC may also result from respiratory muscle weakness with extensive muscle involvement, chest wall discomfort, or sub-maximal effort due to the debilitating effects of systemic disease, although in these extra-pulmonary scenarios, DLco levels are usually relatively less affected. Drug-induced pulmonary toxicity from therapies such as methotrexate and leflunomide should also be considered, although probably less prevalent than in rheumatoid arthritis (based on accumulated clinical experience). Opportunistic infection may also complicate immunosuppressive therapy, and in extensive pulmonary sarcoidosis, immunomodulation may trigger chronic suppurative lung disease. *Aspergillus* infection, which is associated with destructive pulmonary sarcoidosis, is a notorious cause of apparent insidious disease progression, with low-grade systemic symptoms, similar to those of systemic sarcoidosis, a frequent accompaniment. Finally, pulmonary vascular involvement or cardiac disease may be associated with isolated gas transfer trends.

The Optimal Use of Pulmonary Function Variables in Routine Monitoring

It will be obvious, based on the considerations discussed above, that a reliance on serial trends in single pulmonary function variables such as FVC is likely to result in the over-diagnosis of progression of interstitial lung disease. The evaluation of both spirometric variables and measures of gas transfer minimises the confounding effect of measurement variation but does not address the problem of alternative causes of pulmonary function decline. There is no substitute for a wide differential diagnosis for pulmonary function decline and this is especially the case later in the course of disease when disease has stabilised and deterioration is relatively unexpected.

Chest Radiography in Monitoring

For many decades, chest radiography has been routinely used in the evaluation of serial change. Paradoxically, the evaluation of simple global changes in chest radiographic extent has been little studied. As recently as 1990, the fact that deteriorations in pulmonary sarcoidosis with treatment reductions were captured by worsening chest radiographic abnormalities in a small patient cohort was considered to merit publication in a leading international radiographic journal [22], despite the widespread use of chest radiography for this purpose and the documentation of chest radiographic change in a number of short-term studies of corticosteroid therapy.

The search for a reliable approach to the quantification of chest radiographic change in sarcoidosis began with the adaption of complex chest radiographic scoring, which provided detailed information on changes in individual chest radiographic patterns. The ILO pneumoconiosis system, developed to capture the spectrum of chest radiographic findings resulting from exposure to industrial dusts [23], is based on the scoring of the profusion of interstitial opacities in three zones in each lung. Early recognition of the considerable radiological expertise needed for the accurate use of this system led to the licensing of individual radiologists and clinicians as "ILO readers" more than 20 years ago, but very few current practitioners possess this qualification. The major limitations of this approach were well illustrated by one relatively recent series [24], in which changes in ILO profusion scores were evaluated in exacerbations of sarcoidosis. Although there were significant associations between increases in profusion scores and declines in spirometric volumes, inter-observer agreement was only moderate. The authors concluded that this scoring approach was poorly suited to routine clinical evaluation.

Acknowledgement of the limitations of serial ILO scoring prompted the use of a modified ILO system in the British Thoracic Sarcoidosis Study [25]. Radiographic abnormalities were categorised as reticulo-nodular, masses, confluent shadows, and fibrotic change, with each pattern quantified by a score based on extent and profusion [26]. Inter-observer agreement was found to be good. However, chest radiographic change did not correlate well with trends in pulmonary function variables and dyspnoea scores. Only changes in the reticulo-nodular (R) score and fibrosis (F) score were found to be linked to non-radiographic variables and correlation coefficients were disappointingly low. This study did, at least, provide the first validation of a detailed scoring system that could be adopted in later clinical trials.

The Muers system was considered to be the only radiographic scoring system sufficiently referenced in the medical literature to be used in a recent double-blind randomised trial of infliximab in pulmonary sarcoidosis [27]. Crucially, the authors took the opportunity to compare the Muers system with a simple scoring system that reflected the use of serial chest radiography in routine practice, consisting of a simple five-point scale for global chest radiographic change (markedly worsened, worsened, unchanged, improved, markedly improved). Inter-observer agreement between two readers was good for both systems, although it should be stressed that the observations were made by two expert radiologists. However, the simple scoring system was more tightly linked to pulmonary function change. In particular, changes in FVC levels correlated more strongly with changes in global scores ($r=0.35$, $p<0.0001$) than with changes identified using the Muers system ($r=0.24$, $p<0.05$) [27].

From this study, it can be concluded that a minimalist approach to chest radiographic change, centred on global changes in disease extent, is best suited to routine practice. It appears that more detailed scoring of changes in individual chest radiographic patterns results in greater discrepancies with pulmonary function trends, underlining the fact that the chest radiograph is essentially an insensitive tool in the detection of change. This view was underlined in a study of over 350 patients with pulmonary sarcoidosis in which it was demonstrated that serial change in the radiographic extent of lung disease (scored simply as more extensive, stable, or less extensive) was much more frequent than change in radiographic stage [28]. Change in disease extent on chest radiography was linked to PFT trends ($p<0.0005$ for FEV1, FVC, DLco), whereas change in radiographic stage was not.

However, even with the use of a relatively simple approach to serial chest radiographic evaluation, the reconciliation of serial chest radiographic and pulmonary function data is often problematic in individual patients. The correlation between chest radiographic abnormalities and pulmonary function impairment is notoriously poor in pulmonary sarcoidosis. In advanced disease, morphologic abnormalities are superimposed due to the two-dimensional nature of chest radiography, but in other cases, change occurs predominantly in the upper zones which are notoriously functionally silent.

Serial HRCT in Monitoring

In principle, it might be assumed that the sensitivity of HRCT should allow it to be utilised effectively in the clinical monitoring of pulmonary sarcoidosis. However, this use of HRCT remains contentious. In order to use serial HRCT effectively, it is first of all necessary that baseline HRCT images are available. However, the use of HRCT in initial staging varies greatly. While HRCT is routinely performed in some centres, in patients with clinically significant interstitial lung disease, other clinicians have taken a strictly utilitarian view. It has been argued that thoracic HRCT is useful in 30 % of patients with pulmonary sarcoidosis when chest radiographic findings are inconclusive and in patients with atypical sarcoidosis, in whom HRCT patterns "pathognomonic" of sarcoidosis may be diagnostically valuable [29].

Even when serial HRCT images are available, their integration in a routine monitoring algorithm has proven elusive. A number of scoring systems have been used to quantify HRCT abnormalities of sarcoidosis, similar to the system of Remy-Jardin [30] in which each abnormal pattern was scored for extent in the upper, mid, and lower zones by visual estimation and summed to give an overall HRCT severity score. However, these systems have never been validated in serial evaluation and this applies equally to relative simple severity scoring [31], adapted from a more complex system [32]. The cardinal difficulty lies in ascribing clinical significance to serial HRCT change. It must sometimes be concluded that HRCT is too sensitive, as it allows the identification of minor regional change which may have little or no correlation with pulmonary function trends. Moreover, in occasional cases, significant pulmonary function trends may be seen without major HRCT change. Even in therapeutic trials of sarcoidosis and IPF, in which it might be expected that cohort change in morphologic variables should add value to current end-points, this use of HRCT has proven elusive. Thus, at present, serial HRCT cannot be recommended in routine monitoring.

However, based on accumulated clinical experience, serial HRCT has an occasional role when other serial data are conflicting and need to be reconciled. In general, this does not apply to the short-term evaluation of responsiveness to therapy as it is difficult to argue that subtle regression of disease on HRCT is clinically meaningful in the absence of improvements in symptoms and pulmonary function tests. However in occasional patients with insidious progression of fibrotic disease, it is possible to identify a definite increase in disease extent on HRCT when there are worsening symptoms, pulmonary function trends are marginal, and, as is so often the case, chest radiographic evaluation is inconclusive. It should be stressed that the extra information gleaned from HRCT in this context adds value only when it gives rise to changes in therapy.

HRCT is more helpful in routine monitoring when it is suspected that progression is due to infection. Occasionally, when rapid deterioration has occurred, lack of change in the extent of interstitial lung disease on HRCT allows the clinician to treat empirically for infection with greater confidence. In patients with insidious disease progression, in whom supervening chronic suppurative lung disease or *Aspergillus* infection is suspected, HRCT may show bronchiectasis or aspergilloma formation (findings that are equally useful when HRCT is performed for the first time in this clinical scenario). This applies especially to the problem of recurrent major haemoptysis: aspergilloma formation usually occurs in advanced fibrotic lung disease and may not be disclosed by chest radiography. However, these uses of HRCT depend upon the multidisciplinary evaluation of symptoms, pulmonary function trends, and chest radiographic data. It can be concluded that serial HRCT should not be performed by protocol but only in order to answer clinical questions specific to the individual patient.

Pulmonary "Disease Activity" in Monitoring

As long ago as 1986, it was concluded that there is no universally agreed definition of "active" pulmonary disease [33], and 25 years later, the situation remains the same. Pulmonary "disease activity" can loosely be defined as the presence of clinically significant reversible inflammatory disease. However, major inflammatory disease is reliably identified by clinically significant regression of disease with treatment; many patients with irreversible disease continue to deteriorate. In these cases, a reliable measure of ongoing inflammation, following initial treatment, would be an invaluable aid to routine monitoring. But does such a test exist?

A number of tests, evaluated in the staging of "disease activity", have been discarded. 67-Gallium, once widely used to assess sarcoid activity, is no longer routinely used to assess pulmonary disease and its role in monitoring is hampered by the high prevalence of abnormal uptake in patients with stable disease, the absence of a simple reproducible method of quantifying change in signal, and the radiation burden associated with the test. Serum biomarkers have also been unsatisfactory in the identification of active pulmonary disease. Serum ACE levels are elevated in 30–80 % of patients with sarcoidosis but may be normal in active disease and do not correlate with chest radiographic stage [34] or the extent of nodular change and consolidation on HRCT [35]. In the 2008 British Thoracic Society Guidelines for the diagnosis and management of interstitial lung disease [36], serum ACE levels were not considered to add usefully to pulmonary function tests and chest radiography in the monitoring of pulmonary disease. Amongst other serum biomarkers, attention has focused on soluble interleukin 2 receptors (sIL-2r), released by activated T cells in granulomatous inflammation, but correlations between sIL-2r with the percentage and absolute bronchoalveolar lavage (BAL) lymphocyte counts [37–39] were not reproduced in another study [40]. The role of BAL remains contentious in the initial evaluation of "disease activity" in pulmonary sarcoidosis. Although a BAL neutrophilia was predictive of disease progression in one report [41] and the absence of a neutrophilia was associated with spontaneous disease regression in newly diagnosed steroid naïve patients in another study [42], repeat BAL in order to assess responsiveness to therapy or to identify residual inflammatory disease has not been validated.

No measure of "disease activity" exists that can be reliably integrated in routine monitoring in all patients. In occasional patients with elevated levels, repetition of serum ACE may be useful in the scenario of increasing respiratory symptoms which are difficult to interpret: a significant concurrent rise in serum ACE levels may provide helpful ancillary support for pulmonary disease progression, as opposed to worsening symptoms due to the many confounding factors discussed earlier. However, the converse is not true: in the absence of pulmonary function or chest radiographic evidence of a change in disease severity, serial serum ACE levels have little added value. BAL also has an occasional monitoring role in providing supportive evidence for suppurative lung disease and in the identification of opportunistic infection in patients receiving immunosuppressive therapy.

Based on preliminary promising data, FDG PET scanning may have a future role in selected patients. PET scanning is more sensitive than gallium scanning in detecting active pulmonary disease [43]. Reductions in abnormal pulmonary signal have been observed with steroid therapy [44, 45] and infliximab [46]. If these serial reductions in PET signal are shown to predict the longer term disease stabilisation in fibrotic pulmonary sarcoidosis, their integration in routine monitoring protocols in severe disease may eventually be justifiable. However, without this information, the marginal availability and expense of the test dictate that the use of serial PET scanning will be largely confined to pharmaceutical studies.

The Detection of Pulmonary Hypertension in Monitoring

The problem of disproportionate reductions in DLco levels in pulmonary sarcoidosis in serial monitoring is increasingly recognised [28], and in many cases, there is no other overt evidence of pulmonary vascular disease. The traditional view that pulmonary hypertension (PH) is a rare complication applies to the general population of sarcoidosis patients and was underlined by echocardiographic findings in a large series of Japanese patients [47]. However, in chronic pulmonary sarcoidosis, PH has a surprisingly high prevalence, approaching 50 % in one report [48], in patients with disproportionate exercise intolerance. Based on early encouraging reports of the efficacy of targeted PH therapies in sarcoidosis, and also on the adverse prognostic significance of PH with particular reference to lung transplantation, the detection of PH is an important monitoring consideration in advanced pulmonary disease.

However, in diffuse lung disease in general, the severity of reduction in spirometric and plethysmographic volumes is not reliably predictive of the presence of PH. In sarcoidosis in particular, the identification of PH is further complicated by the fact that PH can arise from a number of mechanisms other than progression of interstitial lung disease. The serial measurement of DLco allows the identification of patients at higher risk of developing PH. A reduction in DLco levels disproportionate to lung volume trends should prompt further investigation for PH [49], including echocardiography, estimation of serum BNP levels, the evaluation of oxygen desaturation on exercise, and, in selected cases, right heart catheterisation. Historically, changes in Kco levels (the DLco/VA ratio) have been used to quantify disproportionate reductions in DLco. More recently, a high FVC/DLco ratio [50, 51] has indicated a higher likelihood of pulmonary hypertension in interstitial lung disease. The two ratios provide approximately equivalent information, although the FVC/DLco ratio is a less reproducible figure as it is affected by the variability of both spirometric and gas transfer measurements (whereas Kco is measured with a single manoeuvre). Importantly, no single threshold value of either ratio has been identified as an optimal diagnostic threshold for PH and, thus, the serial measurement of Kco levels, although useful in triggering further evaluation of suspected PH, does not provide diagnostic information in isolation. The likelihood of underlying PH is further increased when disproportionate serial reductions in Kco are associated with severe resting hypoxia or major arterial oxygen desaturation with minor exertion.

Based on these considerations, serial gas transfer estimation is an essential part of the routine monitoring of advanced pulmonary sarcoidosis. In mild pulmonary disease, it can be argued that serial measures of gas transfer are less helpful in the early detection of PH, but, as discussed earlier, DLco trends have an important role in "validating" the clinical significance of marginal changes in FEV1 and FVC. However, even if an early decision is made not to monitor serial DLco levels in mild apparently stable pulmonary disease, it is essential that DLco levels are measured at initial evaluation, both to identify patients with disproportionate reductions in DLco (which should continue to be monitored) and to serve as a baseline in case there are clinical reasons to suspect the development of PH during follow-up.

Oxygen Desaturation in Monitoring

It is difficult to advance an argument for the routine estimation of arterial gases at rest during follow-up, except in patients with end-stage disease. In the absence of PH, significant resting hypoxia is a feature of severe pulmonary sarcoidosis. However, the identification or exclusion of oxygen desaturation on exercise testing provides useful ancillary information in selected patients. Maximal exercise testing has no validated role in routine monitoring. However, in selected cases, it may be helpful in the assessment of unexplained troublesome dyspnoea, not explained by resting pulmonary and cardiac investigations. In this context, severe desaturation on maximal exercise should lead the clinician to conclude that investigations at rest have understated the degree of cardiopulmonary limitation. Alternatively, if there is no desaturation or widening of the alveolar–arterial oxygen gradient when symptoms cause the premature termination of the test, it is possible to infer that limitation is due to chest discomfort, loss of fitness, or musculoskeletal factors. In general, maximal exercise testing is more often useful in demonstrating the absence of significant cardiopulmonary limitation than in quantifying the impact of pulmonary disease. Maximal exercise testing may be especially helpful when primary hyperventilation is suspected as a cause for increasing exercise intolerance.

Although the 6-min walk test is now widely performed in the routine monitoring of IPF, there are, currently, no compelling data for a similar utility in pulmonary sarcoidosis. In sarcoidosis, in particular, interpretation of 6-min walk data is heavily influenced by musculoskeletal factors, loss of fitness, pulmonary vasculopathy, and separate cardiac involvement. However, the 6-min walk test may provide useful monitoring data in selected patients. The test better reflects normal daily activity than maximal exercise testing, and in patients describing disproportionate exercise intolerance, it provides objective information on the gestalt impact of sarcoidosis in day-to-day life. This is especially helpful when the test demonstrates significantly better exercise tolerance than described by the patient. In the monitoring of advanced disease, the detection of marked desaturation on a 6-min walk test alerts the clinician to the possibility of supervening PH and also serves to identify patients who may benefit from ambulatory oxygen.

Frequency of Monitoring

Early in the course of disease, before the intrinsic progressiveness of pulmonary involvement has become apparent, it is usual to re-evaluate patients at three to four monthly intervals, as is common practice in interstitial lung in general. However, this broad approach must be tailored to individual patients, with earlier re-evaluation if there are rapid symptomatic changes. If pulmonary disease remains stable during the first year and treatment is not instituted, the time interval between assessments can be successively increased with, eventually, annual review. Even in mild stable pulmonary sarcoidosis, it is prudent to continue monitoring for a minimum of 4 years, but more prolonged monitoring is appropriate in moderate to severe disease.

Following the institution of treatment, it is common practice to assess responsiveness to higher dose therapy at 4–6 weeks and to tailor the timing of further monitoring to the treatment plan and initial responsiveness. The severity of disease is an important consideration. If there is major residual disease and further progression would be likely to lead to disability, more frequent monitoring is appropriate than in patients with a good pulmonary reserve. In either event, the severity of disease should be reappraised no longer than 3–4 months after each phase of dose reduction, with the patient warned that early evaluation might be required in the event of worsening symptoms.

Conclusion

No single test stands alone as an arbiter of the evaluation of change in disease severity. Accurate evaluation requires the integration of symptoms, chest radiography, and pulmonary function tests with the use of ancillary tests, including HRCT, serum ACE levels, BAL, and exercise testing in selected patients. Although sometimes an important indicator of disease progression, increasing symptoms are often ascribable to factors other than changes in interstitial lung disease. Pulmonary function tests provide the most reliable data, but it is essential that their limitations are taken into account, including the heterogeneity of pulmonary function patterns in sarcoidosis, the confounding effect of ancillary systemic and cardiopulmonary disease processes, and the problem of measurement variability. The chest radiograph is essentially a blunt instrument in the detection of change, although retaining an important monitoring role. Thus, no single chest radiographic or pulmonary function variable is sufficiently robust to stand alone as the cardinal means of assessing serial change in all patients. A multidisciplinary approach is indispensable in the detection of change in pulmonary sarcoidosis. In routine practice, symptomatic change, the evolution of disease on chest radiography, and pulmonary function trends must be reconciled, although no clear guidance on this process exists in current guidelines. This maxim applies equally to defining responses to treatment, detecting changes in disease severity in other contexts, and the early identification of supervening pulmonary hypertension. In a nutshell, the multidisciplinary evaluation of the evolution of pulmonary sarcoidosis, rather than an undue reliance on any single test, is as important in routine monitoring as it is in the diagnosis of pulmonary sarcoidosis at initial evaluation.

References

1. ATS/ERS/WASOG. Statement on sarcoidosis. Am J Respir Crit Care Med. 1999;160: 736–55.
2. Keogh BA, Crystal RG. Pulmonary function testing in interstitial pulmonary disease. What does it tell us? Chest. 1980;78:856–64.
3. de Kleijn WP, De Vries J, Lower EE, Elfferrich MD, Baughman RP, Drent M. Fatigue in sarcoidosis: a systematic review. Curr Opin Pulm Med. 2009;15:499–506.

4. Pena TA, Soubani AO, Samavati L. Aspergillus lung disease in patients with sarcoidosis: a case series and review of the literature. Lung. 2011;189:167–72.
5. Marcias S, Ledda MA, Perra R, et al. Aspecific bronchial hyperreactivity in pulmonary sarcoidosis. Sarcoidosis. 1994;11:118–22.
6. Latsi PI, du Bois RM, Nicholson AG, et al. Fibrotic idiopathic interstitial pneumonia: the prognostic value of longitudinal functional trends. Am J Respir Crit Care Med. 2003;168:531–7.
7. Flaherty KR, Mumford JA, Murray S, et al. Prognostic implications of physiologic and radiographic changes in idiopathic interstitial pneumonia. Am J Respir Crit Care Med. 2003;168:543–8.
8. Collard HR, King Jr TE, Bartelson BB, Vourlekis JS, Schwarz MI, Brown KK. Changes in clinical and physiologic variables predict survival in idiopathic pulmonary fibrosis. Am J Respir Crit Care Med. 2003;168:538–42.
9. Raghu G, Collard HR, Egan JJ, ATS/ERS/JRS/ALAT Committee on Idiopathic Pulmonary Fibrosis, et al. An official ATS/ERS/JRS/ALAT statement: idiopathic pulmonary fibrosis: evidence-based guidelines for diagnosis and management. Am J Respir Crit Care Med. 2011;183(6):788–824.
10. Cotes JE, Chinn DJ, Miller MR. Lung function. 6th ed. Oxford: Blackwell; 2006. p. 79. ISBN 13:978-0-6320-6493-9.
11. Cotton DJ, Graham BL. The usefulness of Kco is questionable (letter, with response from Hughes JMN, Pride NB). Am J Respir Crit Care Med. 2013;187:660.
12. Neville E, Walker A, James DG. Prognostic factors predicting outcome of sarcoidosis: an analysis of 818 patients. Q J Med. 1983;2:525–33.
13. Romer FK. Presentation of sarcoidosis and outcome of pulmonary changes. Dan Med Bull. 1982;29:27–32.
14. Alhamad EH, Lynch 3rd JP, Martinez FJ. Pulmonary function tests in interstitial lung disease: what role do they have? Clin Chest Med. 2001;22:715–50.
15. Harrison BD, Shaylor JM, Stokes TC, Wilkes AR. Airflow limitation in sarcoidosis: a study of pulmonary function in 107 patients with newly diagnosed disease. Respir Med. 1991;85:59–64.
16. Gleeson FV, Traill ZC, Hansell DM. Evidence of expiratory CT scans of small-airway obstruction in sarcoidosis. AJR Am J Roentgenol. 1996;166:1052–4.
17. Hansell DM, Milne DG, Wilsher ML, Wells AU. Pulmonary sarcoidosis: morphologic associations of airflow obstruction on thin section computed tomography. Radiology. 1998;209:697–704.
18. Carrington CB. Structure and function in sarcoidosis. Ann N Y Acad Sci. 1976;278:265–83.
19. Chambellan A, Turbie P, Nunes H, et al. Endoluminal stenosis of proximal bronchi in sarcoidosis: bronchoscopy, function and evolution. Chest. 2005;127:472–81.
20. Lynch 3rd JP, Kazerooni EA, Gaye SE. Pulmonary sarcoidosis. Clin Chest Med. 1997;18:755–85.
21. Wells AU. Forced vital capacity as a primary end-point in idiopathic pulmonary fibrosis treatment trials: making a silk purse from a sow's ear (editorial). Thorax. 2013;68:309–10.
22. Baumann MH, Strange C, Sahn SA. Do chest radiographic findings reflect the clinical course of patients with sarcoidosis during corticosteroid withdrawal. AJR Am J Roentgenol. 1990;154:481–5.
23. ILO Guidelines for the Use of ILO International Classification of Radiographs of Pneumoconioses. Occupational Safety Series #22. Geneva: International Labor Office; 1980.
24. Judson MA, Gilbert GE, Rodgers JK, Greer CF, Schabel SI. The utility of the chest radiograph in diagnosing exacerbations of pulmonary sarcoidosis. Respirology. 2008;13:97–102.
25. Gibson GJ, Prescott RJ, Muers MF, Mitchell DN. British Thoracic Society Sarcoidosis study: effects of long term corticosteroid treatment. Thorax. 1996;51:238–47.
26. Muers MF, Middleton WG, Gibson GJ, et al. A simple radiographic scoring method for monitoring pulmonary sarcoidosis: relations between radiographic scores, dyspnea grade and respiratory function in the British Thoracic Society Study of Long-Term Corticosteroid Treatment. Sarcoidosis Vasc Diffuse Lung Dis. 1997;14:46–56.
27. Baughman RP, Desai S, Drent M, et al. Changes in chest roentgenogram of sarcoidosis patients during a clinical trial of Infliximab therapy: comparison of different methods of evaluation. Chest. 2009;136:526–35.

28. Zappala CJ, Desai SR, Copley SJ, et al. Optimal scoring of serial change on chest radiography in sarcoidosis. Sarcoidosis Vasc Diffuse Lung Dis. 2011;28:130–8.
29. Costabel U, Guzman M. Bronchoalveolar lavage in interstitial lung disease. Curr Opin Pulm Med. 2001;7:255–61.
30. Remy-Jardin M, Giraud F, Remy J, et al. Pulmonary sarcoidosis: role of CT in the evaluation of disease activity and functional impairment and in prognosis assessment. Radiology. 1994;191:675–80.
31. Drent M, De Vries J, Lenters M, et al. Sarcoidosis: assessment of disease severity using HRCT. Eur Radiol. 2003;13:2462–71.
32. Oberstein A, von Zitzewitz H, Schweden F, Muller-Quernheim J. Non-invasive evaluation of the inflammatory activity in sarcoidosis with high-resolution computed tomography. Sarcoidosis Vasc Diffuse Lung Dis. 1997;14:65–72.
33. Turner-Warwick M, McAllister W, Lawrence R, Britten A, Haslam PL. Corticosteroid treatment in pulmonary sarcoidosis: do serial lavage lymphocyte counts, serum angiotensin converting enzyme measurements, and gallium-67 scans help management? Thorax. 1986;41:9903–13.
34. Shorr AF, Torrington KG, Parker JM. Serum angiotensin converting enzyme does not correlate with radiographic stage at initial diagnosis of sarcoidosis. Respir Med. 1997;91:399–401.
35. Leung AN, Brauner MW, Caillat-Vigneron N, Valeyre D, Grenier P. Sarcoidosis activity: correlation of HRCT findings with those of 67Ga scanning, bronchoalveolar lavage, and serum angiotensin-converting enzyme assay. J Comput Assist Tomogr. 1998;22:229–34.
36. Bradley B, Branley HM, Egan JJ, et al. Interstitial lung disease guideline: the British Thoracic Society in collaboration with the Thoracic Society of Australia and New Zealand and the Irish Thoracic Society. Thorax. 2008;63(Suppl V):v1–58.
37. Ziegenhagen MW, Benner UK, Zissel G, et al. Sarcoidosis: TNF-alpha release from alveolar macrophages and serum level of sIL-2R are prognostic markers. Am J Respir Crit Care Med. 1997;156:1586–92.
38. Keicho N, Kitamura K, Takaku F, Yotsumoto H. Serum concentration of soluble interleukin-2 receptor as a sensitive parameter of disease activity in sarcoidosis. Chest. 1990;98:1125–9.
39. Grutters JC, Fellrath JM, Mulder L, et al. Serum soluble interleukin-2 receptor measurement in patients with sarcoidosis: a clinical evaluation. Chest. 2003;124:186–95.
40. Müller-Quernheim J, Pfeifer S, Strausz J, Ferlinz R. Correlation of clinical and immunologic parameters of the inflammatory activity of pulmonary sarcoidosis. Am Rev Respir Dis. 1991;144:1322–9.
41. Ziegenhagen MW, Rothe ME, Schlaak M, Muller-Quernheim J. Bronchoalveolar and serological parameters reflecting the severity of sarcoidosis. Eur Respir J. 2003;21:407–13.
42. Drent M, Jacobs J, de Vries J, et al. Does the cellular bronchoalveolar lavage fluid profile reflect the severity of sarcoidosis? Eur Respir J. 1999;13:1338–44.
43. Teirstein AS, Machac J, Almeida O, et al. Results of 188 whole-body fluorodeoxyglucose positron emission tomography scans in 137 patients with sarcoidosis. Chest. 2007;132:1949–53.
44. Nishiyama Y, Yamamoto Y, Fukunaga K, et al. Comparative evaluation of 18F-FDG PET and 67 Ga scintigraphy in patients with sarcoidosis. J Nucl Med. 2006;47:1571–6.
45. Braun JJ, Kessler R, Constantinesco A, Imperiale A. 18 F-FDG PET/CT in sarcoidosis management: review and report of 20 cases. Eur J Nucl Med Mol Imaging. 2008;35:1537–43.
46. Keijsers RGM, Verzijbergen JF, van Diepen DM, van den Bosch JMM, Grutters JC. 18 F-FDG PET in sarcoidosis: an observational study in 12 patients treated with Infliximab. Sarcoidosis Vasc Diffuse Lung Dis. 2008;25:143–50.
47. Handa T, Nagai S, Miki S, et al. Incidence of pulmonary hypertension and its clinical relevance in sarcoidosis. Chest. 2006;129:1246–53.
48. Baughman RP, Engel PJ, Meyer CA, Barett AB, Lower EE. Pulmonary hypertension in sarcoidosis. Sarcoidosis Vasc Diffuse Lung Dis. 2006;23:108–16.
49. Burke CM, Glanville AR, Morris AJR, et al. Pulmonary function in advanced pulmonary hypertension. Thorax. 1987;42:151–5.
50. Steen VD, Graham G, Conte C, Owens G, Medsger Jr TA. Isolated diffusing capacity reduction in systemic sclerosis. Arthritis Rheum. 1992;35:765–70.
51. Nathan SD, Shlobin OA, Ahmad S, Urbanek S, Barnett SD. Pulmonary hypertension and pulmonary function testing in idiopathic pulmonary fibrosis. Chest. 2007;131:657–63.

Chapter 8
Extrapulmonary Sarcoidosis

Hidenobu Shigemitsu, Hiren V. Patel, and Matthew P. Schreiber

Abstract Sarcoidosis is a systemic granulomatous disorder that can involve any organ in the body. Although the lungs are the most commonly affected organs, extrapulmonary involvements are not uncommon and contribute to the morbidity. The decision to treat extrapulmonary sarcoidosis is dependent on specific organs as not all organ involvement requires treatment. This chapter is a comprehensive review of the clinical presentation, diagnostic pathways, and therapeutic interventions in extrapulmonary sarcoidosis.

Keywords Sarcoidosis • Extrapulmonary • Diagnosis • Treatment

Introduction

Sarcoidosis is a systemic granulomatous disorder with unclear etiology that can involve any organ in the body. Although the lungs are the most commonly affected organ, concomitant involvement of extrapulmonary organs is common and can be seen in up to 50 % of cases of sarcoidosis [1]. Conversely, only 2 % of cases in A Case–Control Etiologic Study of Sarcoidosis (ACCESS) were found to have

H. Shigemitsu, M.D. (✉)
Division of Pulmonary and Critical Care Medicine, University of Southern California Keck School of Medicine, Los Angeles, CA, USA

Division of Pulmonary and Critical Care Medicine, University of Nevada School of Medicine, 2040 West Charleston Blvd Suite 300, Las Vegas, NV 89102, USA
e-mail: hshigemi@gmail.com

H.V. Patel, M.D. • M.P. Schreiber, M.D.
Division of Pulmonary and Critical Care Medicine, University of Nevada School of Medicine, Las Vegas, NV, USA

M.A. Judson (ed.), *Pulmonary Sarcoidosis: A Guide for the Practicing Clinician,*
Respiratory Medicine 17, DOI 10.1007/978-1-4614-8927-6_8,
© Springer Science+Business Media New York 2014

extrapulmonary involvement without pulmonary disease [1]. Extrapulmonary sarcoidosis is important to recognize as it adds to the morbidity, mortality, and reduction of quality of life in patients with pulmonary sarcoidosis.

The prevalence and the extent of extrapulmonary sarcoidosis vary on the demographic of the population that is affected from this disease. For example, African Americans are typically more likely to be affected from extrapulmonary sarcoidosis than Caucasians. However, dysfunction of calcium metabolism is found more in Caucasians. A study comparing the manifestations of sarcoidosis in Japanese and Finnish subjects revealed the rates of sarcoidosis in the heart and eyes to be significantly higher in Japanese subjects [2]. Additionally, extrapulmonary sarcoidosis appears to be more common in females, especially with ocular sarcoidosis, erythema nodosum, and neurosarcoidosis [1]. Finally, peripheral lymph nodes were more commonly seen in subjects with ages less than 40 as opposed to dysfunction of calcium metabolism were significantly higher with ages greater than 40 [1].

Extrapulmonary sarcoidosis can develop anytime during the course of the disease. A detailed physical examination in addition to basic laboratory tests (complete blood cell count, complete metabolic panel including serum calcium and urinalysis), electrocardiogram, ophthalmic examination, and imaging studies are essential in detecting extrapulmonary disease. In general, the diagnosis of extrapulmonary sarcoidosis is typically based on the combination of these clinical evaluations and diagnostic studies with histologic evidence of noncaseating granulomas. It is important to note that histological evidence is not necessarily required from the particular organ of interest to make the diagnosis of extrapulmonary sarcoidosis as long as sarcoidosis has been histologically confirmed in another organ. As part of ACCESS, Judson and colleagues have proposed criteria that categorize the likelihood of each potential organ to definite, probable, and possible involvement (Table 8.1) [1, 3].

The decision whether to institute treatment in extrapulmonary sarcoidosis is dependent on specific organs involved and the extent of organ involvement as not all extrapulmonary sarcoidosis requires treatment. In fact, asymptomatic extrapulmonary involvement typically does not require treatment. However, neurologic, cardiac, and ocular involvement typically mandates treatment as the sequelae are significant and potentially life threatening.

Neurosarcoidosis

Epidemiology

Neurosarcoidosis is a less common manifestation of sarcoidosis with a prevalence of 5–13 % of sarcoidosis with symptomatic neurologic involvement, although, other studies have quoted up to 26–45 % [4, 5]. A prospective epidemiologic study of 736 patients in the USA (ACCESS) found that only 4.6 % had definite or probable neurosarcoidosis [1]. In another study, almost 25 % of systemic sarcoidosis patients

Table 8.1 Clinical criteria for extrapulmonary sarcoidosis organ involvement in patients with biopsy-confirmed sarcoidosis in another organ[a]

Organ	Definite	Probable	Possible
Skin	1. Lupus pernio 2. Annular lesion 3. Erythema nodosum	1. Macular/popular 2. New nodules	1. Keloids 2. Hypopigmentation
Eyes	1. Lacrimal gland swelling 2. Uveitis 3. Optic neuritis	1. Blindness	1. Glaucoma 2. Cataract
Liver	1. Liver function tests >three times normal	1. Compatible computed tomography (CT) scan 2. Elevated alkaline phosphate	
Hypercalcemia/hypercalciuria/nephrolithiasis	1. Increased serum calcium with no other cause	1. Increased urine calcium 2. Nephrolithiasis analysis showing calcium	1. Nephrolithiasis-no stone analysis 2. Nephrolithiasis with negative family history for stones
Neurological	1. Positive magnetic resonance imaging (MRI) with uptake in meninges or brainstem 2. Cerebrospinal fluid with increased lymphocytes and/or protein 3. Diabetes insipidus 4. Bell's palsy 5. Cranial nerve dysfunction 6. Peripheral nerve biopsy	1. Other abnormalities on magnetic resonance imaging (MRI) 2. Unexplained neuropathy 3. Positive electromyogram	1. Unexplained headaches 2. Peripheral nerve radiculopathy
Renal	1. Treatment responsive renal failure	1. Steroid responsive renal failure in patient with diabetes and/or hypertension	1. Renal failure in absence of other disease

Cardiac	1. Treatment responsive cardiomyopathy
	2. Electrocardiogram showing intraventricular conduction defect or nodal block
	3. Positive gallium scan of heart
		1. No other cardiac problem and either:
		  – Ventricular arrhythmia
		  – Cardiomyopathy
			1. In patient with diabetes and/or hypertension:
			  – Cardiomyopathy
			  – Ventricular arrhythmias

(continued)

Table 8.1 (continued)

Organ	Definite	Probable	Possible
Non-thoracic lymph node		1. Palpable node above the waist 2. Lymph node > 2 cm by CT scan	1. New palpable femoral lymph node
Bone marrow	1. Unexplained anemia 2. Leukopenia 3. Thrombocytopenia		1. Anemia with low mean corpuscular volume (MCV)

Spleen		1. Enlargement by:
		  – Exam
		  – CT scan
		  – Radioisotope scan	

Bone/joints	1. Cystic changes on hand or feet phalanges	1. Asymmetric, painful clubbing	1. Arthritis with no other cause
Ear/nose/throat		1. Unexplained hoarseness with exam consistent with granulomatous involvement	1. New onset sinusitis 2. New onset dizziness
Parotids/salivary glands	1. Symmetric parotitis with syndrome of mumps 2. Positive gallium scan ("Panda Sign")		1. Dry mouth
Muscles	1. Increased creatine phosphokinase (CK)/aldolase, which decrease with treatment	1. Increase CK/aldolase	1. Myalgias responding to treatment

[a]There can be no other explanation for the clinical finding in this table for these criteria to be valid. In addition, biopsy of each of these organs would constitute "definite" involvement. Adapted from Judson et al. [3]

were found to have CNS involvement on autopsy and 10 % had evidence of CNS involvement by imaging studies with or without neurologic manifestations [6].

Furthermore, less than 1 % of sarcoidosis patients have isolated neurosarcoidosis without any clinical evidence of extraneural sarcoid. The true incidence remains elusive as making a diagnosis poses a challenge to clinicians as procedures to obtain histological confirmation can lead to life-threatening circumstances.

Clinical Presentation

Cranial Neuropathies

The most common manifestation in neurosarcoidosis includes cranial neuropathies, especially with optic and facial nerves which accounts for 23–70 % of neurologic manifestations in neurosarcoidosis [7]. Facial nerve palsy is the most commonly affected cranial nerves and it presents more commonly as a unilateral finding, although a third of the facial nerve palsy may involve both facial nerves [4]. In one series of 24 patients with facial nerve palsy from sarcoidosis, a complete recovery of about 23 out of 24 patients was observed with treatment using corticosteroids and/or in combination of nonsteroidal immunomodulators [8]. Optic neuritis is the second most commonly affected cranial nerves and it usually presents with diplopia or visual defects (Fig. 8.1). Bilateral disease portends a poorer prognosis versus unilateral disease. Involvement of the base of the brain is thought to be the cause of cranial neuropathies; however, infiltration or compression of nerves may also cause dysfunction [4, 9].

Meningeal Involvement

The occurrence of acute or chronic meningitis ranges from 8 to 40 % of neurologic manifestation of sarcoidosis. This is usually due to meningeal infiltration involving the basal leptomeninges (Fig. 8.2). Clinically it can manifest with headaches, neck stiffness, hydrocephalus, or cranial nerve palsies. The course can be monophasic, chronic, or relapsing. Acute meningitis responds well to corticosteroids and has favorable outcomes [9]. Chronic meningitis often requires long-term treatment with a tendency to relapse.

Seizures

Seizures can occur in up to 22 % of patients with neurosarcoidosis and can occur secondary to leptomeningeal involvement, parenchymal masses, encephalopathy, vasculopathy, hydrocephalus, and metabolic disturbances related to hypothalamic dysfunction [1, 7, 9]. Prognosis of seizures remains controversial as older studies described a poor prognosis; however, more recent studies suggest no evidence in support of the unfavorable prognosis [8, 10].

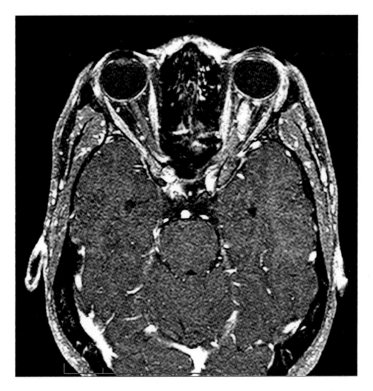

Fig. 8.1 MRI image showing enhancement of optic nerve typical for sarcoid infiltration

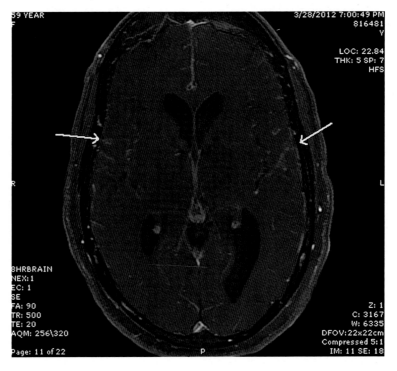

Fig. 8.2 T1-weighted contrast-enhanced MRI image of mild leptomeningeal enhancement and nodules along Sylvian fissures

Hypothalamic/Pituitary Involvement

Endocrinopathies related to neurosarcoidosis are related to granulomatous infiltration of the hypothalamo-hypophyseal region. Hyperprolactinemia (3–32 %) and diabetes insipidus (17–90 %) are the most frequent reported endocrinopathies in neurosarcoidosis. Other clinical features resulting from hypothalamo-pituitary involvement include morbid obesity, dysregulation of body temperature, insomnia, personality changes, syndrome of inappropriate antidiuretic hormone secretion (SIADH), hypothyroidism, hypoadrenalism, growth hormone deficiency, and impaired counter-regulatory response to hypoglycemia [11, 12].

Peripheral Neuropathy

The manifestation of peripheral neuropathy in neurosarcoidosis carries a wide spectrum of symptoms. In a study examining 11 patients with confirmed histologic changes consistent with peripheral nerve involvement from sarcoidosis, Said and colleagues were able to describe Guillain–Barre syndrome like presentation with ascending and progressive muscle weakness with paresthesias, multifocal neuropathies, and sensory polyneuropathies [13].

Small fiber neuropathy is a subtype of peripheral neuropathy or a "paraneuropathy" involving thinly myelinated and unmyelinated nerve fibers causing an aggregate loss of intraepidermal nerve fibers. The typical symptoms consist of pain, dysesthesias (44 %), and abnormal temperature dysfunction (81 %). Additionally, autonomic dysfunction has been described in relation to the small fiber neuropathy [14, 15].

Diagnosis

The process of diagnosing neurosarcoidosis poses a significant challenge to clinicians due to its diverse clinical presentations, nonspecific imaging and laboratory findings, and difficulty in obtaining a neural tissue biopsy. There are two diagnostic criteria that have been summarized by Zajicek et al. [9] (Table 8.2) and Judson et al. [3] (Table 8.1) Both of these criteria have three categories of diagnosis including definite, probable, and possible neurosarcoidosis. For a diagnosis of definite neurosarcoidosis, biopsy of the neural tissue is a prerequisite in the criteria proposed by Zajicek et al., whereas it is not required in the criteria proposed by Judson et al. The latter criteria provide some clinical advantage and practicality in diagnosing patients with a high likelihood of neurosarcoidosis, although there have been no direct comparative studies between these two proposals. As for the diagnosis of probable and possible neurosarcoidosis, various combinations of clinical presentations, imaging studies, and laboratory findings are used to confirm the diagnosis.

Histological confirmation of noncaseating granulomas from neural tissue without any evidence of infectious etiology is the gold standard. However, this option is often impractical due to inherent risks associated with procedures in obtaining neural tissue. If biopsy is considered, it usually involves the meninges or a parenchymal

Table 8.2 Diagnostic criteria for neurosarcoidosis adapted from Zajicek et al. [9]

Definite

Clinical presentation suggestive of neurosarcoidosis with exclusion of other possible diagnoses
  and the presence of positive nervous system histology

Probable

Clinical syndrome suggestive of neurosarcoidosis with laboratory support for CNS inflammation
  (elevated levels of CSF protein and/or cells, the presence of oligoclonal bands and/or MRI
  evidence compatible with neurosarcoidosis) and exclusion of alternative diagnoses together
  with evidence for systemic sarcoidosis (either through positive histology, including Kveim
  test, and/or at least two indirect indicators from Gallium scan, chest imaging and serum ACE)

Possible

Clinical presentation suggestive of neurosarcoidosis with exclusion of alternative diagnoses
  where the above criteria are not met

---

lesion apparent on the imaging study. Accordingly, sampling of tissue from areas that have evidence of involvement by imaging studies improve the sensitivity of the biopsy [16]. Therefore, tissue biopsy is typically obtained from extraneural areas to secure the diagnosis with sarcoidosis which coupled with clinical manifestations can lead to the diagnosis of probable or possible neurosarcoidosis [4].

There is considerable overlap with neurosarcoidosis and other neurologic diseases that mimic neurosarcoidosis based on clinical manifestations. Therefore, the differential diagnoses one must consider in those suspected with neurosarcoidosis include, lymphoma, infections (tuberculous, fungal), Wegener's granulomatosis, Lyme disease, Behcet's disease, and vasculitis. The differential diagnosis for neurosarcoidosis with ocular involvement includes, multiple sclerosis, which typically has more optic nerve involvement than anterior uveitis [4].

Noninvasive test imaging of the brain and spine by MRI with gadolinium contrast is extremely useful with both aiding in diagnosis and in following treatment effect. Common findings on brain MRI are dural involvement (34 %), leptomeningeal enhancement (31 %), cranial nerve enhancement (34 %), and enhancing parenchymal lesions (22 %) [16]. Other areas involved on MRI, include hypothalamus and pituitary involvement (9 %) seen as thickening and enhancement on T1-weighted images [6, 17]. Hydrocephalus occurs in 5–12 % of cases with neurosarcoidosis which can be due to involvement of the dura or leptomeninges by altering the resorption of cerebrospinal fluid (CSF). Common finding on spine MRI are enhancing intramedullary lesions (13 %), enhancing extramedullary lesions (6 %), and cauda equina enhancement (6 %) [16]. MRI findings, however, are nonspecific for neurosarcoidosis as previous studies have shown that lesions seen on MRI can be related to MS (46 %), metastatic disease (36 %), high grade astrocytomas (9 %), and meningioma (5 %) [18].

Other tests that can be used in combination with histology and imaging include cerebrospinal fluid (CSF) analysis. CSF analysis is quite nonspecific as the typical findings for neurosarcoidosis includes lymphocytosis, elevated protein levels, pleocytosis, hypoglycorrhachia, and positive oligoclonal bands. However all of these findings can be seen in a multitude of diseases such as MS, infections, and

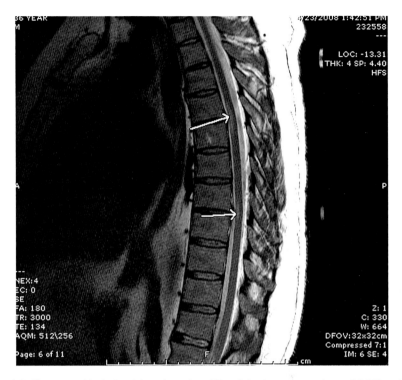

Fig. 8.3 Neurosarcoidosis involving the spine. T2-weighted, contrast-enhanced MRI sagittal images demonstrating two areas of enhancements involving the thoracic spine

vasculitis. CSF analysis may not help with establishing a diagnosis; however, it can exclude possible infectious etiologies such as cryptococcal, tuberculous, and lymphomatous meningitis [4]. The diagnostic utility of CSF angiotensin-converting enzyme (ACE) is uncertain. Elevated CSF ACE levels have a sensitivity and specificity of 55 % and 94 %, respectively [19]. However, other inflammatory diseases such as MS, Bechet's disease, and Guillan–Barre syndrome are also associated with elevated ACE levels [20].

Treatment

Neurosarcoidosis can range from being a self-limiting disease to a chronic and progressive disease. Isolated cranial nerve involvement (i.e., facial nerve palsy) and aseptic meningitis have a good chance of spontaneous recovery or resolution with a short course of corticosteroids [16]. Those with chronic remitting–relapsing course, such as those with parenchymal, leptomeningeal disease, myopathy, or spinal disease will require more intense treatment (Fig. 8.3).

The mainstay of treatment is with the use of corticosteroids. To date, there are no clinical trials to establish initial doses or duration of therapy. However, there is consensus opinion within the field of starting prednisone at doses of 40–80 mg/day [7]. The statement guideline from the American Thoracic Society recommends use of prednisone at 1 mg/kg or its equivalent in severe cases when high dose steroids is necessary [21]. Full recovery with use of corticosteroids or combination of corticosteroids with another immunomodulatory agent varies in range from 29 to 76 % [9, 22–25]. However, Zajicek and colleagues reported that despite treatment with corticosteroids, disease progression or recurring symptoms were observed in about 70 % of patients with neurosarcoidosis during follow-up [9]. Corticosteroid therapy in moderate to severe cases usually mandates prolonged duration of therapy over months to years. As a result, patients become highly susceptible to unwanted side effects from long-term therapy of corticosteroids including osteoporosis, glucose intolerance, weight gain, neuropathy, myopathy, and peptic ulcer disease.

Steroid-sparing immunomodulator therapy may be necessary in patients who are not responding to corticosteroid therapy alone or if they develop intolerance to prolonged corticosteroid therapy. Nonsteroidal immunomodulators include agents such as methotrexate, cyclosporine, azathioprine, cyclophosphamide, chlorambucil, chloroquine, and mycophenolate.

Stern and colleagues were able to lower baseline corticosteroid therapy doses by 30–58 % with the addition of cyclosporine at doses of at 4 mg/kg/day with monitoring of cyclosporine trough levels and for adverse effects of hypertension, renal failure, hypomagnesemia, and neurotoxicity [26].

Methotrexate, another well-known steroid-sparing agent can be started at a dose from 5 to 15 mg/week. The side effects include hepatotoxicity, pulmonary toxicity, and renal toxicity. Hematologic effects such as neutropenia, anemia, and thrombocytopenia can also be seen with methotrexate; however, the side effects can be minimized with the addition of folic acid. Lower and colleagues were able to obtain a beneficial response in 61 % of steroid refractory patients with neurosarcoidosis [8].

Cyclophosphamide is highly toxic with side effects that include bone marrow suppression, teratogenicity, and carcinogenicity. It is usually limited to patients with severe neurosarcoidosis refractory to other agents. One study showed reduction of corticosteroid doses by as much as 58 % with symptomatic and radiologic recovery [27].

Recent case reports using infliximab, a tumor necrosis factor alpha (TNFα) inhibitor, have demonstrated successful treatment of refractory neurosarcoidosis. One case series included seven patients who received infliximab infusion with dramatic improvements in neurologic symptoms after 1–3 infusions; however, symptoms and radiologic abnormalities recurred after cessation of therapy. These patients responded well after reinstitution of infliximab therapy [28].

Prognosis

In general, prognosis in neurosarcoidosis is difficult to predict, although the prognosis to some degree appears to be dependent on the clinical manifestation. Facial nerve palsy and acute meningeal involvement portend a more favorable prognosis [4]. Heerfordt syndrome, which consists of the triad of facial nerve palsy, parotitis, and anterior uveitis, also predicts a favorable prognosis [29].

Myelopathy is associated with poor prognosis based of a case series of 30 cases [30]. In another study that followed 79 patients with seizures and neurosarcoidosis, these patients had more severe, progressive, or relapsing forms of CNS sarcoidosis [10]. Involvement of bilateral optic nerves is also associated with poor prognosis [31].

Cardiac Sarcoidosis

Epidemiology

In the USA, cardiac involvement that is clinically apparent is seen in only minority of patients with sarcoidosis. However approximately 25 % of patients with systemic sarcoidosis had myocardial involvement observed during autopsy [32]. Cardiac sarcoidosis has a poor prognosis with a median survival of less than 2 years following development of clinical signs and symptoms of myocardial involvement [33]. It accounts for about 13–25 % of deaths and is the second most common cause of death from sarcoidosis [34]. In contrast to the USA, up to 85 % of deaths from sarcoidosis in Japan is reported to be from cardiac sarcoidosis, suggesting a geographic and ethnic predilection [33].

Clinical Presentations

The clinical presentation in cardiac sarcoidosis is protean and may be generally categorized into heart failure, conduction abnormalities, and pericardial disease. Only 5 % of patients with cardiac sarcoidosis manifest signs and symptoms that suggest cardiac involvement [34]. The symptoms may be subtle including dyspnea and fatigue. Other symptoms such as palpitations and syncope suggest involvement of the myocardium and conduction system, whereas angina and pleuritic chest pain may raise the suspicion of myocardial and pericardial involvement. In rare instances, sudden cardiac death may occur.

Heart Failure

Heart failure is a significant morbidity in cardiac sarcoidosis and is seen in 23 % of patients with cardiac sarcoidosis [34]. Both restrictive and dilated cardiomyopathy can occur leading to ventricular dysfunction that causes heart failure. In addition, 14–59 % have diastolic dysfunction on echocardiography findings [35, 36]. Furthermore, cor pulmonale as a sequelae of secondary pulmonary hypertension due to sarcoidosis can account for about 5–15 % of heart failure due to sarcoidosis. The functional status of the heart failure is closely related with the prognosis as congestive heart failure is the most common cause of death accounting for approximately 73 % of deaths from cardiac sarcoidosis [36]. In a retrospective study of 95 patients, Yazaki and colleagues demonstrated that worsening of NYHA functional class by one functional class, sustained ventricular tachycardia, and left ventricular end-diastolic diameter were independent predictors of mortality. In the same study, the severity of congestive heart failure was the most powerful prognostic predictor in steroid-treated patients with cardiac sarcoidosis [37].

Conduction Abnormalities

Third-degree heart block or complete heart block is the most common presentation (25–30 %) of conduction abnormalities in cardiac sarcoidosis and it usually presents at a younger age [33]. Bundle branch block occurs in 12–61 % of cases with a predominant presentation of right bundle branch block (RBBB) [38]. These occur as a result of granuloma or scar tissue involving the nodal artery causing ischemia or by direct involvement of the conduction system. The incidence of ventricular tachycardia (VT) is 23 %, with approximately 68 % of the time as a result of reentry mechanisms [33]. Atrial fibrillation/flutter occurs in 19 % of patients due to cardiac sarcoidosis [35]. These supraventricular arrhythmias may be due to atrial dilatation or inflammatory processes involving the atrial foci. Based on an antemortem study of 113 patients, sudden cardiac death was usually caused by arrhythmias with an incidence of about 67 %. Consequently, 35 % of sudden cardiac deaths were the initial manifestation of cardiac sarcoidosis [38].

Pericardial Disease

Pericardial involvement has been demonstrated by echocardiography in about 19 % of patients with sarcoidosis [34]. The clinical presentation for pericardial disease includes pericardial effusion and pericarditis [39]. It is rare for constrictive pericarditis and cardiac tamponade to develop in patients with cardiac sarcoidosis [40, 41]. However, there is significant incidence of asymptomatic pericardial effusion. In a Greek study of 81 histologically confirmed sarcoidosis patients who underwent echocardiogram studies, 21 % of them had mild to moderate pericardial effusions with no clinical evidence of heart disease [42].

Diagnosis

There are multiple diagnostic criteria for cardiac sarcoidosis. The American Thoracic Society (ATS) and World Association for Sarcoidosis and Other Granulomatous Disorders (WASOGD) define cardiac sarcoidosis as cardiac

Table 8.3 Adapted from the Japanese Ministry of Health and Welfare criteria for the diagnosis of cardiac sarcoidosis

Histologic diagnosis: Histologic analysis of endomyocardial biopsy demonstrating epithelioid, noncaseating granulomas

Clinical diagnosis: Histologic confirmation of extracardiac sarcoid demonstrating epithelioid, noncaseating granulomas with the presence of ECG abnormalities (complete RBBB, left axis deviation, AV block, VT, premature ventricular contractions, or abnormal Q or ST-T wave changes) with one or more of the following:

  (a) Abnormal wall motion, regional wall thinning, or dilation of the ventricle

  (b) Perfusion defect by thallium-201 scintigraphy or abnormal accumulation by gallium-67 or technetium-99m scintigraphy

  (c) Depressed ejection fraction, low cardiac output

  (d) Moderate-grade interstitial fibrosis or cellular infiltration on biopsy

dysfunction, ECG abnormalities, and thallium-201 scan defects with or without endomyocardial biopsy [21]. Other criteria adapted from the ACCESS report describe definite cardiac involvement as treatment-responsive cardiomyopathy, ECGs with conduction defects, and positive cardiac gallium scans.

A more widely used standard is from the Japanese Ministry of Health and Welfare (1993) which includes histologic and clinical diagnosis criteria (Table 8.3). Diagnosis of cardiac sarcoidosis is confirmed either by histologic diagnosis or clinical diagnosis group. Histologic diagnosis requires an endomyocardial biopsy demonstrating epithelioid, noncaseating granuloma. Alternatively, diagnosis of cardiac sarcoidosis by the clinical diagnosis group is confirmed on the basis of histologic diagnosis of extracardiac sarcoidosis and the presence of ECG abnormality (complete RBBB, left axis deviation, AV block, VT, premature ventricular contraction, or abnormal Q or ST changes) with the addition of any one of the following criteria: abnormal wall motion, regional wall thinning, or dilation of ventricle; perfusion defect on thallium-201 scintigraphy; decreased ejection fraction or low cardiac output; or moderate interstitial fibrosis or cellular infiltration on endomyocardial biopsy [34].

Endomyocardial Biopsy

Histologic confirmation of myocardial involvement is the gold standard for the diagnosis of cardiac sarcoidosis. However, lack of biopsy confirmation or negative findings do not exclude diagnosis of cardiac sarcoidosis in patients with suspected involvement. The sensitivity of endomyocardial biopsy is variable and reported to be in the range of 25–75 % as opposed to its high specificity of almost 100 % [29, 43, 44]. The wide range of sensitivity is thought to be related with sampling error that is inherent with endomyocardial biopsies and secondary to the patchy distribution of the disease. The procedure itself is performed transvenously and the biopsy is usually obtained from the apical septum whereas the typical distribution of sarcoid granuloma tends to be in the basal areas. Accordingly, sampling accuracy is dependent on the location, where the likelihood of diagnosing sarcoidosis from the right ventricular endomyocardial biopsy was 71 % versus 57 % from the left ventricle [45].

Electrocardiography

Electrocardiography (ECG) abnormalities occur in about 20–50 % of patients with cardiac sarcoidosis. First, second- and third-degree AV blocks may be seen. In a study of 41 patients with long-term corticosteroid therapy, 75 % of subjects experienced resolution of atrioventricular block [46]. Arrhythmias such as ventricular tachycardia and paroxysmal atrial fibrillation can be better assessed with the use of Holter monitor.

Echocardiography

Echocardiography has been useful in the diagnosis of cardiac sarcoidosis as an indirect assessment of the myocardium. Echocardiography can be used for assessment of systolic function, diastolic function, and regional wall motion abnormalities. In cardiac sarcoidosis, granulomatous infiltration can lead to heart failure with segmental wall motion abnormality, global hypokinesis, asymmetric septal hypertrophy, and apical hypertrophy [46]. Thus, echocardiography can be used as a screening tool to detect these abnormalities that may prompt further evaluation with other noninvasive imaging processes such as thallium scanning, gallium scanning, cardiac MRI, or FDG-PET scan to confirm areas of sarcoid involvement.

Noninvasive Nuclear Radiography

Cardiac sarcoidosis has adopted three different nuclear medicine scans to help in the diagnosis of cardiac sarcoidosis. Thallium-201 scintigraphy for diagnosis of cardiac sarcoidosis has been in practice since the 1970s. Thallium scanning can identify focal myocardial defects in uptake of the radio-labeled thallium. On autopsy of patients that have undergone thallium scans, histologic evidence of noncaseating granulomas indicative of granulomatous infiltration of myocardium was evident in areas that were positive on thallium scans [47].

Gallium scanning may also aid in assessing myocardial infiltration from sarcoidosis as uptake of radio-labeled gallium are seen in areas with active inflammation or where rapid cell division is occurring. The sensitivity of 96 % is quite excellent with active inflammation; however, the specificity is 37.5 % [48]. The use of Gallium scan to monitor disease progression is less optimal for two reasons; the first being the radiation exposure which makes for repetition of more often than twice yearly undesirable. Second, prednisone treatment may inhibit gallium uptake which poses difficulty with the practicality of its use as a monitoring tool [47]. Therefore gallium scan may be used as an adjunct modality to aide in difficult diagnostic problems in cases of suspected sarcoidosis, but not as a single tool to diagnose or monitor disease activity in cardiac sarcoidosis.

Recently, FDG-PET scanning has been shown to be useful in cardiac sarcoidosis. In one Japanese study, Yamagishi and colleagues compared thallium and gallium scan against FDG-PET scanning in patients with cardiac sarcoidosis [49]. The authors found that thallium scan and gallium scan were able to detect myocardial defects in

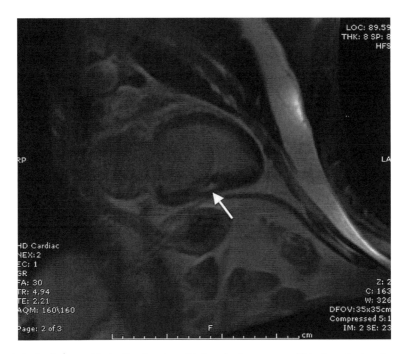

Fig. 8.4 Cardiac sarcoidosis. Focal region of delayed enhancement within the subepicardium and myocardium in the inferior aspect of the left ventricular wall Gadolinium enhanced CMR

35 % and 17 % of the cases, respectively, whereas FDG-PET was able to detect myocardial abnormalities in 82 % of the cases. However, myocardial PET scan abnormalities may represent ischemia and thus a positive finding must be followed with a negative coronary study to confirm the significance of a positive PET scan [50].

Gadolinium-Enhanced Cardiac Magnetic Resonance Imaging

Cardiac magnetic resonance imaging (CMR) is used to assess myocardium in myocardial infarction, hypertrophic cardiomyopathy, and cardiac hypertrophy. It has been adapted in the utility of cardiac sarcoidosis as a noninvasive diagnostic test and to evaluate treatment efficacy.

A prospective study including 58 patients with histologic confirmation of extracardiac sarcoidosis underwent evaluation of cardiac sarcoidosis [51]. This study investigated the accuracy of the various diagnostic modalities outlined by the Japanese Ministry of Health which included ECG, transthoracic echocardiogram, thallium scintigraphy, and CMR. The sensitivity and specificity for CMR were 100 % and 78 %, respectively. CMR had a positive predictive value (PPV) and negative predictive value (NPV) of 55 % and 100 %, respectively. The significant findings seen on CMR included regional contrast enhancement, segmental enhancement, and decreased LVEF (Fig. 8.4).

CMR has also been studied to follow treatment response of cardiac sarcoidosis [44]. One case series followed 16 sarcoidosis patients who underwent CMR for assessment of cardiac involvement of sarcoidosis. The investigators repeated the scan for assessment of treatment efficacy after 1 month of steroid therapy. All eight patients with positive CMR findings showed resolution of abnormal findings on CMR after 1 month of systemic steroid treatment. CMR may prove to be useful in early diagnosis and assessing treatment efficacy in cardiac sarcoidosis.

Treatment

Corticosteroid

Corticosteroid therapy has been the cornerstone therapy in cardiac sarcoidosis supported by case reports and case series which showed resolution of symptoms, such as dyspnea, arrhythmias, and cardiomyopathy. In a study that followed patients with cardiac sarcoidosis treated with prednisone over an average treatment duration of 43 months (range 6–168 months), Chapelon-Abric and colleagues observed signs of clinical resolution in 31 out of 39 patients [46]. Yazaki and colleagues performed a retrospective study demonstrating a 5-year survival of 75 % for those who received steroid treatments, whereas those not treated with steroids had a 5-year survival of 10 % [37]. Unfortunately, much of steroid therapy in cardiac sarcoidosis is based on clinical judgments without guidelines on dose and duration of therapy.

A recent Delphi study attempted to assess if there a consensus existed on the management of cardiac sarcoidosis [52]. They looked for common practices that over 70 % of experts have adapted to their practice. Based on the questionnaire, immunomodulatory therapy was initiated for the presence of ventricular arrhythmias, hypermetabolic activity on a cardiac FDG-PET scan, and/or LV dysfunction. Although prednisone was the choice for initial immunosuppressive therapy, there was no consensus on either the initial dosage of prednisone or the duration of therapy.

There are weak recommendations to use high dose steroids (60–80 mg/day) during the initial treatment phase; however, there was no difference in outcome in patients that had low dose (<30 mg/day) versus high dose (>40 mg/day) [33]. If severe symptoms exist, treatment is typically initiated with intravenous corticosteroids which is switched to oral corticosteroids as the symptoms improve. Once treatment is instituted, continuing lifelong steroid therapy to prevent relapsing cardiac symptoms is recommended as this disease carries high morbidity and mortality. Specifically 23 % of patients have relapse of cardiac sarcoidosis and importantly there is an increased risk of sudden cardiac death due to abrupt discontinuation of steroids [46].

Nonsteroidal Immunomodulators

Several nonsteroidal immunomodulators are being used instead of corticosteroids or as a steroid-sparing agent. Many experts have treated cardiac sarcoid patients successfully with methotrexate and azathioprine based on data from treatment of pulmonary and cutaneous sarcoidosis [53]. Infliximab, a TNFα inhibitor, is a relatively new agent used for treatment of various sarcoidosis organ involvements. There have been case reports of using infliximab as a single agent with complete resolution of cardiac symptoms [54, 55].

Automated Implantable Cardiac Defibrillator

Lethal arrhythmias and sudden cardiac death are a significant morbidity in cardiac sarcoidosis with upwards of 60 % of patients developing sudden cardiac death. Interestingly, the correlation between the patient's left ventricular ejection fraction (LVEF) and the likelihood of sudden cardiac death from ventricular arrhythmias in cardiac sarcoidosis is not clear [56]. The goal to treat ventricular arrhythmias that result in sudden cardiac death has been the major indication for automated implantable cardiac defibrillator (AICD) in these patients. Initially AICDs were placed in patients who demonstrated potentially lethal rhythms in cardiac sarcoidosis with success [57], followed by several reports describing the benefits of prophylactic placement of AICD in cardiac sarcoidosis [56, 58]. An AICD can be placed in cardiac sarcoid patients with either sustained or nonsustained VT. Currently, the American College of Cardiology/American Heart Association/Heart Rhythm Society recommends placement of an implantable defibrillator in infiltrative diseases, such as sarcoidosis (Class IIa recommendation) [59].

Ocular Sarcoidosis

Epidemiology

The prevalence of sarcoidosis is 10–20 per 100,000 of which 25–50 % have ocular involvement [60–62]. The geographic distribution, population samples, duration of follow-up, and the extent of ophthalmologic examination in epidemiologic studies are all closely associated with the true prevalence of ocular sarcoidosis. In a study following 121 patients, uveitis occurred in 24 % of patients with systemic sarcoidosis. Furthermore, 58 % of patients with ocular involvement had uveitis which was the most frequent manifestation of ocular involvement [63]. Rothova and colleagues reported 41 % of sarcoidosis patients developed or had ocular involvement which were more commonly seen in the black population (58 %) and in females (56 %) [63]. Birnbaum and colleagues reported similar demographics for ocular sarcoidosis in which about 68 % of patients with biopsy-proven sarcoidosis and clinical signs of ocular involvement were females and 62 % of these patients were African Americans [64]. Furthermore, genetic studies have demonstrated HLA DRB1*0401 polymorphism to be associated with ocular sarcoidosis [65].

Clinical Presentations

Uveitis

Uveitis is the most common ocular manifestation of sarcoidosis with a prevalence of almost 25–50 %. Uveitis can be compartmentalized into anterior, intermediate, posterior, and panuveitis. Rothova and colleagues studied 582 patients with ocular sarcoidosis and reported that 50 % had anterior uveitis, 22 % had posterior uveitis, followed by 18 % who had panuveitis [66]. Anterior uveitis was predominant in black patients in one study from Amsterdam, whereas posterior and panuveitis were observed more in white patients. Posterior and panuveitis had an increased frequency of complications requiring intraocular surgery and laser coagulation treatment for treatment of glaucoma and severe visual loss [63].

Uveitis typically has a subacute onset early in the course of systemic sarcoidosis and can occur at any time in the disease course of sarcoidosis. In fact patients can present with isolated uveitis followed by eventual development of systemic sarcoidosis. Uveitis can also occur with other symptoms to constitute Lofgren's syndrome (hilar adenopathy, erythema nodosum, and polyarthralgias) and Heerfordt's syndrome (parotitis, uveitis, and cranial nerve palsy) [67].

Characteristics of anterior uveitis that are significant in the diagnosis of ocular sarcoidosis include keratic precipitates (KP) (mutton-fat precipitates), iris nodules found at the papillary margins (Koeppe nodules) or on the surface of the iris (Busacca's nodules), and granulomas on trabecular meshwork (occasionally associated with elevated eye pressure) [66, 67]. Typical characteristics of intermediate uveitis include vitritis and snowballing/string of pearls vitreous opacities. Posterior uveitis is a result of retinal perivasculitis which can manifest as retinal hemorrhage, neovascularization, and choroidal infiltrates surrounding retinal veins with a waxy, yellow appearance described as "candle wax dripping"(Fig. 8.5) [67]. These findings are highly suggestive; however, none of them are pathognomonic to ocular sarcoidosis.

Significant unilateral visual impairment is seen in about 10 % of patients and significant bilateral visual impairment in 14 % of patients with uveitis due to sarcoidosis [60]. Posterior uveitis is usually asymptomatic although it is also considered vision threatening [67]. Thus, the American Thoracic Society recommends that all sarcoidosis patients should have routine ophthalmologic examination on initial evaluation regardless of symptoms [68].

Conjunctival and Lid Involvement

Conjunctival and lid involvement are the next most common manifestation after uveitis in ocular sarcoidosis. In patients with sarcoidosis the prevalence is 19 % and 16 %, respectively [63]. Dacryocystitis (lacrimal gland inflammation), keratoconjunctivitis sicca (KC), and periocular soft tissue inflammation have been described (Fig. 8.6). Both dacrocystitis and KC can occur even without lacrimal gland enlargement, but can be detected using gallium scanning and Schirmer's test, respectively [67].

Fig. 8.5 Candle wax drippings appearance secondary to choroidal infiltrates surrounding retinal veins with a *waxy, yellow* appearance

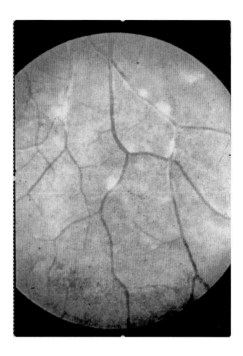

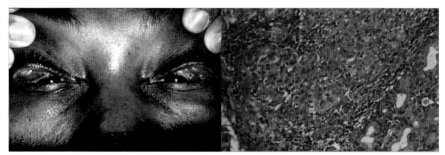

Fig. 8.6 Dacrocystitis presenting as swollen palpebral lobe of the lacrimal glands in both upper eyelids. Biopsy revealed noncaseating granuloma consistent with sarcoidosis

Diagnosis

Diagnosis of ocular sarcoidosis may be challenging as obtaining ocular tissue biopsy can be difficult and the differential diagnosis include entities such as Behcet's disease, ocular tuberculosis, Vogt–Koyanagi–Harada disease, ocular toxoplasmosis, HTLV-1-associated uveitis, leprosy, multiple sclerosis, and syphilis [68].

In 2006, the First International Workshop on Ocular Sarcoidosis (FIWOS) developed criteria for the diagnosis of ocular sarcoidosis [69]. In the guidelines set forth from FIWOS, categories including definite, probable, and possible were incorporated in the diagnosis criteria. These guidelines reflect the difficulty in obtaining

Table 8.4 Clinical signs suggestive of ocular sarcoidosis

1. Mutton-fat/granulomatous KPs and/or iris nodules (Koeppps/Busacca)
2. Trabecular meshwork (TM) nodules and/or tent-shaped peripheral anterior synechiae (PAS)
3. Snowballs/string of pearls vitreous opacities
4. Multiple chorioretinal peripheral lesions (active and/or atrophic)
5. Nodular and/or segmental periphlebitis (± candlewax drippings) and/or retinal macroaneurysm in an inflamed eye
6. Optic disc nodule(s)/granuloma(s) and/or solitary choroidal nodule
7. Bilaterality (assessed by clinical examination or investigational tests showing subclinical inflammation)

Laboratory investigations in suspected ocular sarcoidosis

1. Negative tuberculin test in a BCG vaccinated patient or having had a positive PPD (or Mantoux) skin test previously
2. Elevated serum angiotensin converting enzyme (ACE) and/or elevated serum lysozyme
3. Chest X-ray: bilateral hilar lymphadenopathy (BHL)
4. Abnormal liver enzyme tests [any two of alkaline phosphatase (ALKP), aspartate aminotransferase (AST), alanine aminotransferase (ALT), lactate dehydrogenase (LDH), or gamma glutamyl transpeptidase (GGT)]
5. Chest CT scan in patients with negative chest X-ray

Diagnostic criteria for ocular sarcoidosis

All other causes of uveitis, in particular tuberculous uveitis, have to be ruled out

1. Biopsy supported diagnosis with compatible uveitis	Definite ocular sarcoidosis
2. Biopsy not done; presence of BHL with a compatible uveitis	Presumed ocular sarcoidosis
3. Biopsy not done and BHL negative; presence of three of the suggestive signs and two positive investigational tests	Probable ocular sarcoidosis
4. Biopsy negative, four of the suggestive intraocular signs and two of the investigations are positive	Possible ocular sarcoidosis

ocular tissue biopsy and emphasize the use of seven clinical signs that are characteristic but not pathognomonic for ocular sarcoidosis. It also includes laboratory or radiologic investigations that can be used to support the diagnosis of ocular sarcoidosis. The FIWOS conference utilizes a combination of these factors to establish diagnosis as definite, presumed, probable, and possible ocular sarcoidosis (Table 8.4).

The new guidelines set forth in 2006 were compared to the 1999 criteria to diagnose ocular sarcoidosis [70]. The new guidelines were found to increase the diagnostic specificity from 45.6 to 83 % without sacrificing much on sensitivity which ranged from 80 to 84 %. The newer guidelines were more apt in identifying patients with ocular sarcoidosis versus other etiologies of uveitis.

Treatment

The treatment for ocular sarcoidosis is dependent on the severity of disease. Milder cases of ocular sarcoidosis usually respond well with topical corticosteroids. Most uveitis, especially anterior uveitis, responds well with topical steroids alone or in combination with systemic steroids. However, in one study that followed 75 patients with sarcoid uveitis, almost 49 % of patients eventually required oral steroids for treatment by 5 years into the diagnosis and almost 74 % required oral steroids by year 10 of the diagnosis [71]. Visual acuity returned to normal in about 54 % of patients after treatment with steroids, whereas only 4.6 % developed severe bilateral visual loss.

Treatment with nonsteroidal immunomodulators such as azathioprine, methotrexate, cyclosporine, tacrolimus, and mycophenolate mofetil have been used for steroid refractory or intolerant patients based on weak evidence from case series and case reports with good outcome [60–62, 72]. There is also a role of TNFα inhibitors, such as infliximab in cases of refractory ocular sarcoidosis. The data in the use of infliximab are anecdotal at best but promising [73, 74].

Prognosis

Ocular manifestations of sarcoidosis can be initially asymptomatic and therefore annual ophthalmologic examination is typically recommended in all sarcoidosis patients as the potential consequences are significant. The prognosis is dependent on the compartment involved; anterior ocular involvement typically portends a better prognosis as opposed to posterior ocular involvement and panuveitis are associated with poorer prognosis.

Skin Sarcoidosis

Epidemiology

Sarcoidosis has been described as one of the greatest mimickers in dermatology due to its wide range of presentation [75]. Cutaneous involvement of systemic sarcoidosis is classified as specific or nonspecific based upon the presence or absence of noncaseating granulomas on histopathologic examination [76–78]. The most common specific lesions include lupus pernio (LP), infiltrated plaques, macular and papular lesions, and subcutaneous nodules. Less common manifestations include hypopigmented patches, ulcers, alopecia, verrucous lesions, and erythroderma [76–80]. The most common nonspecific lesion of sarcoidosis is erythema nodosum (EN) [76, 78, 79].

Recently, the ACCESS trial reported an incidence of cutaneous involvement in the overall sarcoidosis population to be 24.2 % with the African-American population demonstrating an increased incidence of skin involvement other than in cases of erythema nodosum [1]. These findings are consistent with other studies [81], although other reports including the American Thoracic Society's position statement have reported slightly higher incidences with additional evidence that skin sarcoidosis may occur more commonly in females [10, 82]. Cutaneous manifestations of

Fig. 8.7 Erythema nodosum
presenting as tender
erythematous lesion on the
pretibial areas of lower
extremities

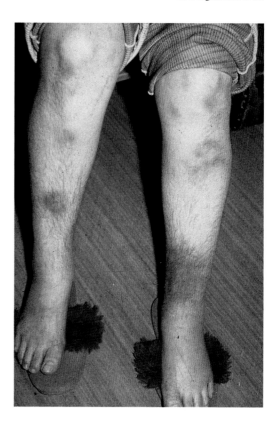

sarcoidosis can be the lone sign of disease and the severity of these lesions can be variable in relation to the degree of systemic disease [83]. Roughly 20 % of patients will have skin lesions prior to the presentation of signs of systemic disease, 50 % will have simultaneous manifestations, and 30 % will experience their first skin involvement several years after their initial diagnosis of systemic sarcoidosis [84].

Erythema Nodosum

EN is found to occur more commonly in European, Puerto Rican, and Mexican patients as well as women of child-bearing age. Furthermore, EN occurs commonly in females with a prevalence between 2 and 20 % [7, 85]. EN is considered a hallmark of acute sarcoidosis. Typical lesions are raised, red, tender, and commonly seen on the anterior aspect of the lower extremities (Fig. 8.7). Additional locations can include the trunk and other limb areas [79, 86]. Adjacent joints are frequently involved with clinically evident swelling or pain. Hallmarks of EN are that granulomas are not seen on skin biopsies, the lesions may resolve with treatment in 6–8 weeks, and that EN serves as a herald of a good overall prognosis [87, 88]. Löfgren's syndrome is a specific syndrome observed in sarcoidosis when EN is combined with fever, hilar

Fig. 8.8 Lupus pernio with indurated plaque involving the forehead, cheeks, and nose

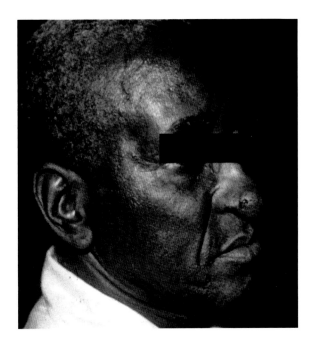

lymphadenopathy, and arthralgia [89]. Löfgren's syndrome's incidence is variable and can be as high as of 20–30 % in Caucasians but less frequent in other races/ethnicities [87, 90]. Löfgren's syndrome typically portends good prognosis. Accordingly, a study that examined the genetic background of Löfgren's syndrome in northern European population found HLA-DRB1*0301 to be associated with higher likelihood of spontaneous remission and good prognosis with this syndrome [91].

Lupus Pernio

In contrast, lupus pernio is an indurated disfiguring plaque with violaceous discoloration typically of the nose, cheeks, lips, ears, and nasal mucosa (Fig. 8.8). Lupus pernio is seen with a higher incidence in African-American females [86, 87] and typically progress to chronic disease without spontaneous remission with worse prognosis. Lupus pernio is often associated with bone cysts, pulmonary fibrosis, and sarcoidosis of upper respiratory tract (SURT) [87, 88].

Macular Skin Lesions, Papules, Nodules, Plaques

Macules can present as hypopigmented, atrophic, or an erythematous variety [92, 93] and lichenoid papules presenting on generalized, localized, or perifollicular areas [94]. Subcutaneous sarcoidosis (Darier–Roussy syndrome), which carries a good prognosis, is a rare condition predominantly affecting middle-aged Caucasian

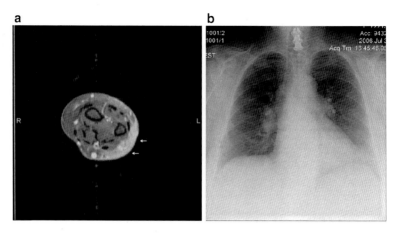

Fig. 8.9 (**a**) Gadolinium-enhanced subcutaneous lesion consistent with Darier–Roussy syndrome. (**b**) Chest radiograph revealed classic bilateral hilar adenopathy consistent with the diagnosis of sarcoidosis

patients. Most cases occur as firm, painless, mobile, round nodules in the upper extremities that demonstrate classic noncaseating epithelioid-cell granulomas on biopsy (Fig. 8.9) [95]. Plaques may present as a morpheaform sarcoidosis that is clinically indistinguishable from true morphea (prominent dermal sclerosis with induration) [96] or erythematous annular lesions with central hypopigmentation [97]. Many of these lesions have been reported to experience high degrees of resolution with various therapies and typically carry a better clinical prognosis than lupus pernio [87].

Other Forms of Skin Sarcoidosis

Additional forms of cutaneous sarcoidosis include ichthyosiform sarcoidosis characterized by noncaseating granulomas in areas of fine scaling on the distal extremities [76], tattoo sarcoid that results as a localized reaction in cosmetic tattoos with systemic spread of tattoo pigment causing reaction in distant systemic sites [98–100], and psoriasiform eruptions that can be indistinguishable from typical forms of psoriasis in the absence of biopsy [101].

Treatment

Treatment of cutaneous sarcoidosis depends on clinical severity and the type of lesion as not all skin lesions require treatment [87]. Topical therapy with corticosteroids in the form of creams, drops, or sprays is a reasonable initial regimen for isolated skin lesions and for lesions of the lip or mucous membranes [87, 102].

Topical regimens may also include the calcineurin inhibitor immunosuppressant tacrolimus. Therapy with 0.1 % tacrolimus ointment twice daily has shown to lead to complete resolution of some skin lesions within a few months and can be used as a single agent or in combination therapy [100, 103–105]. Systemic corticosteroids are the treatment of choice and typically started at a dose between 20 and 40 mg/day. Every effort should be made to taper the corticosteroids to the lowest dose that would provide effect. Alternative treatments including methotrexate, leflunomide, and antimalarial drugs can used as an adjunct to corticosteroid treatment or alone as monotherapy [106, 107]. Thalidomide known for its anti-TNF-α activity has also been used successfully as monotherapy for cutaneous sarcoidosis [108]. Furthermore, other anti-TNF-α medications such as Infliximab or Adalimumab have had success with isolated cases including cases of lupus pernio and other treatment resistant skin lesions, providing hope to patients with lesions that generally carry a relentless clinical course [97, 106, 109–115].

Hepatic Sarcoidosis

Epidemiology

The frequency of hepatic involvement of sarcoidosis is reported with great variability and is dependent on the methods used in these investigations. Autopsy studies have demonstrated liver involvement in up to 44.6 % of patients with sarcoidosis [116] and a case series of needle biopsies in suspected sarcoidosis reported an incidence of granuloma consistent with sarcoidosis in 24–79 % of patients [117, 118]. A number of other studies using a variety of diagnostic modalities have also described hepatic involvement of systemic sarcoidosis with ranges from 50 to 90 % [119–121]. Recently, the ACCESS trial observed an incidence of only 11.5 % for hepatic involvement in sarcoidosis [1] with African Americans being twice as likely to have involvement of the liver than Caucasians ($p < 0.0001$) [1].

Clinical Presentations

Clinical symptoms of hepatic sarcoidosis are often absent and can be highly nonspecific. Manifestations such as fatigue, pruritis, and right upper quadrant pain have only been described in 15.9 % of patients [120]. Weight loss, jaundice, and fever due to hepatic sarcoid are less common and seen in only 5 % of patients [119, 120]. Less than 20 % of patients with hepatic sarcoidosis will have clinically appreciable hepatomegaly [122] and in most cases, liver or spleen involvement is only detected incidentally on radiographic investigations in the absence of clinical or laboratory abnormalities [123].

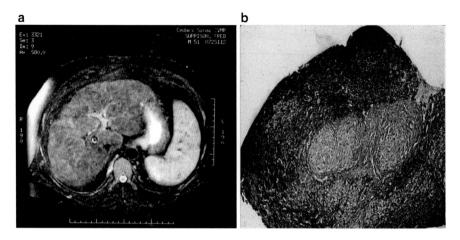

Fig. 8.10 (a) Contrast-enhanced axial CT image of multiple low attenuation lesions that appears to be coalescing throughout the liver. (b) Biopsy revealing noncaseating granuloma

Cirrhosis is seen in 6 % hepatic sarcoidosis that can further lead to portal hypertension in 3 % of patients [120]. The most common cause is from granulomatous infiltration of the portal areas leading to reduced flow to the hepatic sinusoids. Other known sequelae with portal hypertension such as variceal disease in the esophagus and stomach can be a cause of gastrointestinal bleed [124, 125].

Diagnosis

Laboratory Studies

Reports of abnormal serologic tests in hepatic sarcoidosis range from only 4 to 24.4 % [122, 126]. When abnormal, serum liver tests typically reveal a cholestatic pattern with elevation of serum alkaline phosphatase and only mild elevations in transaminases [119, 127–129]. Laboratory studies may be useful in differentiating hepatic sarcoidosis from other hepatic pathologies like primary biliary cirrhosis (PBC) through evidence of an elevated angiotensin-converting enzyme, hypercalcemia, or a negative anti-mitochondrial antibody titer.

CT Imaging

Radiographically, there are no distinct lesions specific to hepatic sarcoidosis. Most granulomata are less than 2 mm in diameter which cannot be adequately assessed using the resolution of abdominal CT scans [130]. The most common findings on CT imaging are diffuse hepatic heterogeneity with hepatomegaly and splenomegaly seen on CT imaging (Fig. 8.10) [131]. Hepatic nodules representing coalescent

Table 8.5 Differential diagnosis of hepatic granulomas

Differential	Granuloma histology	Extrahepatic manifestations	Serologic findings
Sarcoidosis	Sharply circumscribed, discrete granulomata, predominantly in the portal triad, but occasionally elsewhere in the lobules. Lobular architectures are typically well preserved with absence of necrosis	Pulmonary, neurologic, cardiac, ocular, cutaneous, splenic, or other extrapulmonary sarcoid manifestations	Elevated ACE Hypercalcemia
Primary biliary cirrhosis	May be indistinguishable from sarcoidosis	Delayed-type hypersensitivity reactions (i.e., Sjogren's syndrome, fibrosing alveolitis, ulcerative colitis) [31]	Anti-mitochondrial antibodies Anti-GP210
Drug-induced granulomas	Granulomas in the presence of eosinophilic infiltrates	Specific manifestations with drug	None
Mechanical biliary obstruction	Poorly formed granulomas in close association with necrotic hepatocytes with bile pigment	Disease specific manifestations (i.e., weight loss or B-signs of malignancy, Murphy Sign, or jaundice of acute obstruction)	None
Infectious etiologies	May be indistinguishable from sarcoidosis, but often more irregular or lobulated with more peri-granuloma inflammation	Varies with infectious etiology	Viral hepatitis titers Quantiferon gold + Cultures Gastric washings
Idiopathic	May be indistinguishable from sarcoidosis	Diagnosis of exclusion from above etiologies	

granulomas are less commonly observed and are seen in about 5 % of patients [131]. These lesions are typically well defined with low attenuation on CT imaging.

Histopathology

Klatskin described the characteristic histology of hepatic sarcoid as scattered, sharply circumscribed, discrete granulomata, predominantly in the portal triad, but occasionally elsewhere in the lobules. Lobular architectures are typically well preserved with absence of necrosis. Typically, the diagnosis of hepatic sarcoidosis is pursued after identifying evidence of extrahepatic organ involvement.

The presence of granulomas in the liver can also occur from diseases other than sarcoidosis (Table 8.5). In fact when granulomas are observed on biopsy, the frequency of etiologies has been shown to be more commonly due to PBC (23.8 %) than sarcoidosis (11.1 %) [132]. Both sarcoidosis and PBC can lead to chronic cholestasis and biliary cirrhosis which pose difficulty in distinguishing the two diseases [133]. While hepatic sarcoidosis and PBC may be indistinguishable from one another histologically, serologic testing can aid in the differentiation. Positive anti-mitochondrial antibody is commonly detected in PBC but is absent in sarcoidosis [118]. Additionally, anti-GP210 is observed in up to 47 % of patients without anti-mitochondrial antibodies with PBC, but not in sarcoidosis [118, 134].

Other potential diseases with hepatic granulomas include drug induced granulo-mas, mechanical biliary obstruction, tuberculosis, brucellosis, and idiopathic hepatic granulomas. The presence of eosinophilic infiltrates in association with culprit medi-cations (glibenclamide, metronidazole, baclofen, nitrofurantoin, and allopurinol) sug-gests drug-induced granulomas [132]. Granulomas secondary to mechanical biliary obstruction can persist for more than 6 months and are often seen with poorly formed granulomas in close association with necrotic hepatocytes with bile pigment [132]. Infectious etiologies such should be evaluated by additional serologic testing. Finally, in the absence of other supporting elements to conclude the diagnosis of hepatic sar-coidosis or other etiologies, the presence of granulomas can be idiopathic.

Treatment

The vast majority of hepatic sarcoidosis usually do not necessitate treatment as most liver abnormalities spontaneously improve without treatment [135]. Thus asymp-tomatic patients with abnormal liver function tests can be followed closely with serial tests to document improvement over time.

Corticosteroids is the first-line treatment with hepatic sarcoidosis and may be considered in patients who experience fever, nausea, vomiting, weight loss, or right upper quadrant abdominal pain [12]. In most patients with hepatic sarcoidosis, cor-ticosteroids appear to be effective, although the response to corticosteroids can be variable. Furthermore, systemic corticosteroids have not been shown to definitively prevent progression to portal hypertension [119, 136, 137]. In fact, a retrospective study in patients with hepatic sarcoidosis showed corticosteroids to be associated with higher likelihood to develop recurrent active disease [138].

While corticosteroids may improve hepatomegaly and liver function abnormali-ties, symptoms associated with cholestasis may not necessarily show improvement. Alternatively, treatment with ursodeoxycholic acid (UDCA), compared to systemic corticosteroids, has been shown to have improvement with Pruritus, fatigue, jaundice, and serologic improvement and may be used in hepatic sarcoidosis [127, 139–141].

Methotrexate (MTX) also has clinical benefit in the treatment of hepatic sarcoid-osis. However, given the risk for hepatic toxicity, careful assessment of risks and benefits to the patient must be considered before its use especially with hepatic sarcoidosis. The work-up for patients starting MTX should include clinical and serologic assessment of risk factors for MTX toxicity (including alcohol intake), patient education, aspartate aminotransferase (AST), alanine aminotransferase (ALT), albumin, complete blood cell (CBC), creatinine, and chest X-ray. Additionally, it is important to consider that exacerbation of hepatic disease carries additional risk in obesity, diabetes, and both viral and alcoholic hepatitis. While liver function test abnormalities may be due to either hepatic sarcoidosis or MTX, lab values 2–4 times the upper limit of normal should lead to a MTX dose reduction, additional folate supplementation, withdrawal of MTX, or a liver biopsy to evaluate for MTX toxicity [142].

Finally, when patients fail to respond to systemic corticosteroids or MTX or develop severe toxicities, alternate therapies should be considered. Azathioprine, leflunomide, or biologicals can be considered [143, 144]. Although end-stage liver disease (significant liver dysfunction, chronic cholestasis, cirrhosis, portal hypertension) from hepatic sarcoidosis is uncommon, transplant may be required in rare instances [120, 137, 145]. In such cases, there are reports of recurrence of hepatic sarcoidosis in the transplanted liver with no increase in hepatic related mortality [146–148].

Splenic Sarcoidosis

Epidemiology

The incidence of splenic involvement from sarcoidosis is highly variable. Older studies have reported incidences to be 38–77 % based on autopsy reports and 24–59 % with fine needle aspiration biopsies [117, 149–151]. Another older study reported the spleen to be the second most common site of organ involvement in sarcoidosis after the lung [152]. However, the rate of splenic involvement in the recent ACCESS study [1] reported splenic involvement to be only 6.7 %, similar to more recent studies among all sarcoidosis patients [153, 154].

Clinical Signs and Symptoms

Splenic sarcoidosis can present in a variety of ways from asymptomatic radiographic findings to abdominal pain, signs of portal hypertension, pancytopenia, and rarely, acute splenic infarct or rupture [87, 155, 156]. Some patients may experience constitutional symptoms including night sweats, fever, and malaise [157]. In patients with systemic sarcoidosis, less than 20 % have any evidence of hepatosplenomegaly [158], 10–15 % have a palpable spleen on examination [149], and only 3 % can be classified as massive splenomegaly [149].

Diagnosis

The diagnosis of splenic sarcoidosis is often made in a patient with known sarcoidosis and radiographic evidence of splenomegaly, which is more common than hepatomegaly [123, 131, 159]. Focal areas of granulomas seen as multiple lesions with low attenuation on CT imaging may also be seen [160]. However, there may be value in the use of contrast-enhanced ultrasound for the visualization of distinct lesions [154]. Pursuing a potential diagnosis of splenic sarcoidosis is indicated in the setting of abdominal pain, early satiety, leukopenia, anemia, thrombocytopenia, poikilocytosis, or Howell Jolly bodies [161]. Additionally, while not of diagnostic value, spleen size has been shown to be in close correlation with serum markers such as increased angiotensin converting enzyme and relative counts of CD4+ and non-CD4+, non-CD8+ lymphocytes [162, 163].

Treatment

Treatment for splenic involvement of sarcoidosis is not well defined. Case studies have demonstrated spontaneous resolution of the condition with close monitoring and symptom management [164]. Although systemic corticosteroid therapy has been the standard of treatment in regimens for sarcoidosis, its impact on resolution or progression of splenic sarcoidosis has been mixed [155]. Furthermore, splenic involvement has been noted to predict poor efficacy of corticosteroids in treatment of sarcoidosis in other organ systems [157, 165].

Definitive therapy for splenic sarcoidosis is splenectomy and is typically considered when there is concern for, or evidence of, splenic rupture or refractory systemic complications (i.e., thrombocytopenia). Spontaneous rupture of the spleen is extremely rare [166–168] and is not directly associated with the degree of splenomegaly on clinical or radiographic assessment but rather with blood vessel involvement within the spleen with granulomas and fibrinous clots seen on pathologic specimens [169]. Splenectomy has been shown to result in complete resolution of thrombocytopenia in patients with severe disease and repeated episodes of bleeding, but success is limited in patients with only mild disease [170]. Additionally, patient outcomes after splenectomy are impacted by the risk for postoperative death or death from complications of sarcoidosis in additional organs [155]. Therefore, diligent trial of corticosteroid must be pursued and surgical risks must always be weighed with the potential benefits during consideration of splenectomy.

Calcium Dysregulation

The granulomatous disease in sarcoidosis can cause increased 1-α hydroxylase activity leading to increased conversion of 25-hydroxyvitamin D to 1, 25-dihydroxyvitamin D, an active form of vitamin D. As a result, hypercalcemia and hypercalciuria can occur in sarcoidosis [171]. The reported incidence of hypercalcemia can be highly variable ranging from 2 to 63 %, depending on the referenced literature [171]. Hypercalciuria is more commonly seen compared to hypercalcemia and can cause nephrocalcinosis, nephrolithiasis, and renal failure

[172, 173]. Furthermore, hypercalciuria can be the presenting feature of sarcoidosis and occur before hypercalcemia [173]. Therefore serum calcium, creatinine, and urinalysis must be performed as part of the evaluation for sarcoidosis.

Treatment of hypercalcemia must be instituted if serum calcium is greater than 11 mg/dl or there is evidence of renal failure or nephrolithiasis. Milder cases of hypercalcemia may be monitored closely if no other indications for treatment with sarcoidosis exist. Corticosteroids remain the mainstay of treatment and used at a dose between 20 and 40 mg/day. Other treatments such as hydroxychloroquine and ketoconazole have been reported with success [174, 175]. If calcium dysregulation does not improve with treatment, careful evaluation of other disorders that cause hypercalcemia such as parathyroid disease and hematologic and solid organ malignancy must be explored.

Miscellaneous

Sarcoidosis can affect the bones in up to 13 % of patients [176]. African Americans are more commonly affected and it typically involves the bones of the hands and feet, although other bones may be affected. Patients are typically asymptomatic, although some can present as painful lesions with or without adjacent arthritis. Radiographic imaging studies can show cystic or punched-out lesions [177]. Treatment involves using systemic corticosteroids, although alternatives such as methotrexate or azathioprine may be used as an adjunct treatment in addition to corticosteroids [176].

Peripheral lymphadenopathy, with presence of noncaseating granulomas within the affected lymph nodes may be seen in sarcoidosis as part of the involvement of the lymphatic system. However, if noncaseating granulomas are found without other systemic involvement, careful evaluation for infection or malignancy must be undertaken. Findings of granuloma from a lymph node may be seen in the draining lymph nodes of a cancer, as part of "sarcoid-like reaction" [178].

Renal involvement can occur in up to 20 % of patients with sarcoidosis, although clinical manifestations stemming from the granulomas are not common. Interstitial nephritis, membranous glomerulonephritis, mesangioproliferative glomerulonephritis, immunoglobulin A nephropathy, and crescentic glomerulonephritis are rare but have been reported [179].

References

1. Baughman RP, Teirstein AS, Judson MA, et al. Clinical characteristics of patients in a case control study of sarcoidosis. Am J Respir Crit Care Med. 2001;164:1885–9.
2. Pietinalho A, Ohmichi M, Hirasawa M, et al. Familial sarcoidosis in Finland and Hokkaido, Japan – a comparative study. Respir Med. 1999;93:408–12.
3. Judson MA, Baughman RP, Teirstein AS, et al. Defining organ involvement in sarcoidosis: the ACCESS proposed instrument. ACCESS Research Group. A Case Control Etiologic Study of Sarcoidosis. Sarcoidosis Vasc Diffuse Lung Dis. 1999;16:75–86.

4. Nozaki K, Judson MA. Neurosarcoidosis: clinical manifestations, diagnosis and treatment. Presse Med. 2012;41:e331–48.
5. Allen RK, Sellars RE, Sandstrom PA. A prospective study of 32 patients with neurosarcoidosis. Sarcoidosis Vasc Diffuse Lung Dis. 2003 Jun;20(2):118–25.
6. Smith JK, Matheus MG, Castillo M. Imaging manifestations of neurosarcoidosis. AJR Am J Roentgenol. 2004;182:289–95.
7. Lacomis D. Neurosarcoidosis. Curr Neuropharmacol. 2011;9:429–36.
8. Lower EE, Broderick JP, Brott TG, et al. Diagnosis and management of neurological sarcoidosis. Arch Intern Med. 1997;157:1864–8.
9. Zajicek JP, Scolding NJ, Foster O, et al. Central nervous system sarcoidosis – diagnosis and management. QJM. 1999;92:103–17.
10. Krumholz A, Stern BJ, Stern EG. Clinical implications of seizures in neurosarcoidosis. Arch Neurol. 1991;48:842–4.
11. Porter N, Beynon HL, Randeva HS. Endocrine and reproductive manifestations of sarcoidosis. QJM. 2003;96:553–61.
12. Langrand C, Bihan H, Raverot G, et al. Hypothalamo-pituitary sarcoidosis: a multicenter study of 24 patients. QJM. 2012;105:981–95.
13. Said G, Lacroix C, Planté-Bordeneuve V, et al. Nerve granulomas and vasculitis in sarcoid peripheral neuropathy: a clinicopathological study of 11 patients. Brain. 2002;125:264–75.
14. Hoitsma E, Marziniak M, Faber CG, et al. Small fibre neuropathy in sarcoidosis. Lancet. 2002;359:2085–6.
15. Hoitsma E, Reulen JP, de Baets M, et al. Small fiber neuropathy: a common and important clinical disorder. J Neurol Sci. 2004;227:119–30.
16. Gullapalli D, Phillips LH. Neurologic manifestations of sarcoidosis. Neurol Clin. 2002;20:59–83, vi.
17. Shah R, Roberson GH, Curé JK. Correlation of MR imaging findings and clinical manifestations in neurosarcoidosis. AJNR Am J Neuroradiol. 2009;30:953–61.
18. Lower EE, Weiss KL. Neurosarcoidosis. Clin Chest Med. 2008;29:475–92, ix.
19. Tahmoush AJ, Amir MS, Connor WW, et al. CSF-ACE activity in probable CNS neurosarcoidosis. Sarcoidosis Vasc Diffuse Lung Dis. 2002;19:191–7.
20. Sharma OP. Neurosarcoidosis: a personal perspective based on the study of 37 patients. Chest. 1997;112:220–8.
21. Hunninghake GW, Costabel U, Ando M, et al. ATS/ERS/WASOG statement on sarcoidosis. American Thoracic Society/European Respiratory Society/World Association of Sarcoidosis and other Granulomatous Disorders. Sarcoidosis Vasc Diffuse Lung Dis. 1999;16:149–73.
22. Chapelon C, Ziza JM, Piette JC, et al. Neurosarcoidosis: signs, course and treatment in 35 confirmed cases. Medicine (Baltimore). 1990;69:261–76.
23. Wiederholt WC, Siekert RG. Neurological manifestations of sarcoidosis. Neurology. 1965;15:1147–54.
24. Stern BJ, Krumholz A, Johns C, et al. Sarcoidosis and its neurological manifestations. Arch Neurol. 1985;42:909–17.
25. Scott TF, Yandora K, Valeri A, et al. Aggressive therapy for neurosarcoidosis: long-term follow-up of 48 treated patients. Arch Neurol. 2007;64:691–6.
26. Stern BJ, Schonfeld SA, Sewell C, et al. The treatment of neurosarcoidosis with cyclosporine. Arch Neurol. 1992;49:1065–72.
27. Doty JD, Mazur JE, Judson MA. Treatment of corticosteroid-resistant neurosarcoidosis with a short-course cyclophosphamide regimen. Chest. 2003;124:2023–6.
28. Moravan M, Segal BM. Treatment of CNS sarcoidosis with infliximab and mycophenolate mofetil. Neurology. 2009;72:337–40.
29. Costabel U. Sarcoidosis: clinical update. Eur Respir J Suppl. 2001;32:56s–68.
30. Joseph FG, Scolding NJ. Neurosarcoidosis: a study of 30 new cases. J Neurol Neurosurg Psychiatry. 2009;80:297–304.
31. Pawate S, Moses H, Sriram S. Presentations and outcomes of neurosarcoidosis: a study of 54 cases. QJM. 2009;102:449–60.

32. Doughan AR, Williams BR. Cardiac sarcoidosis. Heart. 2006;92:282–8.
33. Ayyala US, Nair AP, Padilla ML. Cardiac sarcoidosis. Clin Chest Med. 2008;29:493–508, ix.
34. Silverman KJ, Hutchins GM, Bulkley BH. Cardiac sarcoid: a clinicopathologic study of 84 unselected patients with systemic sarcoidosis. Circulation. 1978;58:1204–11.
35. Fahy GJ, Marwick T, McCreery CJ, et al. Doppler echocardiographic detection of left ventricular diastolic dysfunction in patients with pulmonary sarcoidosis. Chest. 1996;109:62–6.
36. Sköld CM, Larsen FF, Rasmussen E, et al. Determination of cardiac involvement in sarcoidosis by magnetic resonance imaging and Doppler echocardiography. J Intern Med. 2002;252:465–71.
37. Yazaki Y, Isobe M, Hiroe M, et al. Prognostic determinants of long-term survival in Japanese patients with cardiac sarcoidosis treated with prednisone. Am J Cardiol. 2001;88:1006–10.
38. Roberts WC, McAllister HA, Ferrans VJ. Sarcoidosis of the heart. A clinicopathologic study of 35 necropsy patients (group 1) and review of 78 previously described necropsy patients (group 11). Am J Med. 1977;63:86–108.
39. Imazio M. Pericardial involvement in systemic inflammatory diseases. Heart. 2011;97:1882–92.
40. Sharma OP, Maheshwari A, Thaker K. Myocardial sarcoidosis. Chest. 1993;103:253–8.
41. Garrett J, O'Neill H, Blake S. Constrictive pericarditis associated with sarcoidosis. Am Heart J. 1984;107:394.
42. Angomachalelis N, Hourzamanis A, Salem N, et al. Pericardial effusion concomitant with specific heart muscle disease in systemic sarcoidosis. Postgrad Med J. 1994;70 Suppl 1:S8–12.
43. Uemura A, Morimoto S, Hiramitsu S, et al. Histologic diagnostic rate of cardiac sarcoidosis: evaluation of endomyocardial biopsies. Am Heart J. 1999;138:299–302.
44. Ardehali H, Qasim A, Cappola T, et al. Endomyocardial biopsy plays a role in diagnosing patients with unexplained cardiomyopathy. Am Heart J. 2004;147:919–23.
45. Sekiguchi M, Yazaki Y, Isobe M, et al. Cardiac sarcoidosis: diagnostic, prognostic, and therapeutic considerations. Cardiovasc Drugs Ther. 1996;10:495–510.
46. Chapelon-Abric C, de Zuttere D, Duhaut P, et al. Cardiac sarcoidosis: a retrospective study of 41 cases. Medicine (Baltimore). 2004;83:315–34.
47. Bulkley BH, Hutchins GM, Bailey I, et al. Thallium 201 imaging and gated cardiac blood pool scans in patients with ischemic and idiopathic congestive cardiomyopathy. A clinical and pathologic study. Circulation. 1977;55:753–60.
48. Israel HL, Gushue GF, Park CH. Assessment of gallium-67 scanning in pulmonary and extrapulmonary sarcoidosis. Ann N Y Acad Sci. 1986;465:455–62.
49. Yamagishi H, Shirai N, Takagi M, et al. Identification of cardiac sarcoidosis with (13) N-NH(3)/(18)F-FDG PET. J Nucl Med. 2003;44:1030–6.
50. Okumura W, Iwasaki T, Toyama T, et al. Usefulness of fasting 18F-FDG PET in identification of cardiac sarcoidosis. J Nucl Med. 2004;45:1989–98.
51. Smedema JP, Snoep G, van Kroonenburgh MP, et al. Evaluation of the accuracy of gadolinium-enhanced cardiovascular magnetic resonance in the diagnosis of cardiac sarcoidosis. J Am Coll Cardiol. 2005;45:1683–90.
52. Hamzeh NY, Wamboldt FS, Weinberger HD. Management of cardiac sarcoidosis in the United States: a Delphi study. Chest. 2012;141:154–62.
53. Bussinguer M, Danielian A, Sharma OP. Cardiac sarcoidosis: diagnosis and management. Curr Treat Options Cardiovasc Med. 2012;14:652–64.
54. Uthman I, Touma Z, Khoury M. Cardiac sarcoidosis responding to monotherapy with infliximab. Clin Rheumatol. 2007;26:2001–3.
55. Barnabe C, McMeekin J, Howarth A, et al. Successful treatment of cardiac sarcoidosis with infliximab. J Rheumatol. 2008;35:1686–7.
56. Winters SL, Cohen M, Greenberg S, et al. Sustained ventricular tachycardia associated with sarcoidosis: assessment of the underlying cardiac anatomy and the prospective utility of programmed ventricular stimulation, drug therapy and an implantable antitachycardia device. J Am Coll Cardiol. 1991;18:937–43.
57. Bajaj AK, Kopelman HA, Echt DS. Cardiac sarcoidosis with sudden death: treatment with the automatic implantable cardioverter defibrillator. Am Heart J. 1988;116:557–60.

58. Paz HL, McCormick DJ, Kutalek SP, et al. The automated implantable cardiac defibrillator. Prophylaxis in cardiac sarcoidosis. Chest. 1994;106:1603–7.
59. Kedia R, Saeed M. Implantable cardioverter-defibrillators: indications and unresolved issues. Tex Heart Inst J. 2012;39:335–41.
60. Bodaghi B, Touitou V, Fardeau C, et al. Ocular sarcoidosis. Presse Med. 2012;41:e349–54.
61. Mayers M. Ocular sarcoidosis. Int Ophthalmol Clin. 1990;30:257–63.
62. James DG, Anderson R, Langley D, et al. Ocular sarcoidosis. Br J Ophthalmol. 1964;48: 461–70.
63. Rothova A, Alberts C, Glasius E, et al. Risk factors for ocular sarcoidosis. Doc Ophthalmol. 1989;72:287–96.
64. Birnbaum AD, Oh FS, Chakrabarti A, et al. Clinical features and diagnostic evaluation of biopsy-proven ocular sarcoidosis. Arch Ophthalmol. 2011;129:409–13.
65. Rossman MD, Thompson B, Frederick M, et al. HLA-DRB1*1101: a significant risk factor for sarcoidosis in blacks and whites. Am J Hum Genet. 2003;73:720–35.
66. Rothova A. Ocular involvement in sarcoidosis. Br J Ophthalmol. 2000;84:110–6.
67. Rose AS, Tielker MA, Knox KS. Hepatic, ocular, and cutaneous sarcoidosis. Clin Chest Med. 2008;29:509–24.
68. Cowan CL. Review for disease of the year: differential diagnosis of ocular sarcoidosis. Ocul Immunol Inflamm. 2010;18:442–51.
69. Herbort CP, Rao NA, Mochizuki M, et al. International criteria for the diagnosis of ocular sarcoidosis: results of the first International Workshop On Ocular Sarcoidosis (IWOS). Ocul Immunol Inflamm. 2009;17:160–9.
70. Asukata Y, Ishihara M, Hasumi Y, et al. Guidelines for the diagnosis of ocular sarcoidosis. Ocul Immunol Inflamm. 2008;16:77–81.
71. Edelsten C, Pearson A, Joynes E, et al. The ocular and systemic prognosis of patients presenting with sarcoid uveitis. Eye (Lond). 1999;13(Pt 6):748–53.
72. Bhat P, Cervantes-Castañeda RA, Doctor PP, et al. Mycophenolate mofetil therapy for sarcoidosis-associated uveitis. Ocul Immunol Inflamm. 2009;17:185–90.
73. Cruz BA, Reis DD, Araujo CA, et al. Refractory retinal vasculitis due to sarcoidosis successfully treated with infliximab. Rheumatol Int. 2007;27:1181–3.
74. Orum M, Hilberg O, Krag S, et al. Beneficial effect of infliximab on refractory sarcoidosis. Dan Med J. 2012;59:A4535.
75. Gautam M, Patil S, Munde P. Skin as a marker of internal disease: a case of sarcoidosis. Indian J Dermatol. 2011;56:439–41.
76. Cather JC, Cohen PR. Ichthyosiform sarcoidosis. J Am Acad Dermatol. 1999;40:862–5.
77. Matarasso SL, Bruce S. Ichthyosiform sarcoidosis: report of a case. Cutis. 1991;47:405–8.
78. Mountcastle ME, Lupton GP. An ichthyosiform eruption on the legs. Sarcoidosis. Arch Dermatol. 1989;125:1415–6, 1419.
79. Mana J, Marcoval J, Graells J, et al. Cutaneous involvement in sarcoidosis. Relationship to systemic disease. Arch Dermatol. 1997;133:882–8.
80. Banse-Kupin L, Pelachyk JM. Ichthyosiform sarcoidosis. Report of two cases and a review of the literature. J Am Acad Dermatol. 1987;17:616–20.
81. Mutlu GM, Rubinstein I. Clinical manifestations of sarcoidosis among inner-city African-American dwellers. J Natl Med Assoc. 2006;98:1140–3.
82. Sharma OP. Cutaneous sarcoidosis: clinical features and management. Chest. 1972;61: 320–5.
83. Odom R. Andrews' diseases of the skin. 9th ed. Philadelphia: W.B. Saunders; 2000. p. 896.
84. Gawkrodger D. Rook's text book of dermatology. 7th ed. Massachusetts: Blackwell; 2004. p. 1–23.
85. Cozier YC, Berman JS, Palmer JR, et al. Sarcoidosis in black women in the United States: data from the Black Women's Health Study. Chest. 2011;139:144–50.
86. Sharma O. Sarcoidosis of the skin: Fitzpatrick's dermatology in general medicine. 5th ed. New York: McGraw-Hill; 1999. p. 2099–106.
87. Statement on sarcoidosis. Joint Statement of the American Thoracic Society (ATS), the European Respiratory Society (ERS) and the World Association of Sarcoidosis and Other

Granulomatous Disorders (WASOG) adopted by the ATS Board of Directors and by the ERS Executive Committee, February 1999. Am J Respir Crit Care Med. 1999;160:736–55.

88. Wu JJ, Schiff KR. Sarcoidosis. Am Fam Physician. 2004;70:312–22.

89. Löfgren SH. Erythema nodosum: studies on etiology and pathogenesis in 185 adult cases. Norstedt Acta Med Scand. 1946;124 Suppl 174:1–197.

90. Siltzbach LE, James DG, Neville E, et al. Course and prognosis of sarcoidosis around the world. Am J Med. 1974;57:847–52.

91. Idali F, Wiken M, Wahlstrom J, et al. Reduced Th1 response in the lungs of HLA-DRB1*0301 patients with pulmonary sarcoidosis. Eur Respir J. 2006;27:451–9.

92. Alexis JB. Sarcoidosis presenting as cutaneous hypopigmentation with repeatedly negative skin biopsies. Int J Dermatol. 1994;33:44–5.

93. Kang MJ, Kim HS, Kim HO, et al. Cutaneous sarcoidosis presenting as multiple erythematous macules and patches. Ann Dermatol. 2009;21:168–70.

94. Fujii K, Okamoto H, Onuki M, et al. Recurrent follicular and lichenoid papules of sarcoidosis. Eur J Dermatol. 2000;10:303–5.

95. Shigemitsu H, Yarbrough CA, Prakash S, et al. A 65-year-old woman with subcutaneous nodule and hilar adenopathy. Chest. 2008;134:1080–3.

96. Choi SC, Kim HJ, Kim CR, et al. A case of morpheaform sarcoidosis. Ann Dermatol. 2010;22:316–8.

97. Kaiser CA, Cozzio A, Hofbauer GF, et al. Disfiguring annular sarcoidosis improved by adalimumab. Case Rep Dermatol. 2011;3:103–6.

98. Lubeck G, Epstein E. Complications of tattooing. Calif Med. 1952;76:83–5.

99. Rorsman H, Brehmer-Andersson E, Dahlquist I, et al. Tattoo granuloma and uveitis. Lancet. 1969;2:27–8.

100. Landers MC, Skokan M, Law S, et al. Cutaneous and pulmonary sarcoidosis in association with tattoos. Cutis. 2005;75:44–8.

101. Yanardag H, Pamuk ON, Karayel T. Cutaneous involvement in sarcoidosis: analysis of the features in 170 patients. Respir Med. 2003;97:978–82.

102. Ji R, Koh MS, Irving LB. Cutaneous sarcoidosis. Ann Acad Med Singapore. 2007;36:1044–5, 1057.

103. De Francesco V, Cathryn AS, Piccirillo F. Successful topical treatment of cutaneous sarcoidosis with macrolide immunomodulators. Eur J Dermatol. 2007;17:454–5.

104. Gutzmer R, Volker B, Kapp A, et al. [Successful topical treatment of cutaneous sarcoidosis with tacrolimus]. Hautarzt. 2003;54:1193–7.

105. Katoh N, Mihara H, Yasuno H. Cutaneous sarcoidosis successfully treated with topical tacrolimus. Br J Dermatol. 2002;147:154–6.

106. Badgwell C, Rosen T. Cutaneous sarcoidosis therapy updated. J Am Acad Dermatol. 2007;56:69–83.

107. Baughman RP, Lower EE. Leflunomide for chronic sarcoidosis. Sarcoidosis Vasc Diffuse Lung Dis. 2004;21:43–8.

108. Antoniu SA. Targeting the TNF-alpha pathway in sarcoidosis. Expert Opin Ther Targets. 2010;14:21–9.

109. Heffernan MP, Anadkat MJ. Recalcitrant cutaneous sarcoidosis responding to infliximab. Arch Dermatol. 2005;141:910–1.

110. Noor A, Knox KS. Immunopathogenesis of sarcoidosis. Clin Dermatol. 2007;25:250–8.

111. Baughman RP, Lower EE. Infliximab for refractory sarcoidosis. Sarcoidosis Vasc Diffuse Lung Dis. 2001;18:70–4.

112. Meyerle JH, Shorr A. The use of infliximab in cutaneous sarcoidosis. J Drugs Dermatol. 2003;2:413–4.

113. Mallbris L, Ljungberg A, Hedblad MA, et al. Progressive cutaneous sarcoidosis responding to anti-tumor necrosis factor-alpha therapy. J Am Acad Dermatol. 2003;48:290–3.

114. Roberts SD, Wilkes DS, Burgett RA, et al. Refractory sarcoidosis responding to infliximab. Chest. 2003;124:2028–31.

115. Haley H, Cantrell W, Smith K. Infliximab therapy for sarcoidosis (lupus pernio). Br J Dermatol. 2004;150:146–9.

116. Iwai K, Takemura T, Kitaichi M, et al. Pathological studies on sarcoidosis autopsy. II. Early change, mode of progression and death pattern. Acta Pathol Jpn. 1993;43:377–85.

117. Lehmuskallio E, Hannuksela M, Halme H. The liver in sarcoidosis. Acta Med Scand. 1977;202:289–93.

118. Hercules HD, Bethlem NM. Value of liver biopsy in sarcoidosis. Arch Pathol Lab Med. 1984;108:831–4.

119. Maddrey WC, Johns CJ, Boitnott JK, et al. Sarcoidosis and chronic hepatic disease: a clinical and pathologic study of 20 patients. Medicine (Baltimore). 1970;49:375–95.

120. Devaney K, Goodman ZD, Epstein MS, et al. Hepatic sarcoidosis. Clinicopathologic features in 100 patients. Am J Surg Pathol. 1993;17:1272–80.

121. Ebert EC, Kierson M, Hagspiel KD. Gastrointestinal and hepatic manifestations of sarcoidosis. Am J Gastroenterol. 2008;103:3184–92, quiz 3193.

122. Scadding JG, Mitchell DN. Sarcoidosis. London: Chapman and Hall; 1985. p. 704.

123. Kataoka M, Nakata Y, Hiramatsu J, et al. Hepatic and splenic sarcoidosis evaluated by multiple imaging modalities. Intern Med. 1998;37:449–53.

124. Vilinskas J, Joyeuse R, Serlin O. Hepatic sarcoidosis with portal hypertension. Am J Surg. 1970;120:393–6.

125. Melissant CF, Smith SJ, Kazzaz BA, et al. Bleeding varices due to portal hypertension in sarcoidosis. Favorable effect of propranolol and prednisone. Chest. 1993;103:628–9.

126. Cremers J, Drent M, Driessen A, et al. Liver-test abnormalities in sarcoidosis. Eur J Gastroenterol Hepatol. 2012;24:17–24.

127. Alenezi B, Lamoureux E, Alpert L, et al. Effect of ursodeoxycholic acid on granulomatous liver disease due to sarcoidosis. Dig Dis Sci. 2005;50:196–200.

128. Israel HL, Margolis ML, Rose LJ. Hepatic granulomatosis and sarcoidosis. Further observations. Dig Dis Sci. 1984;29:353–6.

129. Baughman RP. Sarcoidosis. Usual and unusual manifestations. Chest. 1988;94:165–70.

130. Nakata K, Iwata K, Kojima K, et al. Computed tomography of liver sarcoidosis. J Comput Assist Tomogr. 1989;13:707–8.

131. Warshauer DM, Dumbleton SA, Molina PL, et al. Abdominal CT findings in sarcoidosis: radiologic and clinical correlation. Radiology. 1994;192:93–8.

132. Gaya DR, Thorburn D, Oien KA, et al. Hepatic granulomas: a 10 year single centre experience. J Clin Pathol. 2003;56:850–3.

133. Farouj NE, Cadranel JF, Mofredj A, et al. Ductopenia related liver sarcoidosis. World J Hepatol. 2011;3:170–4.

134. Bandin O, Courvalin JC, Poupon R, et al. Specificity and sensitivity of gp210 autoantibodies detected using an enzyme-linked immunosorbent assay and a synthetic polypeptide in the diagnosis of primary biliary cirrhosis. Hepatology. 1996;23:1020–4.

135. Judson M. Hepatic and splenic sarcoidosis. New York: Marcel Dekker; 2006. p. 571–92.

136. Blich M, Edoute Y. Clinical manifestations of sarcoid liver disease. J Gastroenterol Hepatol. 2004;19:732–7.

137. Valla D, Pessegueiro-Miranda H, Degott C, et al. Hepatic sarcoidosis with portal hypertension. A report of seven cases with a review of the literature. Q J Med. 1987;63:531–44.

138. Gottlieb JE, Israel HL, Steiner RM, et al. Outcome in sarcoidosis. The relationship of relapse to corticosteroid therapy. Chest. 1997;111:623–31.

139. Becheur H, Dall'osto H, Chatellier G, et al. Effect of ursodeoxycholic acid on chronic intrahepatic cholestasis due to sarcoidosis. Dig Dis Sci. 1997;42:789–91.

140. Baratta L, Cascino A, Delfino M, et al. Ursodeoxycholic acid treatment in abdominal sarcoidosis. Dig Dis Sci. 2000;45:1559–62.

141. Bakker GJ, Haan YC, Maillette de Buy Wenniger LJ, et al. Sarcoidosis of the liver: to treat or not to treat? Neth J Med. 2012;70:349–56.

142. Cremers JP, Drent M, Bast A, Shigemitsu H, et al. Multinational evidence-based World Association of Sarcoidosis and Other Granulomatous Disorders recommendations for the use of methotrexate in sarcoidosis: integrating systematic literature research and expert opinion of sarcoidologists worldwide. Curr Opin Pulm Med. 2013;19(5):545–61.

143. Muller-Quernheim J, Kienast K, Held M, et al. Treatment of chronic sarcoidosis with an azathioprine/prednisolone regimen. Eur Respir J. 1999;14:1117–22.
144. Sahoo DH, Bandyopadhyay D, Xu M, et al. Effectiveness and safety of leflunomide for pulmonary and extrapulmonary sarcoidosis. Eur Respir J. 2011;38:1145–50.
145. Tekeste H, Latour F, Levitt RE. Portal hypertension complicating sarcoid liver disease: case report and review of the literature. Am J Gastroenterol. 1984;79:389–96.
146. Fidler HM, Hadziyannis SJ, Dhillon AP, et al. Recurrent hepatic sarcoidosis following liver transplantation. Transplant Proc. 1997;29:2509–10.
147. Hunt J, Gordon FD, Jenkins RL, et al. Sarcoidosis with selective involvement of a second liver allograft: report of a case and review of the literature. Mod Pathol. 1999;12:325–8.
148. Pescovitz MD, Jones HM, Cummings OW, et al. Diffuse retroperitoneal lymphadenopathy following liver transplantation – a case of recurrent sarcoidosis. Transplantation. 1995;60:393–6.
149. Fordice J, Katras T, Jackson RE, et al. Massive splenomegaly in sarcoidosis. South Med J. 1992;85:775–8.
150. Taavitsainen M, Koivuniemi A, Helminen J, et al. Aspiration biopsy of the spleen in patients with sarcoidosis. Acta Radiol. 1987;28:723–5.
151. Selroos O, Koivunen E. Usefulness of fine-needle aspiration biopsy of spleen in diagnosis of sarcoidosis. Chest. 1983;83:193–5.
152. Friedman M. Sarcoidosis of the spleen: report of a case with autopsy and a study of intracellular "asteroid bodies". Am J Pathol. 1944;20:621–35.
153. James DG, Turiaf J, Hosoda Y, et al. Description of sarcoidosis: report of the Subcommittee on Classification and Definition. Ann N Y Acad Sci. 1976;278:742.
154. Grzelak P, Augsburg L, Majos A, et al. Use of contrast-enhanced ultrasonography in hepatosplenic sarcoidosis: report of 2 cases. Pol J Radiol. 2012;77:60–3.
155. Webb AK, Mitchell DN, Bradstreet CM, et al. Splenomegaly and splenectomy in sarcoidosis. J Clin Pathol. 1979;32:1050–3.
156. Robertson F, Leander P, Ekberg O. Radiology of the spleen. Eur Radiol. 2001;11:80–95.
157. Kataria YP, Whitcomb ME. Splenomegaly in sarcoidosis. Arch Intern Med. 1980;140:35–7.
158. Scadding JG. A 'burnt-out' case of sarcoidosis. Postgrad Med J. 1968;44:105–8.
159. Kessler A, Mitchell DG, Israel HL, et al. Hepatic and splenic sarcoidosis: ultrasound and MR imaging. Abdom Imaging. 1993;18:159–63.
160. MacArthur KL, Forouhar F, Wu GY. Intra-abdominal complications of sarcoidosis. J Formos Med Assoc. 2010;109:484–92.
161. Stone RW, McDaniel WR, Armstrong EM, et al. Acquired functional asplenia in sarcoidosis. J Natl Med Assoc. 1985;77(930):935–6.
162. Warshauer DM, Semelka RC, Ascher SM. Nodular sarcoidosis of the liver and spleen: appearance on MR images. J Magn Reson Imaging. 1994;4:553–7.
163. Chorostowska-Wynimko J, Leśniewska-Radomska D, Krychniak-Soszka A, et al. Cellular components of the bronchoalveolar lavage correlate with lung function impairment and extrapulmonary involvement markers in active sarcoidosis. J Physiol Pharmacol. 2004;55 Suppl 3:41–7.
164. Ali Y, Popescu NA, Woodlock TJ. Extrapulmonary sarcoidosis: rapid spontaneous remission of marked splenomegaly. J Natl Med Assoc. 1996;88:714–6.
165. Israel HL, Karlin P, Menduke H, et al. Factors affecting outcome of sarcoidosis. Influence of race, extrathoracic involvement, and initial radiologic lung lesions. Ann N Y Acad Sci. 1986;465:609–18.
166. Phillips AK, Luchette AA. Rupture of the spleen due to sarcoidosis. Ohio Med. 1952;48:617–9.
167. Sharma OP. Splenic rupture in sarcoidosis. Report of an unusual case. Am Rev Respir Dis. 1967;96:101–2.
168. James I, Wilson AJ. Spontaneous rupture of the spleen in sarcoidosis. Br J Surg. 1946;33:280–2.
169. Nusair S, Kramer MR, Berkman N. Pleural effusion with splenic rupture as manifestations of recurrence of sarcoidosis following prolonged remission. Respiration. 2003;70:114–7.

170. Dickerman JD, Holbrook PR, Zinkham WH. Etiology and therapy of thrombocytopenia associated with sarcoidosis. J Pediatr. 1972;81:758–64.
171. Sharma OP. Vitamin D, calcium, and sarcoidosis. Chest. 1996;109:535–9.
172. Sharma OP, Trowell J, Cohen N, et al. Abnormal calcium metabolism in sarcoidosis. In: Turiaf J, Chabot J, editors. La sarcoidose: Rapp IV Conf Intern. Paris: maison de Cie; 1967. p. 627–32.
173. Rizato G, Columbo P. Nephrocalcinosis as a presenting feature of chronic sarcoidosis: a prospective study. Sarcoidosis Vasc Diffuse Lung Dis. 1996;13:167–72.
174. Barre PE, Gascon-Barre M, Meekins JL, et al. Hydroxychloroquine treatment of hypercalcemia in a patient with sarcoidosis undergoing hemodialysis. Am J Med. 1987;82:1259–62.
175. Conron M, Beynon HLC. Ketoconazole for the treatment of refractory hypercalcemic sarcoidosis. Sarcoidosis Vasc Diffuse Lung Dis. 2000;17:277–80.
176. Jansen TLTA, Geusens PPMM. Sarcoidosis: joint, muscle, and bone involvement. Eur Respir J Monogr. 2005;10:210–9.
177. Wilcox A, Bharadwaj P, Sharma OP. Bone sarcoidosis. Curr Opin Rheumatol. 2000;12:321–9.
178. Shigemitsu H. Is sarcoidosis frequent in patients with cancer? Curr Opin Pulm Med. 2008;14(5):478–80.
179. Sharma OP. Renal sarcoidosis and hypercalcemia. Eur Respir J Monogr. 2005;10:220–32.

Chapter 9
Instructive Cases of Pulmonary Sarcoidosis

Andrew J. Goodwin and Carlos E. Kummerfeldt

Abstract The respiratory system is the organ system most commonly affected by sarcoidosis. The most common finding is mediastinal and/or hilar lymphadenopathy, however involvement of the upper and lower airways, lung parenchyma, and pulmonary vasculature are also seen with varying frequencies. This chapter utilizes a case-based format in order to highlight different presentations of pulmonary sarcoidosis with which clinicians should be familiar. The accompanying discussions are designed to review the existing literature regarding each presentation as well as provide a historical view of pulmonary sarcoidosis for the practicing clinician. While there are many different presentations of pulmonary sarcoidosis that could have been discussed here, these cases were selected specifically for their instructive potential and not because of their frequency. Our hope is that these cases will enhance clinicians' understanding of different pulmonary sarcoidosis presentations as well as improve their comfort level with the management of this disease.

Keywords Respiratory system • Mediastinal lymphadenopathy • Hilar lymphadenopathy • Lung parenchyma • Pulmonary vasculature

A.J. Goodwin, M.D., M.S.C.R. (✉) • C.E. Kummerfeldt, M.D.
Division of Pulmonary, Critical Care, Allergy, and Sleep Medicine,
Medical University of South Carolina, Charleston, SC, USA
e-mail: goodwian@musc.edu

M.A. Judson (ed.), *Pulmonary Sarcoidosis: A Guide for the Practicing Clinician*,
Respiratory Medicine 17, DOI 10.1007/978-1-4614-8927-6_9,
© Springer Science+Business Media New York 2014

Sarcoidosis with Associated Pulmonary Hypertension

Case Presentation

Mrs. D is a 52-year-old African-American female with a history of sarcoidosis characterized by pulmonary and ocular involvement who was seen in follow-up for increasing fatigue. Aside from sarcoidosis, her medical history is notable for essential hypertension and she has a first cousin with sarcoidosis. She had previously worked in a factory manufacturing electrical wires but currently works as an administrative assistant in an office environment. She has a 12 pack-year smoking history and quit 10 years ago. She was initially diagnosed with sarcoidosis 7 years earlier when she presented with a nonproductive cough, dyspnea, and bilateral eye redness. Chest imaging at the time of her initial presentation revealed hilar lymphadenopathy with bilateral micronodular infiltrates with a bronchovascular and subpleural predominance. She underwent bronchoscopy with transbronchial biopsy that demonstrated non-caseating granulomas without evidence of acid-fast bacilli or fungal organisms. She was also noted to have evidence of uveitis on dedicated eye exam. Her pulmonary function testing at that time revealed a mixed mild obstructive and restrictive deficit with a corresponding mild decrease in the carbon monoxide diffusing capacity (DLCO) (Table 9.1). She was treated with prednisone 20 mg daily for approximately 3 months with improvement in her symptoms after which she was tapered off of prednisone over the next 3 months. She reported no symptoms and had normal pulmonary function testing at a 6 month follow-up visit.

During the following year, she moved to a new state for employment reasons and did not seek follow-up for sarcoidosis for the next 5 years. Then, a year ago, she moved back to the area and was referred back to the pulmonary clinic after presenting to the emergency department with progressive dyspnea and fatigue. At her first visit, she complained of nonproductive cough and exertional dyspnea that is roughly equivalent to New York Heart Association (NYHA) class II symptoms. Her examination was notable for an oxygen saturation of 93 %, no adventitious breath sounds, and trace lower extremity edema. Pulmonary function testing revealed a moderate restrictive deficit with a mild concomitant obstructive deficit with a severely reduced DLCO (Table 9.1). A 6-min walk test (6MWT) demonstrated exertional desaturation to 87 % and mild exercise limitation. During her recent emergency room

Table 9.1 Pulmonary function testing at the time of initial diagnosis and at initial visit when patient re-established care

	7 Years ago	Return to care
FVC (L)	2.44 (83 %)	1.86 (59 %)
FEV1 (L)	1.62 (70 %)	1.24 (54 %)
FEV1/FVC	66 %	66 %
TLC (L)	4.00 (69 %)	3.31 (57 %)
DLCO (mL/mmHg/min)	15.8 (65 %)	7.6 (30 %)

(Percent predicted), *FVC* forced vital capacity, *FEV1* forced expiratory volume in 1 s, *TLC* total lung capacity, *DLCO* carbon monoxide diffusing capacity

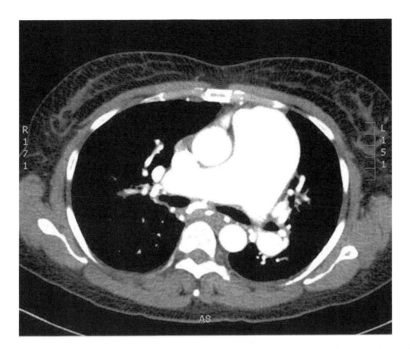

Fig. 9.1 Soft tissue window of the chest CT angiogram performed at the time of presentation to the emergency department. No pulmonary embolism is identified. There is enlargement of the main pulmonary artery, the right and left pulmonary artery branches, and the left lower lobar branch

evaluation, she underwent a chest computed tomography (CT) angiogram with a representative cut shown in Fig. 9.1. Home exertional and nocturnal oxygen was arranged and she was placed back on prednisone 20 mg daily.

An echocardiogram revealed a normal appearing left ventricle with an ejection fraction of 74 %. The right ventricle and atrium were normal in size; however, the right ventricular systolic pressure was estimated from the tricuspid regurgitant jet to be 72 mmHg. She was subsequently scheduled for a right heart catheterization which revealed the following data: right atrial pressure 8 mmHg, pulmonary artery pressure 68/33 (46) mmHg, pulmonary capillary wedge pressure 14 mmHg, and cardiac index 2.78 L/min/m^2 (thermodilution). Inhalation of nitric oxide 40 ppm decreased her pulmonary artery pressures to 50/24 (35) mmHg, while her cardiac index remained stable at 2.81 L/min/m^2. She was prescribed sildenafil 20 mg three times per day as well as Lasix 10 mg daily. As she had normal appearing heart chambers at this time, anticoagulation was not prescribed. A sleep study, ventilation/perfusion scan, and autoimmune serology panel were all performed and are all found to be within normal limits. She was seen in the office 2 months later and reports significantly improved fatigue. Her oxygenation saturation nadir was 91 % on room air during her 6MWT and she walked 85 m longer than previous testing. Over the course of the next several months, her prednisone is tapered down to 5 mg daily with stable spirometry and 6MWT.

Discussion

Epidemiology of Pulmonary Hypertension in Sarcoidosis

Although sarcoidosis was likely first described in 1877 by Sir Jonathan Hutchinson [1], its association with pulmonary hypertension was not published until some 74 years later when Austrian and colleagues described two patients with pulmonary sarcoidosis and elevated pulmonary artery pressures [2]. Since this important observation was made, much has been uncovered about the association between sarcoidosis and pulmonary hypertension; however, there is clearly much that is still incompletely understood. The true prevalence of sarcoidosis-associated pulmonary hypertension (SAPH) is unknown. Published reports vary widely and are largely dependent upon the subject selection criteria. In a Japanese study which screened 212 sarcoidosis patients without other inclusion criteria, 5.7 % had echocardiographic evidence of SAPH [3]. Another study determined that in patients with sarcoidosis and a clinical indication for echocardiography, the prevalence of SAPH was as high as 51 % [4]. Furthermore, an analysis of the United Network for Organ Sharing (UNOS) database revealed that in patients with sarcoidosis listed for lung transplantation who had undergone right heart catheterization, the prevalence of SAPH was as high as 74 % [5]. Clearly, the potential for selection bias in these three studies influences the reported prevalence rates. In reality, the prevalence of SAPH appears to increase with increasing radiographic stage and decreasing lung function [3, 4] but occasionally can be found in the absence of significant parenchymal compromise [6].

Mechanisms of Sarcoidosis-Associated Pulmonary Hypertension

The etiologies of pulmonary hypertension have historically been divided into different functional groups in a classification scheme endorsed by the World Health Organization (WHO). This scheme was most recently updated in 2008 at the 4th World Symposium on Pulmonary Hypertension [7] and divides the etiologies of pulmonary hypertension into five broad groups: Group 1, Arterial causes of pulmonary hypertension (PH); Group 2, Venous causes of PH; Group 3, PH secondary to hypoxemia; Group 4, Chronic thromboembolic PH; and Group 5, Multifactorial causes of PH. Sarcoidosis-associated PH continues to be included in Group 5 as there are a variety of ways in which the disease can cause pulmonary pressure elevations.

While sarcoid granulomata are most commonly found in the pulmonary lymphatics, granulomatous inflammation has been visualized directly in the walls of pulmonary arterioles and venules. This is likely facilitated by the proximity of the lymphatics to the bronchovascular bundle in the lung. The resulting vascular inflammation can lead to an occlusive vasculopathy of both the arteriolar and venular systems [8]. If the venous system is significantly compromised, a pulmonary veno-occlusive disease (PVOD)-like syndrome can occur [6]. Alternatively, the correlation of SAPH and progressive parenchymal sarcoid disease [3, 4] suggests that destruction of vascular beds by fibrosis may also contribute to the pathogenesis of PH in this population. Hepatic sarcoidosis with resultant cirrhosis and portopulmonary hypertension has also been described [9]. As these examples suggest, the various etiologies of SAPH can bear some resemblance to the WHO Group 1.

Myocardial involvement can occur in sarcoidosis and when it does, can lead to both systolic and diastolic dysfunction of the left ventricle. If severe enough, patients can develop SAPH secondary to pulmonary venous hypertension in a manner similar to the WHO Group 2. An echocardiogram and/or right heart catheterization will help to differentiate this etiology by assessing left ventricular function and filling pressures. Hypoxemia related to parenchymal fibrosis in advanced sarcoidosis can result in hypoxemic vasoconstriction and subsequent vascular remodeling. Similarly, the high prevalence rate of obstructive sleep apnea (OSA) in sarcoidosis [10] may further contribute to the relationship between PH and sarcoidosis through repetitive episodes of hypoxemia (akin to WHO Group 3). Finally, a more unique etiology of PH in sarcoidosis has been described in which large, central pulmonary vessels have been stenosed by lymphadenopathy [11, 12] or mediastinal fibrosis [13, 14].

Effects of Pulmonary Hypertension on Sarcoidosis Outcomes

Pulmonary hypertension is known to worsen clinical outcomes when it complicates advanced lung diseases such as idiopathic pulmonary fibrosis (IPF) and chronic obstructive pulmonary disease (COPD) [15–18]. Similarly, the presence of SAPH has been shown to increase the risk of mortality in patients with advanced sarcoidosis who are listed for lung transplant [19–21]. In fact, Baughman and colleagues found that patients with SAPH had a >10-fold mortality risk increase compared to patients without SAPH. In a separate study, right-sided cardiac dysfunction, as defined by a right atrial pressure > 15 mmHg, was the best predictor of death while awaiting transplant in patients with advanced sarcoidosis [21]. In addition to the effect on mortality, the presence of SAPH has also been associated with reduced functional status, inability to work, and need for supplemental oxygen [5].

Diagnosis of Sarcoidosis-Associated Pulmonary Hypertension

One of the most challenging aspects of managing a patient with SAPH can be making the diagnosis. The most common presenting complaint is dyspnea which is often attributed to the underlying sarcoidosis. Certain clinical, functional, or radiographic characteristics may help to identify patients with concomitant PH and, therefore, should be identified when possible.

As with any patient with PH, the physical exam can raise suspicion for SAPH. The presence of resting or exertional hypoxemia could be an important clue to the presence of PH. Indeed, one study reported that if a sarcoidosis patient desaturates to below 90 % during a 6MWT, he or she is 12 times more likely to have SAPH than somebody without desaturation [22]. Likewise classic clinical exam findings consistent with PH such as an accentuated P2 or peripheral edema could represent important clues but may not be specific to SAPH. Pulmonary function testing may be another way to quickly screen for the presence of SAPH. While there is no good data to suggest that spirometry or lung volumes accurately predict the presence or absence of PH in sarcoidosis patients, a significantly reduced DLCO has some predictive ability for SAPH. Bourbannais and Samavati demonstrated that sarcoidosis patients with a DLCO < 60 % predicted had a >7-fold increase in the risk of having coexisting PH [22].

Most patients with sarcoidosis undergo chest imaging. While chest X-ray is still perhaps the most common modality used, its ability to detect signs of pulmonary hypertension may be limited in sarcoidosis due to the common finding of hilar adenopathy which can obscure the evaluation of the proximal pulmonary arteries. In today's practice, however, more and more patients with sarcoidosis are receiving CT scans of the chest. As it is well validated that the size of the diameter of the pulmonary artery (PA) as well as the ratio of the PA diameter to the aortic diameter are sensitive predictors for the presence of PH [23], chest CT scans can also be useful tools for screening for SAPH.

In those patients in whom there is a reasonable suspicion for SAPH, a Doppler transthoracic echocardiogram (TTE) is the least invasive and most appropriate next step in the evaluation. While the possibility of both over and underestimation of pulmonary arterial pressures by TTE is well described in advanced lung disease [24], this modality is often very useful in ruling out significant PH and can also be used to identify other cardiac causes of dyspnea. In patients who have echocardiographic evidence of PH, a right heart catheterization is appropriate to both confirm the diagnosis as well as to assess for left heart dysfunction and pulmonary vasoreactivity. As there is a known risk of pulmonary venous obliteration secondary to granulomatous inflammation in SAPH, patients should be monitored carefully for clinical deterioration during vasodilator trials.

Treatment of Sarcoidosis-Associated Pulmonary Hypertension

The appropriate treatment strategy for SAPH remains controversial largely because of a lack of reliable data. Perhaps the only treatment that would be uniformly recommended for this condition would be the use of supplemental oxygen to maintain exertional and resting oxygen saturations above 90 % to ameliorate any contribution from hypoxic pulmonary vasoconstriction. Additionally, any secondary contributors such as left-sided ventricular or valvular dysfunction should also be managed with appropriate therapies. There is no clear consensus as to which pulmonary vasodilators provide optimal benefit for patients with SAPH because there have been insufficient randomized controlled trials to date. Much of the existing literature includes case series or small randomized trials of endothelin receptor antagonists, phosphodiesterase inhibitors, and prostanoids. These data are reviewed elsewhere in this text in detail. There does not appear to be a consistent role for the use of steroids to treat SAPH unless it is clearly related to extrinsic compression of proximal arteries by lymphadenopathy.

Summary

Sarcoidosis can be frequently complicated by pulmonary hypertension, particularly in advanced disease, and its presence portends higher morbidity and mortality. Clinicians should maintain a high index of suspicion for SAPH in patients with disproportionate dyspnea, signs of right heart failure, or signs of pulmonary vascular disease by CT or DLCO. Several different mechanisms for the development of SAPH have been described and because treatment strategies may differ based on etiology, these mechanisms should be identified in each patient when possible. Pulmonary vasodilators appear to be a safe option in most patients with SAPH, however, efficacy and effectiveness data is still lacking at this time.

The Etiology of Sarcoidosis

Case Presentation

A 49-year-old female was referred to our clinic for evaluation of incidentally found hilar, mediastinal, and retroperitoneal lymphadenopathy. Five years earlier she was diagnosed with invasive ductal carcinoma of her left breast and underwent bilateral mastectomy with four cycles of adjuvant chemotherapy with cyclophosphamide and docetaxel. She subsequently underwent breast reconstruction using silicone implants. One year later, she noted swelling of her left breast and she was found to have a ruptured left implant, which was subsequently replaced. Four years after the discovery of her implant rupture, she noticed intermittent arthralgias and myalgias. Around this time she developed left lower quadrant abdominal pain which was clinically suspicious for diverticulitis. An abdominal computed tomography was performed, which not only confirmed sigmoid diverticulitis but also revealed retroperitoneal lymphadenopathy and a 4-mm round nodule in the lower lobe of the left lung. She was treated with antibiotics with improvement in her abdominal pain. Given her history of breast cancer, a whole body positron-emission computed tomography was performed to better evaluate the incidentally found nodule and adenopathy. This demonstrated hypermetabolic hilar, mediastinal, and retroperitoneal lymphadenopathy (Fig. 9.2). Additionally, there was metabolic activity surrounding the posteromedial aspect of the right breast implant as well as a right peri-implant fluid collection suspicious for rupture. The new left breast implant did not show metabolic activity surrounding the capsule but demonstrated findings consistent with prior implant rupture. She was referred to a thoracic surgeon at another institution who performed mediastinoscopy with paratracheal lymph node resection (Fig. 9.3) as well as right breast capsule biopsies (Fig. 9.4) which all revealed non-caseating granulomas. Cultures and staining were negative for mycobacterial or fungal microorganisms. No silica particles were seen on her biopsies. She was referred to our institution for further evaluation and management of presumed sarcoidosis.

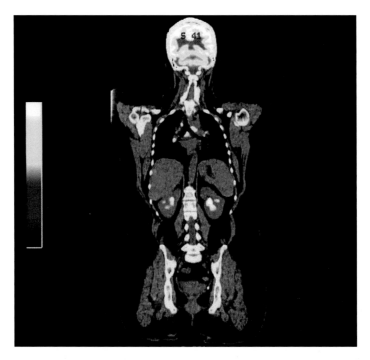

Fig. 9.2 Whole body positron-emission computed tomography showing hypermetabolic mediastinal, hilar, and subcarinal lymphadenopathy

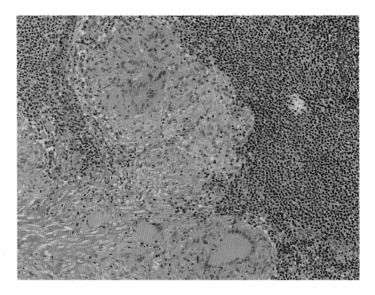

Fig. 9.3 Mediastinal lymph node biopsy demonstrating multiple non-caseating granulomas with giant cell formation (H & E, 100×2)

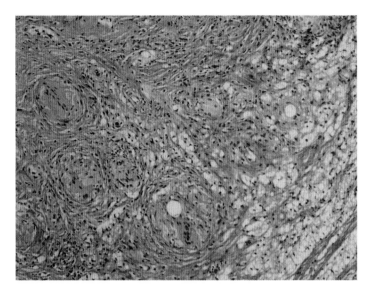

Fig. 9.4 Breast capsule biopsy showing multiple granulomas surrounded by fibrous tissue (H & E, 100×1)

At her initial clinic visit, her arthralgias and myalgias had completely resolved. Her joints and the rest of her physical exam were normal. Her spirometry showed a forced expiratory volume in 1 s over forced vital capacity ratio (FEV1/FVC) of 0.85. Her FVC was 3.09 L (94 % of predicted) and her FEV1 was 2.62 L (100 % of predicted). Total lung volume obtained via nitrogen washout technique was 3.82 L (83 % of predicted). Her carbon monoxide diffusion capacity was 19.6 mL/mmHg/min (80 % of predicted). Her complete blood count, blood urea nitrogen, serum creatinine, calcium, albumin, liver function tests, and alkaline phosphatase were normal. Since she did not have any symptoms, systemic therapy was deferred in favor of further monitoring.

Discussion

A Historical Perspective on the Etiology of Sarcoidosis

Since the first accounts of sarcoidosis, there have been numerous attempts to discover its underlying etiology. Along the way, many different theories have been put forth although, to date, the exact etiology remains elusive. In January 1869, Dr. Jonathan Hutchinson, a British "Medical Renaissance Man" working at the Blackfriars Hospital for Skin Diseases in London, described the first case of what is thought to have been sarcoidosis. A 58-year-old coal-wharf worker presented with purple, symmetrical skin plaques on the legs and hands that had developed over the past 2 years. Dr. Hutchinson attributed the skin lesions to the patient's underlying gout [1]. That same year, however, while visiting a Norwegian university, he was shown drawings of a patient with similar skin manifestations who did not have gout raising the question of an alternative diagnosis [25].

In 1889, the French dermatologist Ernest Besnier described a patient with violaceous skin lesions of the nose, ears, and fingers, coining the term "lupus pernio" [26] suggesting a belief that this disorder was related to lupus erythematosus. Eight years later, Caesar Boeck, a Norwegian physician, became the first person to describe the histology of sarcoidosis. He coined the term "sarkoid" in 1897 after describing the case of a patient with multiple benign sarcoma-like lesions of the skin with well-defined foci of epithelioid cells with giant cells [27]. While he acknowledged that the lesions were not malignant, Dr. Boeck's description suggested a belief that this disorder was neoplastic in origin. After the turn of the twentieth century, the Danish ophthalmologist Christian Heerfordt described uveitis, parotid gland hypertrophy, and cranial nerve palsies as one condition that he called "febris uveoparotidea subchronica" [28]. He attributed this syndrome to mumps, and another 28 years passed before it was eventually established that febris uveoparotidea subchronica was actually a manifestation of sarcoidosis [29, 30].

After it had been demonstrated that sarcoidosis encompassed a broad range of clinical presentations including involvement of many different organ systems, the Swedish dermatologist Jorgen Schaumann provided a common pathologic basis for diverse clinical aspects of the disease and called it "lymphogranulomatosis benigna." He hypothesized that the condition was related to a benign lymphatic tissue proliferation triggered by a nonacid-fast variant of tubercle bacillus or an attenuated form of bovine tubercle bacillus [31]. Lucien-Marie Paultrier, a French dermatologist, also believed that sarcoidosis was caused by "atypical cutaneous tuberculosis" early in his career; however, later changed his views and, instead, attributed the disease to "reticuloendotheliosis" [25]. Sven Löfgren was another Swedish dermatologist who linked erythema nodosum and bilateral hilar adenopathy as a manifestation of sarcoidosis through tissue biopsies. Löfgren favored the notion that sarcoidosis had a viral etiology [32, 33].

Interestingly, despite the significant advances in diagnostic technology that have occurred since the time of the early descriptions of sarcoidosis, the causative mechanisms of the disease remain unclear. Investigative efforts over the last several decades have focused on identifying both organic and inorganic environmental exposures, including occupational exposures, as well as exploring genetic susceptibility. We will briefly summarize some of the seminal studies in this field below.

Environmental Exposures

For many years, the search for a cause of sarcoidosis has been focused on environmental exposures. As the most common presentations of sarcoidosis typically involve the respiratory tract, skin, and eyes, an airborne exposure has long been suspected as the most likely cause. Previous studies have utilized case–control, epidemiologic methodology as well as translational methodologies including the analysis of serum or tissue biopsies with molecular diagnostics such as polymerase chain reaction (PCR). The result of this work has been the identification of several possible associations between environmental antigens and sarcoidosis but no clear proof of causation.

Organic Antigen Exposures

As previously mentioned, since the early days of the study of sarcoidosis, scientists recognized the clinical and pathologic similarity between sarcoidosis and mycobacterial disease including tuberculosis. Naturally, this led many to believe that sarcoidosis was, in fact, a manifestation of mycobacterial infection and resulted in numerous studies attempting to establish this connection. In the 1950s and 1960s Riley and Scadding each described the presence of *Mycobacterium tuberculosis* bacilli inside of granulomas that were felt to be caused by sarcoidosis [34, 35]. Some suggested that sarcoidosis with its non-caseating granulomas was a "transition" point before development of tuberculosis with caseating granulomas [35]. What is not clear from Riley and Scadding's reports, of course, is whether the subjects of their studies truly had sarcoidosis or whether they had tuberculosis with non-caseating granulomas seen on biopsy. Nonetheless, the numerous reports in the literature describing sarcoidosis occurring either after [36–41] or concurrently with tuberculosis [42–45] or with non-tuberculous mycobacterial infections [46–49] raise the question of whether sarcoidosis could develop in response to infection with this family of organisms. Furthermore, studies using PCR have detected the presence of *M. tuberculosis* and non-tuberculous mycobacterial DNA in sarcoid granulomas [50–54], while antibodies against *M. tuberculosis* heat shock protein 70 and *M. tuberculosis* catalase-peroxidase (mKatG) have been identified in the serum of patients with sarcoidosis [55, 56]. Evidence that immune cells from both the blood [57, 58] and the bronchoalveolar lavage (BAL) [57] of patients with sarcoidosis exhibit heightened responses to mycobacterial antigens further supports an association between sarcoidosis and mycobacterial infections.

Another organism which has garnered recent attention in the sarcoidosis arena is *Propionibacterium acnes*. In the 1980s Abe and colleagues described an increased prevalence of *P. acnes* growth in the lung and lymph node tissues of sarcoidosis patients as compared to controls. Subsequent studies have used PCR on sarcoidosis lung tissue to support this finding [59] as well as to demonstrate that *P. acnes* DNA levels are higher in BAL fluid from patients with sarcoidosis as compared to controls [60]. Alternatively, recent data suggest that *P. acnes* may be more common in normal lung than previously estimated, calling into question whether its presence is actually specific to sarcoidosis or whether it is a commensal organism in all humans [61]. Recent efforts in this direction have begun to focus on heterogeneities of the innate immune system and how such heterogeneities could result in *P. acnes* colonization leading to sarcoidosis [62].

In addition to bacterial and mycobacterial organisms, mold has been recognized as possible causative agent in sarcoidosis. The ACCESS study was a large case–control study with the objective of identifying causative exposures of sarcoidosis. The study demonstrated statistically significant associations between sarcoidosis and work environments with mold/mildew exposure as well as work in areas with musty odors [63]. In another study, a high prevalence of new-onset sarcoidosis was seen among the occupants of an office building with water damage [64]. Additionally, in a separate, smaller case–control study [65], measurement of *N*-acetylhexosaminidase, a marker for concentration of fungal cell elements, was performed in the bedrooms of patients with clinically established sarcoidosis as well as controls. Subjects with active and recurrent sarcoidosis had significantly higher levels of fungal elements. A small, prospective study compared treatment of sarcoidosis patients with antifungals versus corticosteroids versus combination therapy. Using the clinical endpoints of serum angiotensin-converting enzyme level and X-ray scores, the authors argued that patients treated with antifungal therapy had better response rates [66]. More rigorous study is necessary, however, before this approach can be widely recommended.

In addition to microbial associations, prior studies have also suggested associations between sarcoidosis and nonmicrobial organic antigens. Classic studies by Buck et al. and Terris et al. revealed that smoke from wood burning stoves is associated with sarcoidosis [67, 68]. Exposure to tree pollen [69, 70] and soil [71, 72] has also been described as having associations with this disease. Additionally, the ACCESS study demonstrated an association between sarcoidosis and agricultural employment as well as occupational insecticide exposure [63]. Conceptually, these nonmicrobial organic exposures would likely serve as antigens which trigger granulomatous inflammation in the absence of true infection.

Inorganic Antigen Exposures

Just as nonmicrobial organic material can serve as antigens, it is equally possible that inorganic material can play a similar role. Indeed, multiple inorganic exposures have been associated with sarcoid granuloma formation, although the majority have been described as case reports or small case series. Several of these are described below with a particular emphasis on silicone and its possible association with sarcoidosis.

Silicone is a synthetic polymer with the favorable property of being "biodurable," which led to its use in a wide range of medical devices. For decades silicone could be found in catheters, drains, joint prostheses, needles, syringes, and extracorporeal circuits and is still used in some of these devices today. Perhaps the most publically known use of silicone in medical technology has been its use in breast implants. Silicone breast implants came under fire in the early 1990s after a series of ruptures generated concern over possible health consequences. Ultimately, the US Food and Drug Administration allowed their continued use in the USA. Since 1994 there have been at least 9 reports of a sarcoidosis-like syndrome occurring after exposure to medical device-related silicone (Table 9.2). Five of the nine were associated with breast implants.

Teuber and colleagues described the first documented case of sarcoidosis related to silicone gel breast implants [73]. The patient's debilitating multisystem sarcoidosis improved following removal of the implants. Similar to the case described in this chapter, capsular breast tissue showed foreign-body granulomas in Teuber's patient. Yoshida and colleagues described a case of neurosarcoidosis that developed 22 years after silicone breast implantation [74]. The implants were not removed but the patient's symptoms improved after steroid administration. Breast biopsy of the patient also showed granulomas. The development of Löfgren's syndrome after silicone breast implantation was reported in one case [75], while Miyashita et al. described a case of pulmonary sarcoidosis that developed 7 months after silicone breast implant rupture [76]. Two cases of cutaneous sarcoidosis due to silicone injections have also been reported [77, 78]. Silica was detected within the

Table 9.2 Medical silicone exposure cases associated with sarcoidosis

Case	Year	Age (years)	Gender	Location	Exposure	Onset after initial exposure	Clinical presentation	Target organs	Pathological findings
Teuber et al.	1994	44	Female	USA	Breast implants	8 years	Chest pain, dyspnea, uveitis, arthralgias	Lung, skin, LAD, oral mucosa	Non-caseating granulomas
Yoshida et al.	1996	55	Female	Japan	Breast implants	22 years	Vestibular ataxia, 8–9th left-sided cranial nerve palsies	LAD; nervous system	Granulomas containing polydimethyl-siloxane (silicone)
Barzo et al.	1998	30	Female	Hungary	Breast implants	10 months	Löfgren's syndrome[a]	LAD, skin, arthritis	Granulomas
Chang et al.	2003	54	Female	Hong Kong (China)	Breast implants	4 years	Facial and neck erythematous lesions	Skin, lung, pleura, LAD	Granulomas with occasional central caseous necrosis (skin); non-caseating granulomas (lung)
Miyashita et al.	2011	54	Female	Japan	Breast implants	5 years (7 months after right implant ruptured)	Fever, dyspnea, jaundice, DIC	Lung, liver	Non-caseating granulomas (liver)
Descamps	2008	48, 64	Both	France	Cosmetic facial fillers (hyaluronic acid and silicone)	Case 1: 5 years Case 2: 2 years	Skin nodules	Skin	Granulomas
Stroh	2009	29, 52	Both	Germany	Adjustable silicone gastric banding	Case 1: 1 year Case 2: 1 year	Enlarged mediastinum; pulmonary infiltrates	Lung	Granulomas
Pimentel et al.	2002	45	Female	Spain	Facial silicone injections	7 years	Facial papules and nodules; right knee and elbow plaques	Cutaneous	Granulomas; silicone confirmed by polarized light
Andrews et al.	2005	65	Female	USA	Facial silicone injections	15 years	Facial, knee and right forearm subcutaneous nodules	Cutaneous	Granulomas

LAD lymphadenopathy, *DIC* disseminated intravascular coagulation, *BAL* bronchoalveolar lavage, *MTB Mycobacterium tuberculosis*
[a] Löfgren syndrome is characterized by the triad of erythema nodosum, arthritis, and hilar lymphadenopathy

granulomas via polarized light in these cases. Similarly, a case of cutaneous granulomas occurred after injection of an industrial lubricating oil containing silicone, however, the authors argue that the patient did not have sarcoidosis [79]. Two cases of systemic sarcoidosis associated with cutaneous facial filler injections, one of which might have been with silicone, were reported by Descamps and colleagues. It is worth noting, however, that both patients were being treated with interferon for chronic hepatitis C [80]. Stroh et al. reported two cases of pulmonary sarcoidosis after implantation of silicone gastric banding [81].

Overall, the detection of silica or silicone-derived particles by polarized light within biopsies in the cases described above is inconsistent. Similarly, Kim and colleagues found polarizable foreign bodies in 12 of 50 patients (24 %) with cutaneous sarcoidosis, all of which had at least one other granulomatous systemic lesion [82]. As such, it is difficult to say definitively that medical silicone is truly a causative agent in sarcoidosis. The accumulation of more evidence will be required to make this determination in the future.

The World Trade Center (WTC) catastrophe has resulted in the report of several cases of sarcoid-like granulomatous lung disease. Izbicki and colleagues reported 26 cases among firefighters with new-onset sarcoidosis, six of which had extrathoracic disease [83]. Thirteen patients were identified during the first year after 9/11 and the rest during the next 4 years following the disaster. A separate study also identified 38 cases among WTC non-firefighter disaster responders [84]. Bowers and colleagues reported two cases, both of whom had direct exposure to ground zero during rescue operations [85]. In a nested case–control study, Jordan and et al. identified a total of 43 sarcoidosis cases after the WTC catastrophe. They concluded that working on the WTC debris pile was associated with an elevated risk (Odds Ratio = 9.1) of developing sarcoidosis [86].

Other inorganic environmental exposures associated with sarcoidosis or sarcoidosis-like syndromes have been described in the literature. For example, it is known that several different metals can promote granuloma formation [87]. Furthermore, in a study conducted in Switzerland, Deubelbeiss and colleagues found an increased prevalence of granulomatous disease in workers in the metal industry [88]. Individual case reports have also described sarcoidosis after exposure to inorganic dusts related to dental surgery and tunnel excavation [89, 90]. Recently, Song and colleagues [91] reported a case series of seven factory workers exposed to silica nanoparticles that developed respiratory symptoms. Two of the cases were fatal and biopsies performed showed pleural-based foreign-body granulomas. Nanoparticles to which the patients had been exposed were recovered from the biopsies.

The Role of Genetics

While there is substantial evidence suggesting that environmental exposures contribute to the development of sarcoidosis, a pertinent question becomes: "Why doesn't everyone with a particular exposure develop sarcoid?" The most likely answer is that genetic heterogeneity affects a person's susceptibility to the disease.

This hypothesis is supported by a study which demonstrated an increased risk of developing sarcoidosis in siblings of patients with the disease [92] as well as the apparent higher concordance rate in monozygotic twins compared to dizygotic twins [93].

To date, numerous candidate genes have been associated with sarcoidosis. Early work identified an association between sarcoidosis and class I HLA-B8 antigens [94], whereas subsequent studies discovered that specific regions of HLA-DQ and HLA-DR are linked to developing the disease [95]. Genome-wide association scans (GWAS) have identified regions on chromosomes 3p and 6p in white Europeans [96] and regions on 5p and 5q on black Americans that are related to sarcoidosis [97]. Validation studies have confirmed that genes in each of these regions influence susceptibility to sarcoidosis [98–100]. More recently, polymorphisms in matrix metalloproteinases and their inhibitors have also been associated with development of sarcoidosis [101].

Interestingly, the literature also suggests the existence of specific genes which modify the course of the disease. Specifically, Rybicki et al. described an association between a gene on chromosome 1p and radiographic resolution of disease as well as a gene on 18q associated with cardiac or renal involvement [102]. Veltkamp et al. analyzed the different haplotypes of the Toll-like receptor (TLR) gene cluster (TLR10-TLR1-TLR6) and found that distinct haplotypes were associated with chronic sarcoidosis and that these haplotypes differed from those associated with self-remitting disease [103]. Similarly, Pabst and colleagues reported polymorphisms in the TLR9 promoter region that are associated with chronic disease [104].

At this time, we still do not possess a complete understanding of the role of genetics in the development and maintenance of sarcoidosis. Future work will likely focus on further exploration of known candidate genes in the hope of identifying both prognostic biomarkers as well as therapeutic targets. An analysis of whether specific genetic polymorphisms preferentially predispose people to reacting to some exposures but not others would also help to clarify the heterogeneous nature of this disease.

Summary

Ultimately, the search for a single cause of sarcoidosis has yet to yield a satisfying, single answer. This has led many to propose a multifactorial etiology including both an environmental exposure and a "second hit," likely due to genetic susceptibility. Just as multiple infectious agents can cause granulomatous inflammation (mycobacterium species, fungal organisms, etc.); it is equally likely that multiple environmental exposures can cause the clinical phenotype of sarcoidosis. In fact, the possibility of multiple environmental exposures may help to explain the variable clinical phenotypes that have been described in the literature. Likewise, it is probable that more than one genetic predisposition exists. Distinct evolutionary pressures would suggest that a genetic predisposition in a Northern European sarcoidosis population may differ from a genetic predisposition in African Americans in the Southeastern USA. Furthermore, it is possible that certain genotypes only predispose people to developing sarcoidosis from specific environmental exposures. This may explain why case–control studies have failed to replicate certain promising exposures that were identified in other populations. Hopefully, future studies will help us to better understand and treat this fascinating disease.

Fibrocystic Sarcoidosis

Case Presentation

Mrs. B is a 49-year-old African-American female with a history of pulmonary sarcoidosis who was referred to the clinic by an emergency room physician after she presented the previous week with progressively worsening cough productive of brown sputum as well as right-sided pleuritic chest pain. In addition to sarcoidosis, she has been diagnosed with hyperlipidemia in the past. She has worked in housekeeping in the hotel industry for most of her adult life and she denies any known occupational or hobby-related inhalational exposures. She can recall no personal exposures to tuberculosis, nor does she admit to any risk factors for tuberculosis. She was diagnosed with sarcoidosis 15 years earlier when she was seen by a physician for chronic cough and dyspnea. She reports that a chest X-ray at that time was abnormal, stating "They thought I had cancer." She subsequently underwent a bronchoscopy with transbronchial biopsy which revealed non-caseating granulomatous inflammation without evidence of acid-fast bacilli or fungi. She was treated with prednisone for "a few years" but ultimately was lost to follow up about 10 years ago and stopped all therapy. In the interim, she again developed a chronic cough and mild dyspnea both of which have become progressively more severe over the last 2 years. She has noted that over the last 18 months, the cough has gone from being nonproductive to productive of dark brown sputum. Ultimately, she developed right-sided pleuritic chest pain in addition to these symptoms which prompted her to present to the emergency room. An electrocardiogram and a CT angiogram were both performed and she was discharged with an appointment in the pulmonary clinic.

In the office, she was noted to be afebrile with a normal respiratory pattern and no increased work of breathing. Her respiratory rate was 14 and her oxygen saturation was 99 % on room air. Her ocular and skin exams were normal. Her chest exam was notable for amphoric breath sounds in the upper lung zones bilaterally. Her pulmonary function testing revealed reduction in her FVC (74 % predicted), FEV1 (70 % predicted), TLC (57 % predicted), and DLCO (44 % predicted) with a normal FEV1/FVC ratio (0.76) suggesting a restrictive deficit with an accompanying gas exchange abnormality. Her CT angiogram (Fig. 9.5) revealed no evidence of

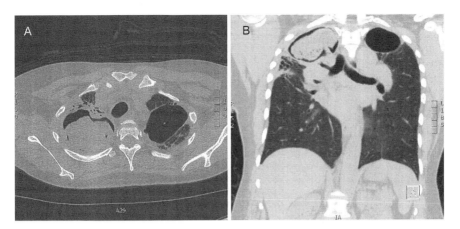

Fig. 9.5 Chest CT scan demonstrating fibrocystic sarcoidosis with an associated mycetoma. (**a**) Transverse cut; (**b**) coronal cut

pulmonary embolism but does reveal bilateral upper lobe predominant bronchiectasis with adjacent fibrosis and volume loss. Additionally, a 7.6 cm×6.0 cm right upper lobe bulla was seen which is nearly completely filled by a solid mass. A smaller left upper lobe bulla was also visualized. Mediastinal and hilar adenopathy were present. Taken together, the image suggested fibrocystic sarcoidosis complicated by a right upper lobe mycetoma. A trial of prednisone 20 mg was prescribed in an attempt to improve any symptoms that may be due to active sarcoid inflammation. Additionally, she was referred to a thoracic surgeon for consideration of bullectomy/mycetoma resection.

During the thoracic surgery consultation, she was deemed not to be a surgical candidate due to poor pulmonary reserve and deconditioning. One week after this consultation, she called the pulmonary clinic reporting hemoptysis. She described coughing up "a cup" of bright red blood. She was instructed to come to the emergency room and was subsequently admitted to the intensive care unit for close observation. She proceeded to cough up several more tablespoons of blood overnight but did not experience respiratory decompensation. Treatment options including bronchial arterial embolization (BAE) and intracavitary instillation of amphotericin B (ICAB) were considered and ultimately ICAB was chosen. The patient was taken to interventional radiology where a transcutaneous catheter was placed into the right upper lobe bulla. Fifty milligrams of amphotericin B diluted in 20 cc of 5 % dextrose was then instilled into the cavity daily for 10 days. Her hemoptysis resolved by day 3, the catheter was removed without complication after 10 days, and the patient was discharged to home. Her productive cough has lessened in frequency and intensity and her hemoptysis has not recurred to date. There was no marked improvement in her dyspnea or PFTs on prednisone and this was tapered down to 5 mg over the following 6 months.

Discussion

Fibrocystic Sarcoidosis

In addition to a wide variety of extra-pulmonary manifestations, sarcoidosis can also exhibit many different pulmonary presentations. The classic descriptions by Scadding introduced a staging system utilizing chest roentgenograms that seemed to have prognostic capabilities [105]. In this system, a stage II was designated if there were simultaneous adenopathy and "mottled shadowing" of the parenchyma, while "mottled shadowing" in the absence of adenopathy fell into stage III. Stage IV was assigned to patients with radiographic evidence of fibrosis. Over time, published cases have revealed considerable heterogeneity in the potential parenchymal manifestations of sarcoidosis including micronodular, macronodular, reticular, consolidation, bronchiectasis, and fibrosis. Of these possibilities, one of the more common radiographic presentations is fibrocystic sarcoidosis.

Fibrocystic sarcoidosis is characterized by the presence peribronchovascular fibrosis radiating out from the hila with resultant upper lobe traction, and many times cystic, bronchiectasis with bullae formation. The fibrosis often results in an upward retraction of the hila and frequently a clumping of bronchiectatic airways is seen (Fig. 9.6). Histologically, the bullae and cysts seen in fibrocystic sarcoidosis are not true cavities; in fact, actual cavitary sarcoidosis is quite rare [106]. Patients with fibrocystic sarcoidosis will commonly have symptoms that seem relatively mild and out of proportion to the degree of radiographic abnormality. Similarly, despite considerable parenchymal damage, patients with fibrocystic disease commonly have little deficit in resting oxygenation unless they have sarcoidosis associated pulmonary hypertension. This is likely due to the upper lobe predominance of this disease which allows for relatively preserved ventilation–perfusion matching in the well-perfused lower lobes. Pulmonary function testing often reveals either a restrictive or combined restrictive and obstructive deficit with an associated decrease in DLCO. Prognostically, fibrocystic disease indicates progressive disease that seldom remits without therapy [107–109]. Additionally, fibrocystic disease can lead to complications that are unique to this particular form of pulmonary sarcoidosis.

Mycetomas

As with all pulmonary disease which causes cavity or bullae formation, fibrocystic sarcoidosis predisposes patients to the development of mycetomas. Mycetomas are mass-like collections of fungus or bacteria which grow inside abnormal and enlarged spaces in the lung. They likely develop from continuous inhalation of ubiquitous

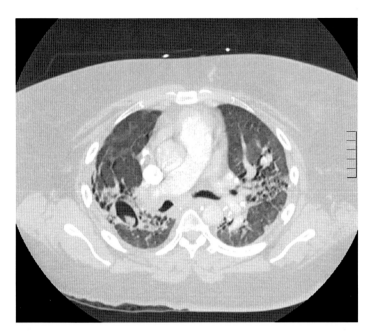

Fig. 9.6 Chest CT scan demonstrating bronchiectatic airway clumping in fibrocystic sarcoidosis. Right-sided mycetoma incidentally seen

environmental microbes which are able to colonize and grow in regions of the lung where mucosal immunity is disrupted. While many different species are known to cause mycetomas including *Candida*, *Streptomyces*, and *Nocardia*, the most commonly seen species is *Aspergillus*.

Often, mycetomas are discovered incidentally and generate no symptoms. Other times, mycetomas can cause a productive cough with dark, sometimes brown, sputum as well as constitutional symptoms including fatigue and weight loss. The most serious sequela of a mycetoma, however, is hemoptysis which occurs when the mycetoma invades the surrounding walls. The hemoptysis can be either persistent or intermittent and can range from small volumes (blood-streaked sputum) to massive hemoptysis which can be a life-threatening complication requiring urgent intervention.

Surgical removal of the affected area is the only definitive therapy for a mycetoma [110, 111]. Unfortunately, patients with mycetomas often have severe underlying lung disease which precludes their candidacy for the procedure [112]. Those who do have sufficient pulmonary reserve to undergo a resection are faced with the perioperative challenges of poor lung incision integrity leading to persistent air leaks, bleeding, and fungal soilage of the remaining lung during the mycetoma removal [113–116]. For the majority of patients who cannot undergo resection, the optimal treatment strategy is unclear. Systemic therapy with azole antifungals seldom leads to resolution of mycetomas [117–119]. Similarly, systemic amphotericin B does not sufficiently penetrate mycetomas [120, 121]. As such, many patients with asymptomatic mycetomas or those with productive cough but no hemoptysis are often managed with observation alone. However, the development of massive hemoptysis usually requires an urgent intervention. In nonsurgical candidates, a traditional approach has been to use BAE in order to control bleeding. While BAE often successfully controls acute bleeding, further mycetoma growth and revascularization result in high rates of recurrence [122–125].

An alternative approach to treating symptomatic pulmonary mycetomas is the instillation of antifungals directly into the cavity or bulla using either a percutaneous or a transbronchial route of delivery. To date, this approach has been described largely on a case report/series level [120, 126–131] but demonstrates promise as a potential effective treatment. In addition to improving hemoptysis, this approach may also provide the added benefit of reducing mycetoma size and improving recurrence rates in some patients [132]—however, this has yet to be definitively proven. At this point, there has been no head to head comparison between BAE and ICAB nor is there a consensus regarding the appropriate regimen for intracavitary therapy.

Pneumothorax

In general, pneumothorax is an uncommon complication of sarcoidosis but it is well described, particularly in patients with advanced fibrocystic disease [133–135]. The etiology of secondary pneumothoraces in fibrocystic sarcoidosis is most likely secondary to subpleural bleb/bulla rupture [135]; however, subpleural granulomatous cavitation may also contribute [34, 136]. Patients with sarcoidosis and spontaneous pneumothoraces present with symptoms similar to other patients with spontaneous secondary pneumothoraces (SSP): pleuritic chest pain and acute dyspnea. As with all SSPs, the initial approach to the patient with a sarcoid-associated pneumothorax includes rapid assessment and stabilization of cardiopulmonary status. If the pneumothorax is small (pleural line <1 cm from chest wall), patients may be observed on supplemental oxygen for signs of clinical deterioration. Larger pneumothoraces and/or pronounced symptoms will often require tube thoracostomy because of the high risk of complications [137].

Patients with SSP, including sarcoid-associated pneumothorax, are at greater risk of developing persistent air leaks as compared to those with primary spontaneous pneumothoraces (PSP) [138]. As such, these patients are frequently considered for interventions aimed at closing the leak. As with mycetoma therapy, a video-assisted thoracoscopic surgery (VATS) procedure to staple or remove a ruptured bleb and simultaneously perform a mechanical or chemical pleurodesis is considered to be optimal therapy. However, as previously discussed, many patients with advanced fibrocystic sarcoidosis are unable to tolerate thoracic surgery. In these patients, chemical pleurodesis or a blood patch [139–141] can be attempted via the existing thoracostomy tube. In non-operable patients who fail pleurodesis/blood patching, conservative management with supplemental oxygen and Heimlich valves is also considered. The emergence of therapeutic endobronchial valves which allow for air to escape bullous lung while simultaneously preventing further inhalation of air into these regions may offer less-invasive alternatives for persistent air leak management in the non-operable patient [142, 143]; however, their effectiveness and their risk-benefit profile is not yet fully characterized.

Summary

Pulmonary sarcoidosis can present with a myriad of patterns ranging from minor amounts of micronodular disease to fibrocystic patterns with extensive lung involvement. In addition to carrying a poor prognosis regarding spontaneous remission, the presence of fibrocystic disease also carries the potential for unique complications including mycetoma formation and spontaneous pneumothorax. Clinicians should be attentive to signs or symptoms of these complications when caring for patients with pulmonary sarcoidosis. While surgical interventions remain the definitive therapies for both of these complications, many patients with advanced sarcoidosis are not surgical candidates. Therefore a familiarity with less-invasive therapies is important for the clinician.

References

1. Hutchinson J, editor. Anomalous diseases of skin and fingers: case of livid papillary psoriasis? Illustrations of clinical surgery. London: J and A Churchill; 1877.
2. Austrian R, McClement JH, Renzetti Jr AD, Donald KW, Riley RL, Cournand A. Clinical and physiologic features of some types of pulmonary diseases with impairment of alveolar-capillary diffusion; the syndrome of "alveolar-capillary block". Am J Med. 1951;11(6):667–85.
3. Handa T, Nagai S, Miki S, Fushimi Y, Ohta K, Mishima M, et al. Incidence of pulmonary hypertension and its clinical relevance in patients with sarcoidosis. Chest. 2006;129(5):1246–52.
4. Sulica R, Teirstein AS, Kakarla S, Nemani N, Behnegar A, Padilla ML. Distinctive clinical, radiographic, and functional characteristics of patients with sarcoidosis-related pulmonary hypertension. Chest. 2005;128(3):1483–9.
5. Shorr AF, Helman DL, Davies DB, Nathan SD. Pulmonary hypertension in advanced sarcoidosis: epidemiology and clinical characteristics. Eur Respir J. 2005;25(5):783–8.
6. Nunes H, Humbert M, Capron F, Brauner M, Sitbon O, Battesti JP, et al. Pulmonary hypertension associated with sarcoidosis: mechanisms, haemodynamics and prognosis. Thorax. 2006;61(1):68–74.
7. Simonneau G, Robbins IM, Beghetti M, Channick RN, Delcroix M, Denton CP, et al. Updated clinical classification of pulmonary hypertension. J Am Coll Cardiol. 2009;54(1 Suppl):S43–54.
8. Shigemitsu H, Nagai S, Sharma OP. Pulmonary hypertension and granulomatous vasculitis in sarcoidosis. Curr Opin Pulm Med. 2007;13(5):434–8.
9. Salazar A, Mana J, Sala J, Landoni BR, Manresa F. Combined portal and pulmonary hypertension in sarcoidosis. Respiration. 1994;61(2):117–9.
10. Turner GA, Lower EE, Corser BC, Gunther KL, Baughman RP. Sleep apnea in sarcoidosis. Sarcoidosis Vasc Diffuse Lung Dis. 1997;14(1):61–4.

11. Damuth TE, Bower JS, Cho K, Dantzker DR. Major pulmonary artery stenosis causing pulmonary hypertension in sarcoidosis. Chest. 1980;78(6):888–91.
12. Morawiec E, Hachulla-Lemaire AL, Chabrol J, Remy-Jardin M, Wallaert B. Venoatrial compression by lymphadenopathy in sarcoidosis. Eur Respir J. 2010;35(5):1188–91.
13. Hamilton-Craig CR, Slaughter R, McNeil K, Kermeen F, Walters DL. Improvement after angioplasty and stenting of pulmonary arteries due to sarcoid mediastinal fibrosis. Heart Lung Circ. 2009;18(3):222–5.
14. Toonkel RL, Borczuk AC, Pearson GD, Horn EM, Thomashow BM. Sarcoidosis-associated fibrosing mediastinitis with resultant pulmonary hypertension: a case report and review of the literature. Respiration. 2010;79(4):341–5.
15. Lettieri CJ, Nathan SD, Barnett SD, Ahmad S, Shorr AF. Prevalence and outcomes of pulmonary arterial hypertension in advanced idiopathic pulmonary fibrosis. Chest. 2006;129(3):746–52.
16. Burrows B, Kettel LJ, Niden AH, Rabinowitz M, Diener CF. Patterns of cardiovascular dysfunction in chronic obstructive lung disease. N Engl J Med. 1972;286(17):912–8.
17. Weitzenblum E, Hirth C, Ducolone A, Mirhom R, Rasaholinjanahary J, Ehrhart M. Prognostic value of pulmonary artery pressure in chronic obstructive pulmonary disease. Thorax. 1981;36(10):752–8.
18. Traver GA, Cline MG, Burrows B. Predictors of mortality in chronic obstructive pulmonary disease. A 15-year follow-up study. Am Rev Respir Dis. 1979;119(6):895–902.
19. Baughman RP, Engel PJ, Taylor L, Lower EE. Survival in sarcoidosis-associated pulmonary hypertension: the importance of hemodynamic evaluation. Chest. 2010;138(5):1078–85.
20. Shorr AF, Davies DB, Nathan SD. Predicting mortality in patients with sarcoidosis awaiting lung transplantation. Chest. 2003;124(3):922–8.
21. Arcasoy SM, Christie JD, Pochettino A, Rosengard BR, Blumenthal NP, Bavaria JE, et al. Characteristics and outcomes of patients with sarcoidosis listed for lung transplantation. Chest. 2001;120(3):873–80.
22. Bourbonnais JM, Samavati L. Clinical predictors of pulmonary hypertension in sarcoidosis. Eur Respir J. 2008;32(2):296–302.
23. Tan RT, Kuzo R, Goodman LR, Siegel R, Haasler GB, Presberg KW. Utility of CT scan evaluation for predicting pulmonary hypertension in patients with parenchymal lung disease. Medical College of Wisconsin Lung Transplant Group. Chest. 1998;113(5):1250–6.
24. Arcasoy SM, Christie JD, Ferrari VA, Sutton MS, Zisman DA, Blumenthal NP, et al. Echocardiographic assessment of pulmonary hypertension in patients with advanced lung disease. Am J Respir Crit Care Med. 2003;167(5):735–40.
25. James DG, Sharma OP. From Hutchinson to now: a historical glimpse. Curr Opin Pulm Med. 2002;8(5):416–23.
26. Bessnier E. Lupus Pernio de la Face. Ann Derm Syph. 1889;10:33–6.
27. Boeck C. Multiple benign sarcoid of the skin. Norsk Mag Laegevid. 1899;14:1321–45.
28. Heerfordt CF. Meber eine "Febris uveo-parotidea subchronica Graefes Arch". Clin Exp Ophthalmol. 1909;70:254.
29. Loncope W, Pierson J. Boeck's sarcoid (sarcoidosis). Bull Johns Hopkins Hosp. 1937;60: 223–96.
30. Pautrier L. Syndrome de Heerfordt et maladie de Besnier-Boeck-Schaumann. Bull Soc Med Hop Paris. 1937;53:1608–20.
31. Schaumann J. Lymphogranuloma benigna in the light of prolonged clinical observations and autopsy findings. Br J Dermatol. 1936;48:399.
32. Lofgren S. Primary pulmonary sarcoidosis. I. Early signs and symptoms. Acta Med Scand. 1953;145(6):424–31.
33. Lofgren S. Primary pulmonary sarcoidosis. II. Clinical course and prognosis. Acta Med Scand. 1953;145(6):465–74.
34. Riley EA. Boeck's sarcoid; a review based upon a clinical study of fifty-two cases. Am Rev Tuberc. 1950;62(3):231–85.
35. Scadding JG. Mycobacterium tuberculosis in the aetiology of sarcoidosis. Br Med J. 1960;2(5213):1617–23.

36. Emerson PA, Young FH. Sarcoidosis following tuberculosis. Tubercle. 1956;37(2):116–9.
37. Lees AW. Transition from open pulmonary tuberculosis to sarcoidosis. Am Rev Tuberc. 1958;78(5):769–72.
38. Hatzakis K, Siafakas NM, Bouros D. Miliary sarcoidosis following miliary tuberculosis. Respiration. 2000;67(2):219–22.
39. Rutherford RM, Gilmartin JJ. A case of sarcoidosis following exposure to Mycobacterium tuberculosis (MTb). Ir Med J. 2003;96(2):58–9.
40. Luk A, Lee A, Ahn E, Soor GS, Ross HJ, Butany J. Cardiac sarcoidosis: recurrent disease in a heart transplant patient following pulmonary tuberculosis infection. Can J Cardiol. 2010;26(7):e273–5.
41. Ganguly S, Ganguly D. Sarcoidosis following sputum positive pulmonary tuberculosis: a rare entity. Indian J Dermatol. 2012;57(1):76–8.
42. Taylor AJ. The association of sarcoidosis, active pulmonary tuberculosis and insensitivity to tuberculin. Br J Tuberc Dis Chest. 1958;52(1):70–3.
43. Giotaki HA, Stefanou DG. Biopsy-documented tuberculous pleural effusion in a patient with biopsy-proven coexisting sarcoidosis. Respiration. 1988;54(3):193–6.
44. Wong CF, Yew WW, Wong PC, Lee J. A case of concomitant tuberculosis and sarcoidosis with mycobacterial DNA present in the sarcoid lesion. Chest. 1998;114(2):626–9.
45. Oluboyo PO, Awotedu AA, Banach L. Concomitant sarcoidosis in a patient with tuberculosis: first report of association in Africa. Cent Afr J Med. 2005;51(11-12):123–5.
46. Greally JF, Manning D, McNicholl B. Sarcoidosis following B.C.G. vaccination in a lymphopaenic boy. Sarcoidosis. 1989;6(2):156–7.
47. el-Zaatari FA, Naser SA, Markesich DC, Kalter DC, Engstand L, Graham DY. Identification of Mycobacterium avium complex in sarcoidosis. J Clin Microbiol. 1996;34(9):2240–5.
48. Osborne GE, Mallon E, Mayou SC. Juvenile sarcoidosis after BCG vaccination. J Am Acad Dermatol. 2003;48(5 Suppl):S99–102.
49. Terzian C, Rahal JJ. Mycobacterial infection as a precursor to sarcoid-like, corticosteroid-responsive, diffuse granulomatous disease. Int J Infect Dis. 2006;10(5):407–8.
50. Saboor SA, Johnson NM, McFadden J. Detection of mycobacterial DNA in sarcoidosis and tuberculosis with polymerase chain reaction. Lancet. 1992;339(8800):1012–5.
51. Schick U, May A, Schwarz M. Detection of mycobacterial DNA in a patient with neurosarcoidosis. Acta Neurol Scand. 1995;91(4):280–2.
52. Richter E, Greinert U, Kirsten D, Rusch-Gerdes S, Schluter C, Duchrow M, et al. Assessment of mycobacterial DNA in cells and tissues of mycobacterial and sarcoid lesions. Am J Respir Crit Care Med. 1996;153(1):375–80.
53. el-Zaatari FA, Graham DY, Samuelsson K, Engstrand L. Detection of Mycobacterium avium complex in cerebrospinal fluid of a sarcoid patient by specific polymerase chain reaction assays. Scand J Infect Dis. 1997;29(2):202–4.
54. Brownell I, Ramirez-Valle F, Sanchez M, Prystowsky S. Evidence for mycobacteria in sarcoidosis. Am J Respir Cell Mol Biol. 2011;45(5):899–905.
55. Song Z, Marzilli L, Greenlee BM, Chen ES, Silver RF, Askin FB, et al. Mycobacterial catalase-peroxidase is a tissue antigen and target of the adaptive immune response in systemic sarcoidosis. J Exp Med. 2005;201(5):755–67.
56. Dubaniewicz A, Dubaniewicz-Wybieralska M, Sternau A, Zwolska Z, Izycka-Swieszewska E, Augustynowicz-Kopec E, et al. Mycobacterium tuberculosis complex and mycobacterial heat shock proteins in lymph node tissue from patients with pulmonary sarcoidosis. J Clin Microbiol. 2006;44(9):3448–51.
57. Oswald-Richter KA, Beachboard DC, Zhan X, Gaskill CF, Abraham S, Jenkins C, et al. Multiple mycobacterial antigens are targets of the adaptive immune response in pulmonary sarcoidosis. Respir Res. 2010;11:161.
58. Carlisle J, Evans W, Hajizadeh R, Nadaf M, Shepherd B, Ott RD, et al. Multiple Mycobacterium antigens induce interferon-gamma production from sarcoidosis peripheral blood mononuclear cells. Clin Exp Immunol. 2007;150(3):460–8.

59. Ishige I, Usui Y, Takemura T, Eishi Y. Quantitative PCR of mycobacterial and propionibacterial DNA in lymph nodes of Japanese patients with sarcoidosis. Lancet. 1999;354(9173): 120–3.

60. Ichikawa H, Kataoka M, Hiramatsu J, Ohmori M, Tanimoto Y, Kanehiro A, et al. Quantitative analysis of propionibacterial DNA in bronchoalveolar lavage cells from patients with sarcoidosis. Sarcoidosis Vasc Diffuse Lung Dis. 2008;25(1):15–20.

61. Ishige I, Eishi Y, Takemura T, Kobayashi I, Nakata K, Tanaka I, et al. Propionibacterium acnes is the most common bacterium commensal in peripheral lung tissue and mediastinal lymph nodes from subjects without sarcoidosis. Sarcoidosis Vasc Diffuse Lung Dis. 2005;22(1):33–42.

62. Tanabe T, Ishige I, Suzuki Y, Aita Y, Furukawa A, Ishige Y, et al. Sarcoidosis and NOD1 variation with impaired recognition of intracellular Propionibacterium acnes. Biochim Biophys Acta. 2006;1762(9):794–801.

63. Newman LS, Rose CS, Bresnitz EA, Rossman MD, Barnard J, Frederick M, et al. A case control etiologic study of sarcoidosis: environmental and occupational risk factors. Am J Respir Crit Care Med. 2004;170(12):1324–30.

64. Laney AS, Cragin LA, Blevins LZ, Sumner AD, Cox-Ganser JM, Kreiss K, et al. Sarcoidosis, asthma, and asthma-like symptoms among occupants of a historically water-damaged office building. Indoor Air. 2009;19(1):83–90.

65. Tercelj M, Salobir B, Harlander M, Rylander R. Fungal exposure in homes of patients with sarcoidosis – an environmental exposure study. Environ Health. 2011;10(1):8.

66. Tercelj M, Salobir B, Zupancic M, Rylander R. Antifungal medication is efficient in the treatment of sarcoidosis. Ther Adv Respir Dis. 2011;5(3):157–62.

67. Buck AA, Sartwell PE. Epidemiologic investigations of sarcoidosis. II. Skin sensitivity and environmental factors. Am J Hyg. 1961;74:152–73.

68. Terris M, Chaves AD. An epidemiologic study of sarcoidosis. Am Rev Respir Dis. 1966; 94(1):50–5.

69. Cummings MM, Hudgins PC. Chemical constituents of pine pollen and their possible relationship to sarcoidosis. Am J Med Sci. 1958;236(3):311–7.

70. Burdick KH. Cutaneous reaction to pine pollen in sarcoidosis. Study of forty cases. J Invest Dermatol. 1964;42:449–51.

71. Gentry JT, Nitowsky HM, Michael Jr M. Studies on the epidemiology of sarcoidosis in the United States: the relationship to soil areas and to urban-rural residence. J Clin Invest. 1955;34(12):1839–56.

72. Hurley HJ, Close HP, English RS. Soil extracts as antigens in sarcoidosis. Am Rev Respir Dis. 1962;86:100–2.

73. Teuber SS, Howell LP, Yoshida SH, Gershwin ME. Remission of sarcoidosis following removal of silicone gel breast implants. Int Arch Allergy Immunol. 1994;105(4):404–7.

74. Yoshida T, Tanaka M, Okamoto K, Hirai S. Neurosarcoidosis following augmentation mammoplasty with silicone. Neurol Res. 1996;18(4):319–20.

75. Barzo P, Tamasi L. [Lofgren syndrome after silicone breast prosthesis implantation]. Orv Hetil. 1998;139(39):2323–6.

76. Miyashita T, Yoshioka K, Nakamura T, Yamagami K. A case of sarcoidosis with unusual radiographic findings that developed 5 years after silicone augmentation mammoplasty complicated by miliary tuberculosis during corticosteroid treatment. Case Rep Pulmonol. 2011;2011:268620.

77. Pimentel L, Barnadas M, Vidal D, Sancho F, Fontarnau R, Alomar A. Simultaneous presentation of silicone and silica granuloma: a case report. Dermatology. 2002;205(2):162–5.

78. Andrews TR, Calamia KT, Waldorf JC, Walsh JS. Subcutaneous nodules on the face – quiz case. Arch Dermatol. 2005;141(1):93–8.

79. Kogushi H, Egawa K, Ono T. Sarcoidal granuloma developing not only at the entry site of industrial lubricating oil, but also at a regional lymph node and entry points of venepuncture. Dermatology. 2006;212(3):250–2.

80. Descamps V, Landry J, Frances C, Marinho E, Ratziu V, Chosidow O. Facial cosmetic filler injections as possible target for systemic sarcoidosis in patients treated with interferon for chronic hepatitis C: two cases. Dermatology. 2008;217(1):81–4.

81. Stroh C, Bottger J, Meyer F, Lippert H, Manger T. Sarcoidosis after adjustable silicone gastric banding – a report of two cases in Germany. Obes Facts. 2009;2(5):332–4.

82. Kim YC, Triffet MK, Gibson LE. Foreign bodies in sarcoidosis. Am J Dermatopathol. 2000;22(5):408–12.

83. Izbicki G, Chavko R, Banauch GI, Weiden MD, Berger KI, Aldrich TK, et al. World Trade Center "sarcoid-like" granulomatous pulmonary disease in New York City Fire Department rescue workers. Chest. 2007;131(5):1414–23.

84. Crowley LE, Herbert R, Moline JM, Wallenstein S, Shukla G, Schechter C, et al. "Sarcoid like" granulomatous pulmonary disease in World Trade Center disaster responders. Am J Ind Med. 2011;54(3):175–84.

85. Bowers B, Hasni S, Gruber BL. Sarcoidosis in World Trade Center rescue workers presenting with rheumatologic manifestations. J Clin Rheumatol. 2010;16(1):26–7.

86. Jordan HT, Stellman SD, Prezant D, Teirstein A, Osahan SS, Cone JE. Sarcoidosis diagnosed after September 11, 2001, among adults exposed to the World Trade Center disaster. J Occup Environ Med Sep. 2011;53(9):966–74.

87. Newman LS. Metals that cause sarcoidosis. Semin Respir Infect. 1998;13(3):212–20.

88. Deubelbeiss U, Gemperli A, Schindler C, Baty F, Brutsche MH. Prevalence of sarcoidosis in Switzerland is associated with environmental factors. Eur Respir J. 2010;35(5):1088–97.

89. Checchi L, Nucci MC, Gatti AM, Mattia D, Violante FS. Sarcoidosis in a dental surgeon: a case report. J Med Case Rep. 2010;4:259.

90. Kawano-Dourado LB, Carvalho CR, Santos UP, Canzian M, Coletta EN, Pereira CA, et al. Tunnel excavation triggering pulmonary sarcoidosis. Am J Ind Med. 2012;55(4):390–4.

91. Song Y, Li X, Wang L, Rojanasakul Y, Castranova V, Li H, et al. Nanomaterials in humans: identification, characteristics, and potential damage. Toxicol Pathol. 2011;39(5):841–9.

92. Rybicki BA, Iannuzzi MC, Frederick MM, Thompson BW, Rossman MD, Bresnitz EA, et al. Familial aggregation of sarcoidosis. A case-control etiologic study of sarcoidosis (ACCESS). Am J Respir Crit Care Med. 2001;164(11):2085–91.

93. Familial associations in sarcoidosis. A report to the Research Committee of the British Thoracic and Tuberculosis Association. Tubercle. 1973;54(2):87–98.

94. Brewerton DA, Cockburn C, James DC, James DG, Neville E. HLA antigens in sarcoidosis. Clin Exp Immunol. 1977;27(2):227–9.

95. Voorter CE, Amicosante M, Berretta F, Groeneveld L, Drent M, van den Berg-Loonen EM. HLA class II amino acid epitopes as susceptibility markers of sarcoidosis. Tissue Antigens. 2007;70(1):18–27.

96. Schurmann M, Reichel P, Muller-Myhsok B, Schlaak M, Muller-Quernheim J, Schwinger E. Results from a genome-wide search for predisposing genes in sarcoidosis. Am J Respir Crit Care Med. 2001;164(5):840–6.

97. Iannuzzi MC, Iyengar SK, Gray-McGuire C, Elston RC, Baughman RP, Donohue JF, et al. Genome-wide search for sarcoidosis susceptibility genes in African Americans. Genes Immun. 2005;6(6):509–18.

98. Valentonyte R, Hampe J, Huse K, Rosenstiel P, Albrecht M, Stenzel A, et al. Sarcoidosis is associated with a truncating splice site mutation in BTNL2. Nat Genet. 2005;37(4):357–64.

99. Rybicki BA, Walewski JL, Maliarik MJ, Kian H, Iannuzzi MC. The BTNL2 gene and sarcoidosis susceptibility in African Americans and Whites. Am J Hum Genet. 2005;77(3):491–9.

100. Gray-McGuire C, Sinha R, Iyengar S, Millard C, Rybicki BA, Elston RC, et al. Genetic characterization and fine mapping of susceptibility loci for sarcoidosis in African Americans on chromosome 5. Hum Genet. 2006;120(3):420–30.

101. Piotrowski WJ, Gorski P, Pietras T, Fendler W, Szemraj J. The selected genetic polymorphisms of metalloproteinases MMP2, 7, 9 and MMP inhibitor TIMP2 in sarcoidosis. Med Sci Monit. 2011;17(10):CR598–607.

102. Rybicki BA, Sinha R, Iyengar S, GrayMcGuire C, Elston RC, Iannuzzi MC, et al. Genetic linkage analysis of sarcoidosis phenotypes: the sarcoidosis genetic analysis (SAGA) study. Genes Immun. 2007;8(5):379–86.

103. Veltkamp M, van Moorsel CH, Rijkers GT, Ruven HJ, Grutters JC. Genetic variation in the Toll-like receptor gene cluster (TLR10-TLR1-TLR6) influences disease course in sarcoidosis. Tissue Antigens. 2012;79(1):25–32.

104. Pabst S, Bradler O, Gillissen A, Nickenig G, Skowasch D, Grohe C. Toll-like receptor-9 polymorphisms in sarcoidosis and chronic obstructive pulmonary disease. Adv Exp Med Biol. 2013;756:239–45.

105. Scadding JG. Prognosis of intrathoracic sarcoidosis In England. BMJ. 1961;4:1165.

106. Rohatgi PK, Schwab LE. Primary acute pulmonary cavitation in sarcoidosis. AJR Am J Roentgenol. 1980;134(6):1199–203.

107. Hunninghake GW, Costabel U, Ando M, Baughman R, Cordier JF, du Bois R, et al. ATS/ERS/WASOG statement on sarcoidosis. American Thoracic Society/European Respiratory Society/World Association of Sarcoidosis and other Granulomatous Disorders. Sarcoidosis Vasc Diffuse Lung Dis. 1999;16(2):149–73.

108. Neville E, Walker AN, James DG. Prognostic factors predicting the outcome of sarcoidosis: an analysis of 818 patients. Q J Med. 1983;52(208):525–33.

109. Hillerdal G, Nou E, Osterman K, Schmekel B. Sarcoidosis: epidemiology and prognosis. A 15-year European study. Am Rev Respir Dis. 1984;130(1):29–32.

110. Kauffman CA. Quandary about treatment of aspergillomas persists. Lancet. 1996;347(9016):1640.

111. Khan MA, Dar AM, Kawoosa NU, Ahangar AG, Lone GN, Bashir G, et al. Clinical profile and surgical outcome for pulmonary aspergilloma: nine year retrospective observational study in a tertiary care hospital. Int J Surg. 2011;9(3):267–71.

112. Israel HL, Lenchner GS, Atkinson GW. Sarcoidosis and aspergilloma. The role of surgery. Chest. 1982;82(4):430–2.

113. Regnard JF, Icard P, Nicolosi M, Spagiarri L, Magdeleinat P, Jauffret B, et al. Aspergilloma: a series of 89 surgical cases. Ann Thorac Surg. 2000;69(3):898–903.

114. Garvey J, Crastnopol P, Weisz D, Khan F. The surgical treatment of pulmonary aspergillomas. J Thorac Cardiovasc Surg. 1977;74(4):542–7.

115. Kaestel M, Meyer W, Mittelmeier HO, Gebhardt C. Pulmonary aspergilloma – clinical findings and surgical treatment. Thorac Cardiovasc Surg. 1999;47(5):340–5.

116. Massard G, Roeslin N, Wihlm JM, Dumont P, Witz JP, Morand G. Pleuropulmonary aspergilloma: clinical spectrum and results of surgical treatment. Ann Thorac Surg. 1992;54(6):1159–64.

117. Campbell JH, Winter JH, Richardson MD, Shankland GS, Banham SW. Treatment of pulmonary aspergilloma with itraconazole. Thorax. 1991;46(11):839–41.

118. De Beule K, De Doncker P, Cauwenbergh G, Koster M, Legendre R, Blatchford N, et al. The treatment of aspergillosis and aspergilloma with itraconazole, clinical results of an open international study (1982-1987). Mycoses. 1988;31(9):476–85.

119. Dupont B. Itraconazole therapy in aspergillosis: study in 49 patients. J Am Acad Dermatol. 1990;23(3 Pt 2):607–14.

120. Hargis JL, Bone RC, Stewart J, Rector N, Hiller FC. Intracavitary amphotericin B in the treatment of symptomatic pulmonary aspergillomas. Am J Med. 1980;68(3):389–94.

121. Hammerman KJ, Sarosi GA, Tosh FE. Amphotericin B in the treatment of saprophytic forms of pulmonary aspergillosis. Am Rev Respir Dis. 1974;109(1):57–62.

122. Mossi F, Maroldi R, Battaglia G, Pinotti G, Tassi G. Indicators predictive of success of embolisation: analysis of 88 patients with haemoptysis. Radiol Med. 2003;105(1-2):48–55.

123. Shin BS, Jeon GS, Lee SA, Park MH. Bronchial artery embolisation for the management of haemoptysis in patients with pulmonary tuberculosis. Int J Tuberc Lung Dis. 2011;15(8): 1093–8.

124. Uflacker R, Kaemmerer A, Neves C, Picon PD. Management of massive hemoptysis by bronchial artery embolization. Radiology. 1983;146(3):627–34.

125. Chun JY, Belli AM. Immediate and long-term outcomes of bronchial and non-bronchial systemic artery embolisation for the management of haemoptysis. Eur Radiol. 2010;20(3): 558–65.

126. Lee KS, Kim HT, Kim YH, Choe KO. Treatment of hemoptysis in patients with cavitary aspergilloma of the lung: value of percutaneous instillation of amphotericin B. AJR Am J Roentgenol. 1993;161(4):727–31.

127. Shapiro MJ, Albelda SM, Mayock RL, McLean GK. Severe hemoptysis associated with pulmonary aspergilloma. Percutaneous intracavitary treatment. Chest. 1988;94(6):1225–31.

128. Rumbak M, Kohler G, Eastrige C, Winer-Muram H, Gavant M. Topical treatment of life threatening haemoptysis from aspergillomas. Thorax. 1996;51(3):253–5.

129. Munk PL, Vellet AD, Rankin RN, Muller NL, Ahmad D. Intracavitary aspergilloma: transthoracic percutaneous injection of amphotericin gelatin solution. Radiology. 1993;188(3):821–3.

130. Giron J, Poey C, Fajadet P, Sans N, Fourcade D, Senac JP, et al. CT-guided percutaneous treatment of inoperable pulmonary aspergillomas: a study of 40 cases. Eur J Radiol. 1998;28(3):235–42.

131. Jackson M, Flower CD, Shneerson JM. Treatment of symptomatic pulmonary aspergillomas with intracavitary instillation of amphotericin B through an indwelling catheter. Thorax. 1993;48(9):928–30.

132. Kravitz JN, Berry MW, Schabel SI, Judson MA. A modern series of percutaneous intracavitary instillation of amphotericin B for the treatment of severe hemoptysis from pulmonary aspergilloma. Chest. 2013;143(5):1414–21.

133. Freiman DG. Sarcoidosis. N Engl J Med. 1948;239:664.

134. Ross RJ, Empey DW. Bilateral spontaneous pneumothorax in sarcoidosis. Postgrad Med J. 1983;59(688):106–7.

135. Froudarakis ME, Bouros D, Voloudaki A, Papiris S, Kottakis Y, Constantopoulos SH, et al. Pneumothorax as a first manifestation of sarcoidosis. Chest. 1997;112(1):278–80.

136. Sharma OP. Sarcoidosis: unusual pulmonary manifestations. Postgrad Med. 1977;61(3):67–73.

137. Schoenenberger RA, Haefeli WE, Weiss P, Ritz RF. Timing of invasive procedures in therapy for primary and secondary spontaneous pneumothorax. Arch Surg. 1991;126(6):764–6.

138. Mathur R, Cullen J, Kinnear WJ, Johnston ID. Time course of resolution of persistent air leak in spontaneous pneumothorax. Respir Med. 1995;89(2):129–32.

139. Rinaldi S, Felton T, Bentley A. Blood pleurodesis for the medical management of pneumothorax. Thorax. 2009;64(3):258–60.

140. Ando M, Yamamoto M, Kitagawa C, Kumazawa A, Sato M, Shima K, et al. Autologous blood-patch pleurodesis for secondary spontaneous pneumothorax with persistent air leak. Respir Med. 1999;93(6):432–4.

141. Aihara K, Handa T, Nagai S, Tanizawa K, Watanabe K, Harada Y, et al. Efficacy of blood-patch pleurodesis for secondary spontaneous pneumothorax in interstitial lung disease. Intern Med. 2011;50(11):1157–62.

142. Travaline JM, McKenna Jr RJ, De Giacomo T, Venuta F, Hazelrigg SR, Boomer M, et al. Treatment of persistent pulmonary air leaks using endobronchial valves. Chest. 2009;136(2):355–60.

143. Greer T, Pastis N, Strange C, Huggins J. Sarcoidosis with secondary spontaneous pneumothorax treated with endobronchial valves. Chest. 2012;142:874A.

Index

Printed by Publishers' Graphics LLC
LMO140430.23.38.26